Radiography and Radiology for Dental Care Professionals

THIRD EDITION

To our families

Content Strategist: Alison Taylor
Content Development Specialist: Barbara Simmons
Project Manager: Caroline Jones
Designer/Design Direction: Miles Hitchen
Illustration Manager: Jennifer Rose

Radiography and Radiology for Dental Care Professionals

Third edition

WRITTEN AND ILLUSTRATED BY

Eric Whaites

MSc BDS(Hons) FDSRCS(Edin) FDSRCS(Eng) FRCR DDRRCR

Senior Lecturer and Honorary Consultant in Dental and Maxillofacial Radiology, Head of the Unit of Dental and Maxillofacial Radiological Imaging, King's College London Dental Institute at Guy's, King's College and St Thomas' Hospitals, London, UK

Nicholas Drage

BDS(Hons) FDSRCS(Eng) FDSRCPS(Glas) DDRRCR

Consultant and Honorary Senior Lecturer in Dental and Maxillofacial Radiology, University Dental Hospital, Cardiff and Vale University Health Board, Cardiff, UK

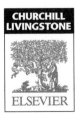

CHURCHILL LIVINGSTONE

ELSEVIER

Edinburgh   London   New York   Oxford   Philadelphia   St Louis   Sydney   Toronto   2013

First edition 2005
Second edition 2009
Third edition 2013
    Reprinted 2014, 2017, 2018

ISBN 9780702045981
eBook ISBN 9780702051678

British Library Cataloguing in Publication Data
A catalogue record for this book is available from the British Library

Library of Congress Cataloging in Publication Data
A catalog record for this book is available from the Library of Congress

Notices
Knowledge and best practice in this field are constantly changing. As new research and experience broaden our understanding, changes in research methods, professional practices, or medical treatment may become necessary.
    Practitioners and researchers must always rely on their own experience and knowledge in evaluating and using any information, methods, compounds, or experiments described herein. In using such information or methods they should be mindful of their own safety and the safety of others, including parties for whom they have a professional responsibility.
    With respect to any drug or pharmaceutical products identified, readers are advised to check the most current information provided (i) on procedures featured or (ii) by the manufacturer of each product to be administered, to verify the recommended dose or formula, the method and duration of administration, and contraindications. It is the responsibility of practitioners, relying on their own experience and knowledge of their patients, to make diagnoses, to determine dosages and the best treatment for each individual patient, and to take all appropriate safety precautions.
    To the fullest extent of the law, neither the Publisher nor the authors, contributors, or editors, assume any liability for any injury and/or damage to persons or property as a matter of products liability, negligence or otherwise, or from any use or operation of any methods, products, instructions, or ideas contained in the material herein.

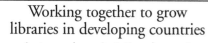

Working together to grow
libraries in developing countries

www.elsevier.com | www.bookaid.org | www.sabre.org

ELSEVIER   BOOK AID International   Sabre Foundation

ELSEVIER   your source for books,
journals and multimedia
in the health sciences
www.elsevierhealth.com

The publisher's policy is to use paper manufactured from sustainable forests

Printed in Great Britain
Last digit is the print number: 10 9 8 7

Contents

Preface

It is now 20 years since the first edition of *Essentials* was published and 7 years since the first edition of this slimmed down, condensed version for Dental Nurses and other Dental Care Professionals, so I felt that the time was right for the injection of new ideas and to bring on board a co-author. I am delighted that my friend and colleague for many years, Nicholas Drage, accepted both the offer and the challenge.

Together we have gone through, revised and updated every chapter. Now that Cone Beam CT is established as the imaging modality of choice in certain clinical situations, this section has been expanded and numerous new examples of advanced imaging have been added. We have also replaced some of the conventional images with new and better examples.

A major change has been the establishment of a website linked to the book. This has allowed us the opportunity to remove from the book the detailed UK legislative details (only relevant to UK Dentists and Dental Care Professionals). We can now update this information as and when necessary and readers from outside the UK are spared unnecessary and irrelevant details. More importantly the linked website has given us the opportunity to include on-line self-assessment questions based on each chapter. We hope this innovation will provide a useful additional teaching and learning resource for Dental Care Professionals.

The aims and objectives of this book remain the same, namely to provide a basic and practical account of what we consider to be the essential subject matter of both dental radiography and radiology required by Dental Care Professionals. As in previous editions some things have inevitably had to be omitted, or sometimes, over-simplified. It therefore remains first and foremost a teaching manual, rather than a comprehensive reference book. We hope the content remains sufficiently broad, detailed and up-to-date to satisfy the requirements of most post-qualification examinations.

We hope that the result is a clear, logical and easily understandable text, that continues to make a positive contribution to the challenging task facing Dental Care Professionals as they embark on broadening their skills to include dental radiography.

EW
London 2013

Acknowledgements

As with previous editions, this edition has only been possible thanks to the enormous amount of help and encouragement that we have received from our families, friends and colleagues (now too numerous to mention them all by name) in both London and Cardiff.

Over the years many people have contributed their help and advice for which we are very grateful, but none more so than Professor Rod Cawson who died in the summer of 2007. Without his help and involvement the first *Essentials* manuscript would never have been completed and, as a consequence, this spin-off book would never have been written. His unfailing support and encouragement will never be forgotten.

For this edition we would like to thank in particular Chris Greenall and Tim Huckstep from the Dental Radiology Department in Cardiff Dental Hospital and Christie Lennox from the Dental Illustration Unit in Cardiff University for their help in producing many of the new radiographic images. We would also like to thank Wil Evans for his help with the section on radiation dose and Arnold Rust for his help with the section on dosemeters.

We are also grateful to the Health Protection Agency (formerly the National Radiological Protection Board) for their permission to again reproduce parts of the 2001 Guidance Notes (that now appear in the on-line section on the book) and to reproduce parts of their specific guidance on the use of CBCT. We are also grateful to Professor Keith Horner and the Faculty of General Dental Practice (UK) for their permission to reproduce sections from their 2013 Selection Criteria booklet and to Professor Horner and SEDENTEX CT project for their permission to reproduce some material from their 2011 guidelines on the clinical use of CBCT.

Special thanks to the team at Elsevier including Alison Taylor, Caroline Jones, Barbara Simmons and Jim Chiazzese for all their help and advice with project – both the book itself and the on-line resource.

Finally, the most special thanks of all to our wives Catriona and Anji and our children Stuart, Felicity and Claudia, and Karisma and Jaimini for their love, encouragement and understanding throughout the production of this edition.

EW
London 2013
ND
Cardiff 2013

List of colour plates

Additional online material

Besides the wealth of information found within *Radiography and Radiology for Dental Care Professionals 3E*, the authors have created a unique website – www.whaitesessentialsdentalradiography. com – to accompany the volume. This site contains two separate sections:

1. A summary of the UK ionising radiation legislation and guidance on good practice for all dental practitioners and dental care professionals

2. Self assessment questions and answers. Questions have been specially prepared for each of the 21 chapters to enable DCPs to assess their own knowledge and understanding. These include a mixture of multiple choice questions and multiple response questions, drag and drop identification of radiological anatomy as well as new examples of various pathological conditions to enable practice of diagnostic skills.

To access the site, go to www.whaitesessentialsdentalradiography.com and follow the simple log-on instructions shown.

Colour plates

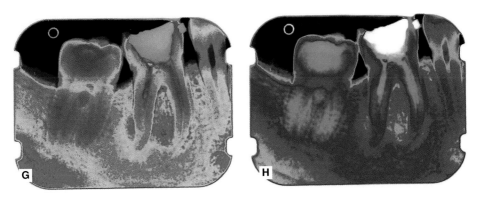

Fig. 3.31 Examples of digital image enhancement. **G** and **H** Pseudocoloured. *(See p. 46)*

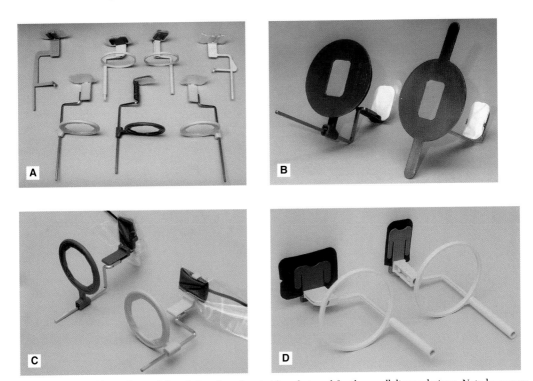

Fig. 7.6 A A selection of film packet and digital phosphor plate holders designed for the paralleling technique. Note how some manufacturers use colour coding to identify holders for different parts of the mouth. **B** Holders incorporating additional rectangular collimation — the Masel Precision all-in-one metal holder and the Rinn XCP holder with the metal collimator attached to the locator ring. **C** Blue anterior and yellow posterior Rinn XCP-DS solid-state digital sensor holders. **D** Green/yellow anterior and red/yellow posterior Hawe–Neos holders suitable for film packets and digital phosphor plates (shown here). *(See p. 82)*

1

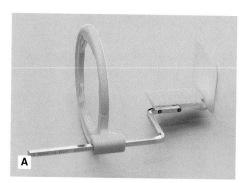

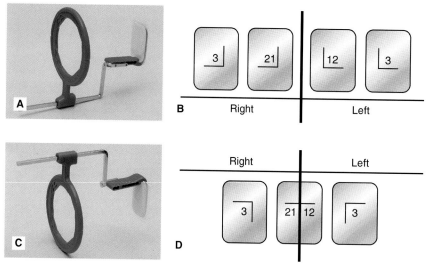

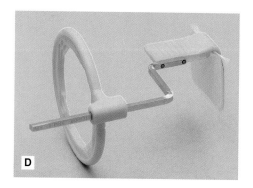

Fig. 7.7 A The anterior Rinn XCP holder suitable for imaging the maxillary incisors and canines. **B** Diagram showing the four small image receptors required to image the right and left maxillary incisors and canines. **C** The same anterior Rinn XCP holder suitable for imaging the mandibular incisors and canines. **D** Diagram showing the three small image receptors required to image the right and left mandibular incisors and canines. (See p. 82)

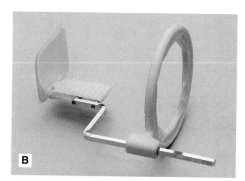

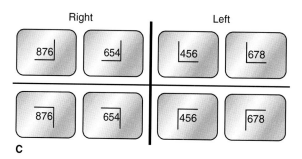

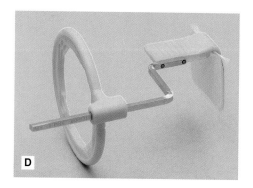

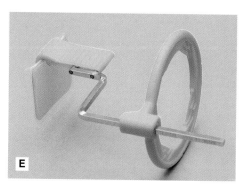

Fig. 7.8 A The posterior Rinn XCP holder assembled for imaging the RIGHT maxillary premolars and molars. **B** The posterior Rinn XCP holder assembled for imaging the LEFT maxillary premolars and molars. **C** Diagram showing the two large image receptors required to image the right and left premolars and molars in each quadrant. **D** The posterior Rinn XCP holder assembled for imaging the RIGHT mandibular premolars and molars. **E** The posterior Rinn XCP holder assembled for imaging the LEFT mandibular premolars and molars. (See p. 83)

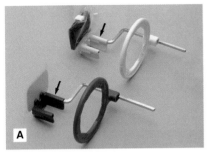

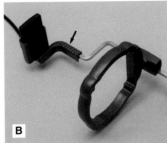

Fig. 7.38 Specially designed image receptor holders and beam-aiming devices for use during endodontics. **A** Rinn Endoray® suitable for film packets and digital phosphor plates (green) and solid-state digital sensors (white). **B** Anterior Planmeca solid-state digital sensor holder. Note the modified designs of the biteblocks (arrowed) to accommodate the handles of the endodontic instruments. Colour coding of holders by some manufacturers is now used to facilitate clinical use. (*See p. 106*)

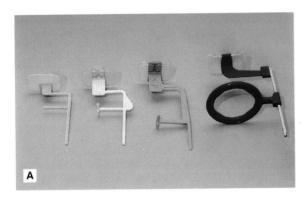

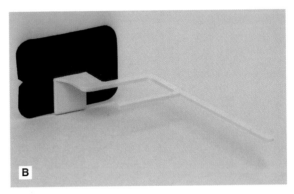

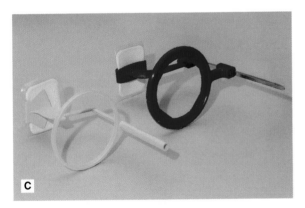

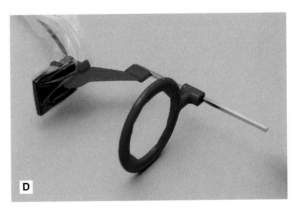

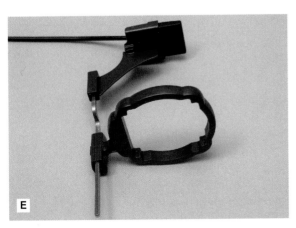

Fig. 8.5 Bitewing image receptor holders with beam-aiming devices. **A** A selection of horizontal bitewing holders set-up using a film packet as the image receptor — note the red colour coding for the Rinn XCP System. **B** The Hawe–Neos Kwikbite horizontal holder set-up using a digital phosphor plate. **C** Vertical bitewing holders — the red Rinn XCP holder and the yellow Hawe–Neos Parobite holder set-up using film packets. **D** The red Rinn XCP-DS horizontal bitewing solid-state digital sensor holder. **E** The Planmeca horizontal bitewing holder designed specifically for use with their dixi2 solid-state digital sensors. (*See p. 115*)

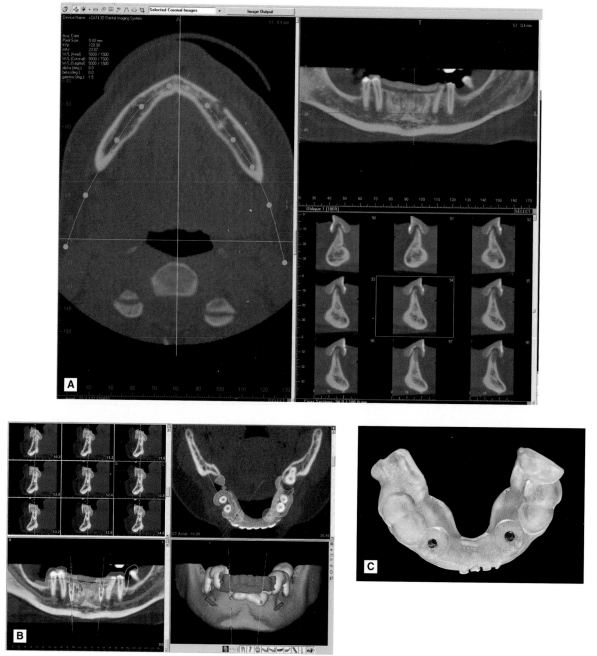

Fig. 20.4 Examples of pre-implant assessment CBCT images of the mandible. **A** Axial, panoramic and a series of cross-sectional images (or transaxial) images. **B** Example of an implant planning software program being used to plan the placement of implants in the lower right and left canine regions. Using the software the ideal position of the implants can be planned in three dimensions. The software is then used to design a drill guide, so the implant fixtures can be placed at the proposed sites (© Materialise Dental NV-SimPlant®). **C** The tooth-borne drill guide constructed to place implants in the lower canine regions. (Kindly provided by Dr Matthew Thomas.) *(See p. 263)*

Introduction

Part 1

The radiographic image

Introduction

The use of X-rays is an integral part of clinical dentistry, with some form of radiographic examination necessary on the majority of patients. As a result, radiographs are often referred to as the clinician's *main diagnostic aid*.

The range of knowledge of dental radiography and radiology thus required can be divided conveniently into four main sections:

- *Basic physics and equipment* – the production of X-rays, their properties and interactions which result in the formation of the radiographic image
- *Radiation protection* – the protection of patients and dental staff from the harmful effects of X-rays
- *Radiography* – the techniques involved in producing the various radiographic images
- *Radiology* – the interpretation of these radiographic images.

Understanding the radiographic image is central to the entire subject. This chapter provides an introduction to the nature of this image and to some of the factors that affect its quality and perception.

Nature of the radiographic image

Traditionally the image was produced by the X-rays passing through an object (the patient) and interacting with the photographic emulsion on a *film*, which resulted in blackening of the film. Film is gradually being replaced by a variety of *digital sensors* with the image being created in a computer. Those parts of the digital sensor that have been hit by X-rays appear black in the computer-generated image. The extent to which the emulsion or the computer-generated image is blackened depends on the number of X-rays reaching the film or the sensor (either device can be referred to as an *image receptor*), which in turn depends on the density of the object.

However the final image is captured, it can be described as a two-dimensional picture made up of a variety of black, white and grey superimposed shadows and is thus sometimes referred to as a *shadowgraph* (see Fig. 1.1).

Understanding the nature of the shadowgraph and interpreting the information contained within it requires a knowledge of:

- The radiographic shadows
- The three-dimensional anatomical tissues
- The limitations imposed by a two-dimensional picture and superimposition.

The radiographic shadows

The amount the X-ray beam is stopped (attenuated) by an object determines the *radiodensity* of the shadows:

- The white or *radiopaque* shadows on a film represent the various dense structures within the object which have totally stopped the X-ray beam.
- The black or *radiolucent* shadows represent areas where the X-ray beam has passed through the object and has not been stopped at all.
- The grey shadows represent areas where the X-ray beam has been stopped to a varying degree.

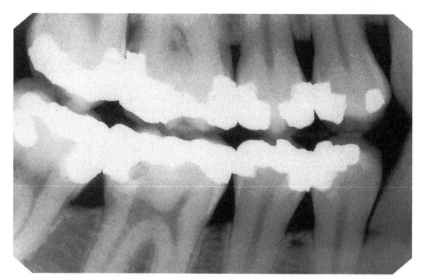

Fig. 1.1 A typical dental radiograph. The image shows the various black, grey and white radiographic shadows. The metallic amalgam fillings have totally stopped the X-ray beam so they appear white or *radiopaque*.

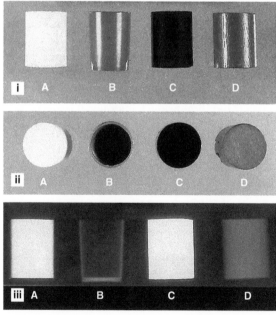

Fig. 1.2 **(i)** Front view and **(ii)** plan view of various cylinders of similar shape but made of different materials: **A** plaster of Paris, **B** hollow plastic, **C** metal, **D** wood. **(iii)** Radiographs of the cylinders show how objects of the same shape, but of different materials, produce different radiographic images.

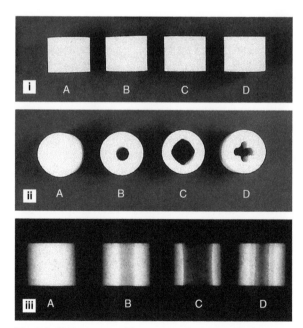

Fig. 1.3 **(i)** Front view of four apparently similar cylinders made from plaster of Paris. **(ii)** Plan view shows the cylinders have varying internal designs and thicknesses. **(iii)** Radiographs of the apparently similar cylinders show how objects of similar shape and material, but of different densities, produce different radiographic images.

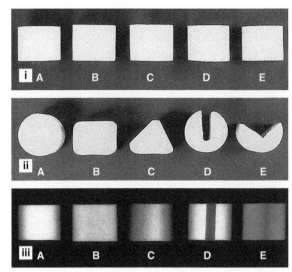

Fig. 1.4 (i) Front view of five apparently similar cylinders made from plaster of Paris. (ii) Plan view shows the objects are in fact different shapes. (iii) Radiographs show how objects of different shape, but made of the same material, produce different radiographic images.

The final *shadow density* of any object is thus affected by:

- The specific type of material of which the object is made
- The thickness or density of the material
- The shape of the object
- The intensity of the X-ray beam used
- The position of the object in relation to the X-ray beam and image receptor
- The sensitivity and type of image receptor.

The effect of different materials, different thicknesses/densities, different shapes and different X-ray beam intensities on the radiographic image shadows is shown in Figs 1.2–1.5.

The three-dimensional anatomical tissues

The shape, density and thickness of the patient's tissues, principally the hard tissues, must also affect the radiographic image. Therefore, when viewing two-dimensional radiographic images, the three-dimensional anatomy responsible for the image must be considered (see Fig. 1.6). A sound anatomical knowledge is obviously a prerequisite for radiological interpretation (see Ch. 16).

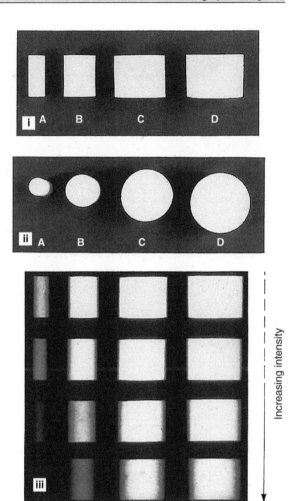

Fig. 1.5 (i) Front view and (ii) plan view of four cylinders made from plaster of Paris but of different diameters. (iii) Four radiographs using different intensity X-ray beams show how increasing the intensity of the X-ray beam causes greater penetration of the object with less attenuation, hence the less radiopaque (white) shadows of the object that are produced, particularly of the smallest cylinder.

The limitations imposed by a two-dimensional image and superimposition

The main limitations of viewing the two-dimensional image of a three-dimensional object are:

- Appreciating the overall shape of the object
- Superimposition and assessing the location and shape of structures *within* an object.

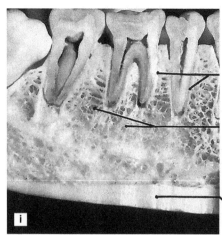

Cortical bone of the socket, producing the radiological lamina dura

Cancellous or trabecular bone, producing the radiological trabecular pattern

Dense compact bone of the lower border

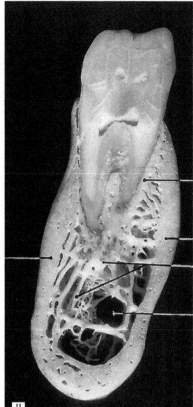

Cortical bone of the socket

Buccal cortical plate

Cancellous or trabecular bone

Inferior dental canal

Lingual cortical plate

A

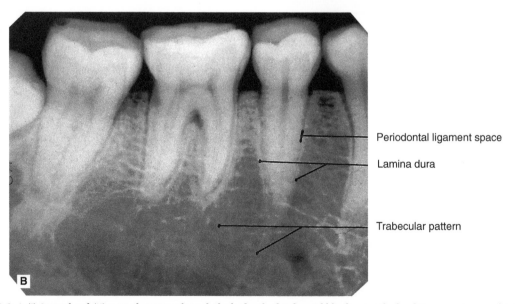

Periodontal ligament space

Lamina dura

Trabecular pattern

B

Fig. 1.6 A **(i)** Sagittal and **(ii)** coronal sections through the body of a dried mandible showing the hard tissue anatomy and internal bone pattern. **B** Two-dimensional radiographic image of the three-dimensional mandibular anatomy.

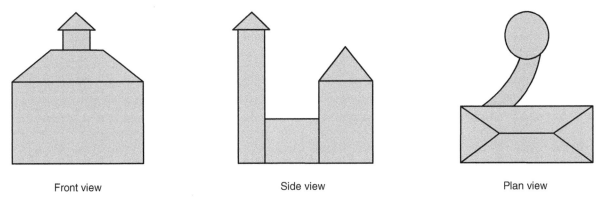

Front view Side view Plan view

Fig. 1.7 Diagram illustrating three views of a house. The side view shows that there is a corridor at the back of the house leading to a tall tower. The plan view provides the additional pieces of information that the roof of the tall tower is round and that the corridor is curved.

Appreciating the overall shape

To visualize all aspects of any three-dimensional object, it must be viewed from several different positions. This can be illustrated by considering an object such as a *house,* and the minimum information required if an architect is to draw all aspects of the three-dimensional building in two dimensions (see Fig. 1.7). Unfortunately, it is only too easy for the observer to forget that teeth and patients are three-dimensional. To expect one radiograph to provide *all* the required information about the shape of a tooth or a patient is like asking the architect to describe the whole house from the front view alone.

Superimposition and assessing the location and shape of structures within an object

The shadows cast by different parts of an object (or patient) are superimposed upon one another on the final radiograph. The image therefore provides limited or even misleading information as to where a particular internal structure lies, or to its shape, as shown in Fig. 1.8.

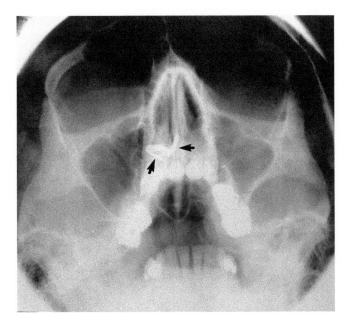

Fig. 1.8 Radiograph of the head from the front (an *occipitomental* view) taken with the head tipped back and the X-ray beam horizontal. This positioning lowers the dense bones of the base of the skull and raises the facial bones so avoiding superimposition of one on the other. A radiopaque (white) object (arrowed) can be seen apparently in the base of the right nasal cavity.

In addition, a dense radiopaque shadow on one side of the head may overlie an area of radiolucency on the other, so obscuring it from view, or a radiolucent shadow may make a superimposed radiopaque shadow appear less opaque.

One clinical solution to these problems is to take two views, at right angles to one another (see Figs 1.9 and 1.10). Unfortunately, even two views may still not be able to provide all the desired information for a diagnosis to be made (see Fig. 1.11).

These limitations of the conventional radiographic image have very important clinical implications and may be the underlying reason for a *negative radiographic report*. The fact that a particular feature or condition is not visible on one radiograph does not mean that the feature or condition does not exist, merely that it cannot be seen. The recently developed advanced imaging modality of cone beam computed tomography (CBCT) has been designed to try to overcome some of these limitations (see Chapter 13).

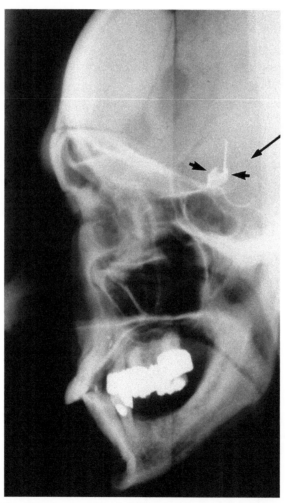

Fig. 1.9 Radiograph of the head from the side (a *true lateral skull view*) of the same patient shown in Fig. 1.8. The radiopaque (white) object (arrowed) now appears intracranially just above the skull base. It is in fact a metallic aneurysm clip positioned on an artery in the Circle of Willis at the base of the brain. The long black arrow indicates the direction of the X-ray beam required to produce the radiograph in Fig. 1.8, illustrating how an intracranial metallic clip can appear to be in the nose.

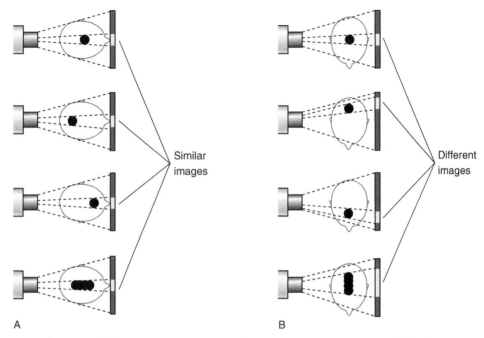

Fig. 1.10 Diagrams illustrating the limitations of a two-dimensional image. **A** Posteroanterior views of a head containing a variable mass. The mass appears as a similar sized opaque image on the radiograph, providing no differentiating information on its position or shape. **B** The side view provides a possible solution to the problems illustrated in **A**.

Quality of the radiographic image

Overall image quality and the amount of detail shown on a radiograph depend on several factors, including:

- Contrast – the visual difference between the various black, white and grey shadows
- Image geometry – the relative positions of the image receptor, object and X-ray tubehead
- Characteristics of the X-ray beam
- Image sharpness and resolution.

These factors are in turn dependent on several variables, relating to the density of the object, the type of image receptor and the X-ray equipment. They are discussed in greater detail in Chapter 14. However, to introduce how the geometrical accuracy and detail of the final image can be influenced, two of the main factors are considered below.

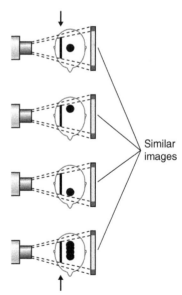

Fig. 1.11 Diagrams illustrating the problems of superimposition. Lateral views of the same masses shown in Fig. 1.10 but with an additional radiodense object superimposed (arrowed). This produces a similar image in each case with no evidence of the mass. The information obtained previously is now obscured and the usefulness of using two views at right angles is negated.

Positioning of the image receptor, object and X-ray beam

The position of the X-ray beam, object and image receptor needs to satisfy certain basic geometrical requirements. These include:

- The object and the image receptor should be in contact or as close together as possible.
- The object and the image receptor should be parallel to one another.
- The X-ray tubehead should be positioned so that the beam meets both the object and the image receptor at right angles.

These ideal requirements are shown diagrammatically in Fig. 1.12. The effects on the final image of varying the position of the object, image receptor or X-ray beam are shown in Fig. 1.13.

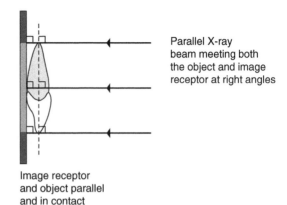

Parallel X-ray beam meeting both the object and image receptor at right angles

Image receptor and object parallel and in contact

Fig. 1.12 Diagram illustrating the ideal geometrical relationship between the object, image receptor and X-ray beam.

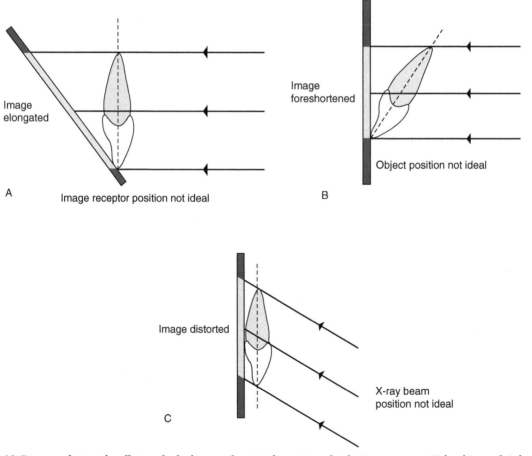

Image elongated

Image receptor position not ideal

A

Image foreshortened

Object position not ideal

B

Image distorted

X-ray beam position not ideal

C

Fig. 1.13 Diagrams showing the effect on the final image of varying the position of **A** the image receptor, **B** the object and **C** the X-ray beam.

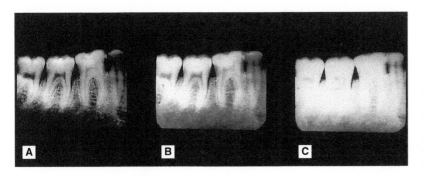

Fig. 1.14 Radiographs of the same area showing variation in contrast – the visual difference in the black, white and grey shadows due to the penetration of the X-ray beam. **A** Increased exposure (overpenetration). **B** Normal exposure. **C** Reduced exposure (underpenetration).

X-ray beam characteristics

The ideal X-ray beam used for imaging should be:

- Sufficiently penetrating, to pass through the patient and react with the film emulsion or digital sensor and produce good *contrast* between the different shadows (Fig. 1.14)
- Parallel, i.e. non-diverging, to prevent magnification of the image
- Produced from a point source, to reduce blurring of the edges of the image, a phenomenon known as the *penumbra* effect.

These ideal characteristics are discussed further in Chapter 3.

Perception of the radiographic image

The verb *to perceive* means *to apprehend with the mind using one or more of the senses.* Perception is the *act* or *faculty of perceiving.* In radiology, we use our sense of sight to perceive the radiographic image, but, unfortunately, we cannot rely completely on what we see. The apparently simple black, white and grey shadowgraph is a form of optical *illusion* (from the Latin *illudere*, meaning *to mock*). The radiographic image can thus mock our senses in a number of ways. The main problems can be caused by the effects of:

- Partial images
- Contrast
- Context.

Effect of partial images

As mentioned already, the radiographic image only provides the clinician with a partial image with limited information in the form of different density shadows. To complete the picture, the clinician fills in the gaps, but we do not all necessarily do this in the same way and may arrive at different conclusions. Three non-clinical examples are shown in Fig. 1.15. Clinically, our differing perceptions may lead to different diagnoses.

Effect of contrast

The apparent density of a particular radiographic shadow can be affected considerably by the density of the surrounding shadows. In other words, the contrast between adjacent structures can alter the perceived density of one or both of them (see Fig. 1.16). This is of particular importance in dentistry, where metallic restorations produce densely white radiopaque shadows that can affect the apparent density of the adjacent tooth tissue. This is discussed again in Chapter 17 in relation to caries diagnosis.

Effect of context

The environment or context in which we see an image can affect how we interpret that image. A non-clinical example is shown in Fig. 1.17. In dentistry, the environment that can affect our perception of radiographs is that created by the patient's description of the complaint. We can imagine that we see certain radiographic changes, because the patient has conditioned our perceptual apparatus.

These various perceptual problems are included simply as a warning that radiographic interpretation is not as straightforward as it may at first appear.

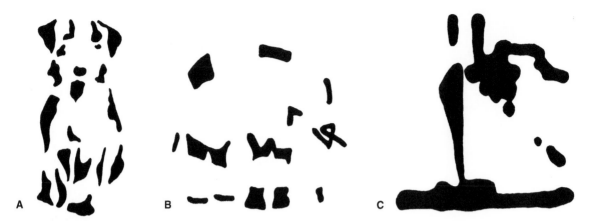

Fig. 1.15 The problem of partial images requiring the observer to fill in the missing gaps. Look at the three non-clinical pictures and what do you perceive? The objects shown are **A** a dog, **B** an elephant and **C** a steam ship. We all *see* the same partial images, but we don't necessarily *perceive* the same objects. Most people perceive the dog, some perceive the elephant while only a few perceive the ship and take some convincing that it is there. Interestingly, once observers have perceived the correct objects, it is impossible to look at the pictures again in the future without perceiving them correctly. (Figures from: Coren S, Porac C, Ward LM 1979 *Sensation and Perception*. Harcourt Brace and Company, reproduced by permission of the publisher.)

Fig. 1.16 The effect of contrast. The four small inner squares are in reality all the same grey colour, but they appear to be different because of the effect of contrast. When the surrounding square is black, the observer perceives the inner square to be very pale, while when the surrounding square is light grey, the observer perceives the inner square to be dark. (Figure from: Cornsweet TN 1970 *Visual Perception*. Harcourt Brace and Company, reproduced by permission of the publisher.)

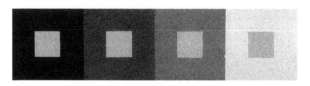

Fig. 1.17 The effect of context. If asked to read the two lines shown here most, if not all, observers would read the letters A,B,C,D,E,F and then the numbers 10,11,12,13,14. Closer examination shows the letter B and the number 13 to be identical. They are perceived as B and 13 because of the context (surrounding letters or numbers) in which they are seen. (Figure from: Coren S, Porac C, Ward LM 1979 *Sensation and Perception*. Harcourt Brace and Company, reproduced by permission of the publisher.)

Common types of dental radiographs

The various radiographic images of the teeth, jaws and skull are divided into two main groups:

- *Intraoral* – the image receptor is placed *inside* the patient's mouth, including:
  - Periapical radiographs (Ch. 7)
  - Bitewing radiographs (Ch. 8)
  - Occlusal radiographs (Ch. 9)
- *Extraoral* – the image receptor is placed *outside* the patient's mouth, including:
  - Oblique lateral radiographs (Ch. 10)
  - Lateral skull radiographs (Ch. 11)
  - Panoramic radiographs (Ch. 12).

These various radiographic techniques are described later, in the chapters indicated. The approach and format adopted throughout these radiography chapters are intended to be straightforward, practical and clinically relevant and are based upon the essential knowledge required. This includes:

- WHY each particular projection is taken – i.e. the main clinical indications
- HOW the projections are taken – i.e. the relative positions of the patient, image receptor and X-ray tubehead
- WHAT the resultant radiographs should look like and which anatomical features they show.

To access the self assessment questions for this chapter please go to www.whaitesessentialsdentalradiography.com

Radiation physics, equipment and radiation protection

Part 2

PART CONTENTS

2 The production, properties and interactions of X-rays

Introduction

X-rays and their ability to penetrate human tissues were discovered by Röentgen in 1895. He called them X-rays because their nature was then unknown. They are in fact a form of high-energy electromagnetic radiation and are part of the electromagnetic spectrum, which also includes low-energy radiowaves, television and visible light (see Table 2.1).

X-rays are described as consisting of *wave packets* of energy. Each packet is called a *photon* and is equivalent to one *quantum* of energy. The X-ray *beam*, as used in diagnostic radiology, is made up of millions of individual photons.

To understand the production and interactions of X-rays a basic knowledge of atomic physics is essential. The next section aims to provide a simple summary of this required background information.

Atomic structure

Atoms are the basic building blocks of matter. They consist of minute particles – the so-called fundamental or elementary particles – held together by electric and nuclear forces. They consist of a central dense *nucleus* made up of nuclear particles – *protons* and *neutrons* – surrounded by *electrons* in specific orbits or shells (see Fig. 2.1).

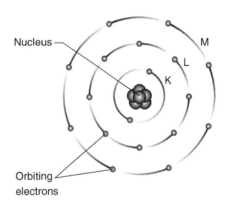

Nucleus

M

L

K

Orbiting electrons

Fig. 2.1 Diagrammatic representation of atomic structure showing the central nucleus and orbiting electrons.

Table 2.1 The electromagnetic spectrum ranging from the low energy (long wavelength) radio waves to the high energy (short wavelength) X- and gamma-rays

Radiation	Wavelength	Photon energy
Radio, television and radar waves	3×10^4 m to 100 µm	4.1×10^{-11} eV to 1.2×10^{-2} eV
Infra-red	100 µm to 700 nm	1.2×10^{-2} eV to 1.8 eV
Visible light	700 nm to 400 nm	1.8 eV to 3.1 eV
Ultra-violet	400 nm to 10 nm	3.1 eV to 124 eV
X-and gamma-rays	10 nm to 0.01 pm	124 eV to 124 MeV

Useful definitions

- *Atomic number* (Z) – The number of protons in the nucleus of an atom
- *Neutron number* (N) – The number of neutrons in the nucleus of an atom
- *Atomic mass number* (A) – Sum of the number of protons and number of neutrons in an atom (A = Z + N)
- *Isotopes* – Atoms with the same atomic number (Z) but with different atomic mass numbers (A) and hence different numbers of neutrons (N)
- *Radioisotopes* – Isotopes with unstable nuclei which undergo radioactive disintegration.

Main features of the atomic particles

Nuclear particles (nucleons)

Protons

- Mass = 1.66×10^{-27} kg
- Charge = positive: 1.6×10^{-19} coulombs.

Neutrons

- Mass = 1.70×10^{-27} kg
- Charge = nil
- Neutrons act as *binding agents* within the nucleus and hold it together by counteracting the repulsive forces between the protons.

Electrons

- Mass = 1/1840 of the mass of a proton
- Charge = negative: -1.6×10^{-19} coulombs
- Electrons move in predetermined circular or elliptical shells or orbits around the nucleus
- The shells represent different *energy levels* and are labelled K,L,M,N,O outwards from the nucleus
- The shells can contain up to a maximum number of electrons per shell:
  K ... 2
  L ... 8
  M ... 18
  N ... 32
  O ... 50
- Electrons can move from shell to shell but cannot exist between shells – an area known as *the forbidden zone*

- To remove an electron from the atom, additional energy is required to overcome the *binding energy* of attraction which keeps the electrons in their shells.

Summary of important points on atomic structure

- In the neutral atom, the number of orbiting electrons is equal to the number of protons in the nucleus. Since the number of electrons determines the chemical behaviour of an atom, the *atomic number* (Z) also determines this chemical behaviour. Each *element* has different chemical properties and thus each *element* has a different *atomic number*. These form the basis of the *periodic table*.
- Atoms in the ground state are electrically neutral because the number of positive charges (protons) is balanced by the number of negative charges (electrons).
- If an electron is removed, the atom is no longer neutral, but becomes positively charged and is referred to as a *positive ion*. The process of removing an electron from an atom is called *ionization*.
- If an electron is displaced from an inner shell to an outer shell (i.e. to a higher energy level), the atom remains neutral but is in an excited state. This process is called *excitation*.
- The unit of energy in the atomic system is the electron volt (eV):

$$1\,\text{eV} = 1.6 \times 10^{-19}\ \text{joules}.$$

X-ray production

X-rays are produced inside machines, so called *X-ray generating equipment*, which are described in more detail in Chapter 3. However, a typical dental X-ray machine is shown in Fig. 2.2A. The X-ray generating part is referred to as the *tube-head* (see Fig. 2.2B), within which is a small evacuated glass envelope called the *X-ray tube* (see Fig. 2.2C and D). X-rays are produced inside the X-ray tube when energetic (high speed) electrons bombard the target and are suddenly brought to rest.

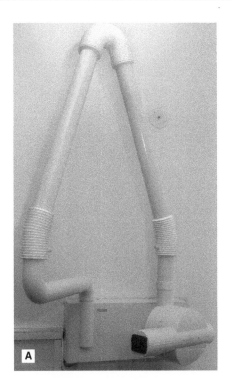

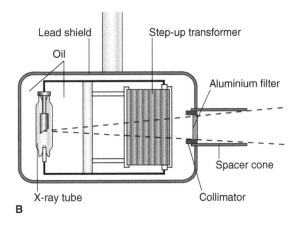

B

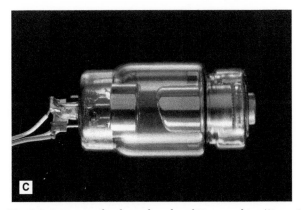

C

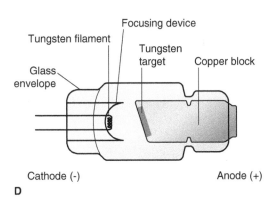

D

Fig. 2.2 **A** An example of a modern dental X-ray machine (Sirona Hediodent® DS). **B** Diagram of a typical *tubehead* showing the main components. **C** An example of an actual dental X-ray *tube*. **D** Diagram of the dental X-ray *tube* showing the main components.

Main features and requirements of an X-ray tube

- The *cathode* (negative) consists of a heated filament of tungsten that provides the source of electrons.
- The *anode* (positive) consists of a *target* (a small piece of tungsten) set into the angled face of a large *copper block* to allow efficient removal of heat.
- A *focusing device* aims the stream of electrons at the *focal spot* on the target.
- A high-voltage (kilovoltage, kV) connected between the cathode and anode accelerates the electrons from the negative filament to the positive target. This is sometimes referred to as kVp or kilovoltage peak, as explained later in Chapter 3.
- A current (milliamperage, mA) flows from the cathode to the anode. This is a measure of the quantity of electrons being accelerated.
- A surrounding *lead casing* absorbs unwanted X-rays as a radiation protection measure since X-rays are emitted in all directions.
- Surrounding *oil* facilitates the removal of heat.

Practical considerations

The production of X-rays can be summarized as the following sequence of events:

1. The filament is electrically heated and a cloud of electrons is produced around the filament.
2. The high-voltage (potential difference) across the tube accelerates the electrons at very high speed towards the anode.
3. The focusing device aims the electron stream at the focal spot on the target.
4. The electrons bombard the target and are brought suddenly to rest.
5. The energy lost by the electrons is transferred into either *heat* (about 99%) or X-rays (about 1%).
6. The heat produced is removed and dissipated by the copper block and the surrounding oil.
7. The X-rays are emitted in all directions from the target. Those emitted through the small

window in the lead casing constitute the *beam* used for diagnostic purposes.

Interactions at the atomic level

The high-speed electrons bombarding the target (Fig. 2.3) are involved in two main types of *collision* with the tungsten atoms:

- Heat-producing collisions
- X-ray-producing collisions.

Heat-producing collisions

- The incoming electron is deflected by the cloud of outer-shell tungsten electrons, with a small loss of energy, in the form of *heat* (Fig. 2.4A).
- The incoming electron collides with an outer shell tungsten electron displacing it to an even more peripheral shell (excitation) or displacing it from the atom (ionization), again with a small loss of energy in the form of *heat* (Fig. 2.4B).

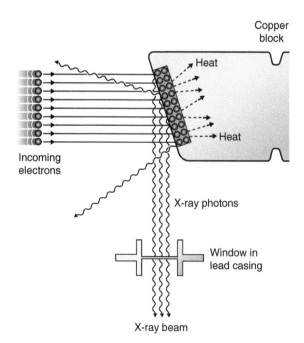

Fig. 2.3 Diagram of the anode enlarged, showing the target and summarizing the interactions at the target.

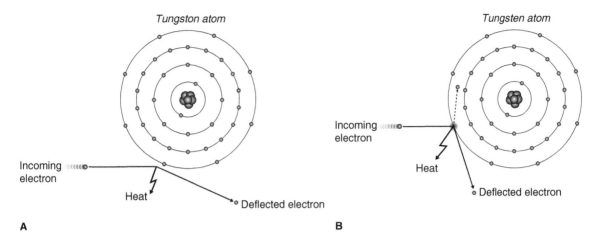

Fig. 2.4 A Heat-producing collision: the incoming electron is deflected by the tungsten electron cloud. **B** Heat-producing collision: the incoming electron collides with and displaces an outer-shell tungsten electron.

Important points to note

- Heat-producing interactions are the most common because there are millions of incoming electrons and many outer-shell tungsten electrons with which to interact.
- Each individual bombarding electron can undergo many heat-producing collisions resulting in a considerable amount of heat at the target.
- Heat needs to be removed quickly and efficiently to prevent damage to the target. This is achieved by setting the tungsten target in the copper block, utilizing the high thermal capacity and good conduction properties of copper.

X-ray-producing collisions

- The incoming electron penetrates the outer electron shells and passes close to the nucleus of the tungsten atom. The incoming electron is dramatically slowed down and deflected by the nucleus with a large loss of energy which is emitted in the form of *X-rays* (Fig. 2.5A).
- The incoming electron collides with an inner-shell tungsten electron displacing it to an outer shell (excitation) or displacing it from the atom (ionization), with a large loss of energy and subsequent emission of *X-rays* (Fig. 2.5B).

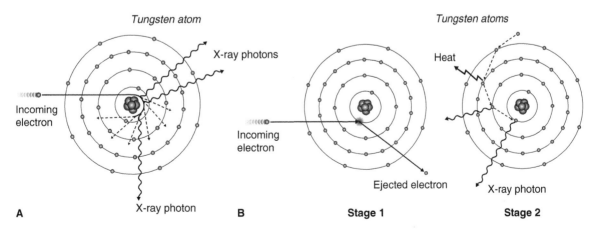

Fig. 2.5 A X-ray-producing collision: the incoming electron passes close to the tungsten nucleus and is rapidly slowed down and deflected with the emission of X-ray photons. **B** X-ray-producing collision: Stage 1 – the incoming electron collides with an inner-shell tungsten electron and displaces it; Stage 2 – outer-shell electrons drop into the inner shells with subsequent emission of X-ray photons.

X-ray spectra

The two X-ray-producing collisions result in the production of two different types of *X-ray spectra:*

- Continuous spectrum
- Characteristic spectrum.

Continuous spectrum

The X-ray photons emitted by the rapid deceleration of the bombarding electrons passing close to the nucleus of the tungsten atom are sometimes referred to as *bremsstrahlung* or *braking radiation.* The amount of deceleration and degree of deflection determine the amount of energy lost by the bombarding electron and hence the energy of the resultant emitted photon. A wide range or *spectrum* of photon energies is therefore possible and is termed the *continuous spectrum* (see Fig. 2.6).

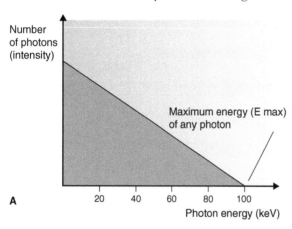

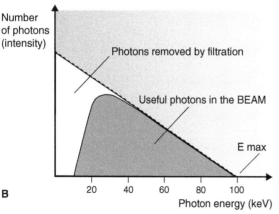

Fig. 2.6 A Graph showing the continuous X-ray spectrum at the target for an X-ray tube operating at 100 kV. **B** Graph showing the continuous spectrum in the emitted beam, as the result *of filtration.*

Summary of important points

- Small deflections of the bombarding electrons are the most common, producing many *low-energy* photons.
- Low-energy photons have little penetrating power and most will not exit from the X-ray tube itself. They will not contribute to the useful X-ray beam (see Fig. 2.6B). This removal of low-energy photons from the beam is known as *filtration* (see later).
- Large deflections are less likely to happen so there are relatively few *high-energy* photons.
- The maximum photon energy possible (Emax) is directly related to the size of the potential difference (kV) across the X-ray tube.

Characteristic spectrum

Following the ionization or excitation of the tungsten atoms by the bombarding electrons, the orbiting tungsten electrons rearrange themselves to return the atom to the neutral or ground state. This involves electron 'jumps' from one energy level (shell) to another, and results in the emission of X-ray photons with specific energies. As stated previously, the energy levels or shells are specific for any particular atom. The X-ray photons emitted from the target are therefore described as *characteristic of tungsten atoms* and form the *characteristic* or *line spectrum* (see Fig. 2.7). The photon lines are named K and L, depending on the shell from which they have been emitted (see Fig. 2.1).

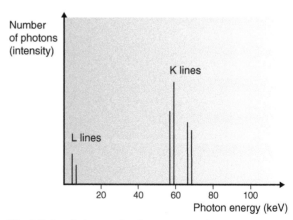

Fig. 2.7 Graph showing the characteristic or line spectrum at the target for an X-ray tube (with a tungsten target) operating at 100 kV.

Summary of important points

- Only the K lines are of diagnostic importance since the L lines have too little energy.
- The bombarding high-speed electron must have sufficient energy (69.5 kV) to displace a K-shell tungsten electron to produce the characteristic K line on the spectrum. (The energy of the bombarding electrons is directly related to the potential difference (kV) across the X-ray tube, see later.)
- Characteristic K-line photons are not produced by X-ray tubes with tungsten targets operating at less than 69.5 kV – referred to as the *critical voltage* (Vc).
- Dental X-ray equipment usually operates between 50 kV and 90 kV (see Ch. 3).

Combined spectra

In X-ray equipment operating above 69.5 kV, the final total spectrum of the useful X-ray *beam* will be the addition of the continuous and characteristic spectra (see Fig. 2.8).

Summary of the main properties and characteristics of X-rays

- X-rays are *wave packets* of energy of electromagnetic radiation that originate at the atomic level.
- Each *wave packet* is equivalent to a *quantum* of energy and is called a *photon*.

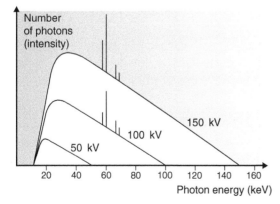

Fig. 2.8 Graphs showing the combination photon energy spectra (in the final beam) for X-ray sets operating at 50 kV, 100 kV and 150 kV.

- An X-ray *beam* is made up of millions of photons of different energies.
- The diagnostic X-ray beam can vary in its *intensity* and in its *quality*:
  - Intensity = the number or quantity of X-ray photons in the beam
  - Quality = the energy carried by the X-ray photons which is a measure of their penetrating power.
- The factors that can affect the intensity and/or the quality of the beam include:
  - Size of the tube voltage (kV)
  - Size of the tube current (mA)
  - Distance from the target (d)
  - Time = length of exposure (t)
  - Filtration
  - Target material
  - Tube voltage waveform (see Ch. 3).
- In free space, X-rays travel in straight lines.
- Velocity in free space = 3×10^8 m s^{-1}.
- In free space, X-rays obey the inverse square law:

$$\text{Intensity} = 1/d^2$$

Doubling the distance from an X-ray source reduces the intensity to ¼ (a very important principle in radiation protection, see Ch. 5).
- No medium is required for propagation.
- Shorter-wavelength X-rays possess greater energy and can therefore penetrate a greater distance.
- Longer-wavelength X-rays, sometimes referred to as *soft X-rays*, possess less energy and have little penetrating power.
- The energy carried by X-rays can be attenuated by matter, i.e. absorbed or scattered (see later).
- X-rays are capable of producing *ionization* (and subsequent biological damage in living tissue, see Ch. 5) and are thus referred to as *ionizing radiation*.
- X-rays are undetectable by human senses.
- X-rays can affect film emulsion to produce a visual image (the radiograph) and can cause certain salts to fluoresce and to emit light – the principle behind the use of intensifying screens in extraoral cassettes and digital sensors (see Ch. 3).

Interaction of X-rays with matter

When X-rays strike matter, such as a patient's tissues, the photons have four possible fates, shown diagrammatically in Fig. 2.9. The photons may be:

- Completely scattered with no loss of energy
- Absorbed with total loss of energy
- Scattered with some absorption and loss of energy
- Transmitted unchanged.

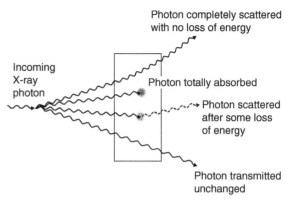

Fig. 2.9 Diagram summarizing the main interactions when X-rays interact with matter.

Definition of terms used in X-ray interactions

- *Scattering* – change in direction of a photon with or without a loss of energy
- *Absorption* – deposition of energy, i.e. removal of energy from the beam
- *Attenuation* – reduction in the intensity of the main X-ray beam caused by absorption and scattering

    Attenuation = Absorption + Scattering

- *Ionization* – removal of an electron from a neutral atom producing a negative ion (the electron) and a positive ion (the remaining atom).

Interaction of X-rays at the atomic level

There are four main interactions at the atomic level, depending on the energy of the incoming photon, these include:

- Unmodified or Rayleigh scattering – pure scatter
- Photoelectric effect – pure absorption
- Compton effect – scatter and absorption
- Pair production – pure absorption.

    Only two interactions are important in the X-ray energy range used in dentistry:

- Photoelectric effect
- Compton effect.

Photoelectric effect

The photoelectric effect is a pure absorption interaction predominating with *low-energy* photons (see Fig. 2.10).

Summary of the stages in the photoelectric effect

1. The incoming X-ray photon interacts with a bound inner-shell electron of the tissue atom.
2. The inner-shell electron is ejected with considerable energy (now called a *photoelectron*) into the tissues and will undergo further interactions (see below).
3. The X-ray photon disappears having deposited all its energy; the process is therefore one of pure *absorption*.
4. The vacancy which now exists in the inner electron shell is filled by outer-shell electrons dropping from one shell to another.
5. This cascade of electrons to new energy levels results in the formation of very low energy radiation (e.g. light) which is quickly absorbed.
6. Atomic stability is finally achieved by the capture of a free electron to return the atom to its neutral state.
7. The high-energy ejected *photoelectron* behaves like the original high-energy X-ray photon, undergoing many similar interactions and ejecting other electrons as it passes through the tissues. It is these ejected high-energy electrons that are responsible for the majority of the ionization interactions within tissue, and the possible resulting damage attributable to X-rays.

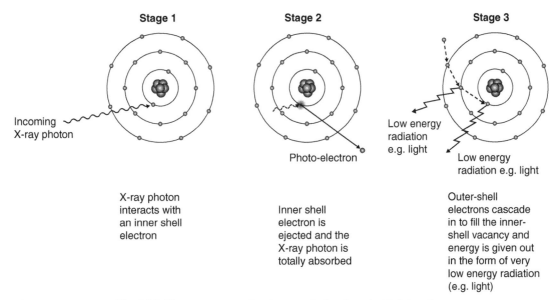

Fig. 2.10 Diagrams representing the stages in the photoelectric interaction.

Important points to note

- The X-ray photon energy needs to be equal to, or just greater than, the binding energy of the inner-shell electron to be able to eject it.
- As the density (atomic number, Z) increases, the number of bound inner-shell electrons also increases. The probability of photoelectric interactions occurring is $\propto Z^3$. Lead has an atomic number of 82 and is therefore a good absorber of X-rays – hence its use in radiation protection (see Ch. 5). The approximate atomic number for soft tissue is 7 ($Z^3 = 343$) and for bone is 12 ($Z^3 = 1728$) – hence their obvious difference in radiodensity, and the *contrast* between the different tissues seen on radiographs.
- This interaction predominates with low energy X-ray photons – the probability of photoelectric interactions occurring is $\propto 1/kV^3$. This explains why low kV X-ray equipment results in high absorption (dose) in the patient's tissues, but provides good contrast radiographs.
- The overall result of the interaction is *ionization* of the tissues.
- Intensifying screens, described in Chapter 3, function by the photoelectric effect – when exposed to X-rays, the screens emit their excess energy as *light,* which subsequently affects the film emulsion.

Compton effect

The Compton effect is an absorption *and* scattering process predominating with *higher-energy* photons (see Fig. 2.11).

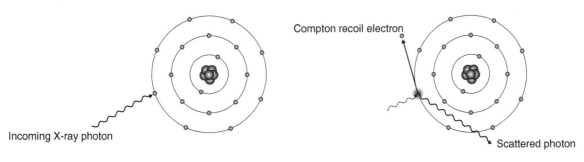

Fig. 2.11 Diagram showing the interactions of the Compton effect.

Summary of the stages in the Compton effect

1. The incoming X-ray photon interacts with a *free* or loosely bound outer-shell electron of the tissue atom.
2. The outer-shell electron is ejected (now called the *Compton recoil electron*) with some of the energy of the incoming photon, i.e. there is some *absorption*. The ejected electron then undergoes further ionizing interactions within the tissues (as before).
3. The remainder of the incoming photon energy is deflected or *scattered* from its original path as a scattered photon.
4. The scattered photon may then:
   - Undergo further Compton interactions within the tissues
   - Undergo photoelectric interactions within the tissues
   - Escape from the tissues – it is these photons that form the *scatter radiation* of concern in the clinical environment.
5. Atomic stability is again achieved by the capture of another free electron.

Important points to note

- The energy of the incoming X-ray photon is much greater than the binding energy of the outer-shell or free electron.
- The incoming X-ray photon cannot distinguish between one free electron and another – the interaction is not dependent on the atomic number (Z). Thus, this interaction provides very little diagnostic information as there is very little discrimination between different tissues on the final radiograph.
- This interaction predominates with high X-ray photon energies. This explains why high-voltage X-ray sets result in radiographs with poor contrast.
- The energy of the scattered photon (Es) is always less than the energy of the incoming photon (E), depending on the energy given to the recoil electron (e):

$$Es = E - e$$

- Scattered photons can be deflected in any direction, but the angle of scatter (θ) depends on their energy. *High-energy* scattered photons produce *forward* scatter; *low-energy* scattered photons produce *back* scatter (see Fig. 2.12).
- Forward scatter may reach the film and degrade the image.
- The overall result of the interaction is ionization of the tissues (see Ch. 5).

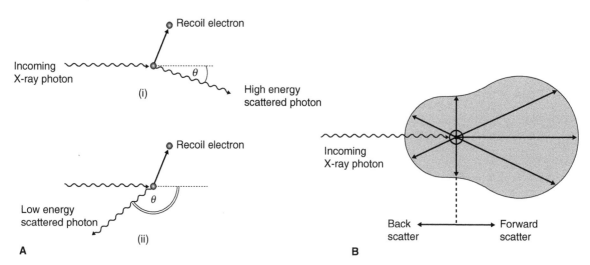

Fig. 2.12 A Diagram showing the angle of scatter θ with **(i)** high- and **(ii)** low-energy scattered photons. **B** Typical scatter distribution diagram of a 70 kV X-ray set. The length of any radius from the source of scatter indicates the relative amount of scatter in that direction. At this voltage, the majority of scatter is in a forward direction.

To access the self assessment questions for this chapter please go to www.whaitesessentialsdentalradiography.com

3

Dental X-ray equipment, image receptors and image processing

This chapter summarizes the more important points of the equipment and the other practical aspects involved in the production of the final radiographic image, namely:

- X-ray generating equipment – required to produce the X-rays
- Image receptors (film and digital) – required to detect the X-rays
- Image processing (chemical or computer) – required to produce the visual black, white and grey image.

Dental X-ray generating equipment

There are several conventional dental X-ray units available from various manufacturers. They vary in appearance, complexity and cost, but all consist of three main components:

- A tubehead
- Positioning arms
- A control panel and circuitry.

These dental units can either be *fixed* (wall, floor or ceiling mounted) or *mobile* (attached to a sturdy frame on wheels), as shown in Figs 3.1A and B. A recent development has been the production of *hand-held* dental units (Fig. 3.1C), particularly useful for domiciliary and forensic radiology.

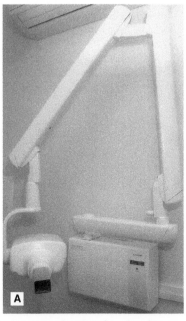

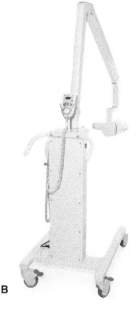

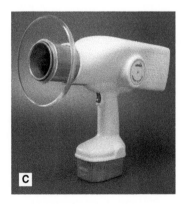

Fig. 3.1 Examples of modern dental X-ray generating equipment. **A** Wall-mounted Prostyle Intra® manufactured by Planmeca. **B** Mobile Kodak 2200. **C** Hand-held Nomad ™ manufactured by Aribex.

Ideal requirements

The equipment should be:

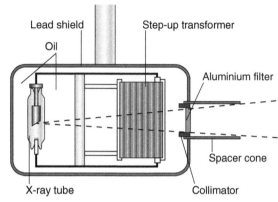

- Safe and accurate
- Capable of generating X-rays in the desired energy range and with adequate mechanisms for heat removal
- Small
- Easy to manoeuvre and position
- Stable, balanced and steady once the tubehead has been positioned
- Easily folded and stored
- Simple to operate and capable of both film and digital imaging
- Robust.

Fig. 3.2 Diagram of the tubehead of a typical dental X-ray set showing the main components.

Main components of the tubehead

A diagram of a typical tubehead is shown in Fig. 3.2. The main components include:

- The *glass X-ray tube*, including the filament, copper block and the target (see Ch. 2)
- The *step-up transformer* required to step-up the mains voltage of 240 volts to the high voltage (kV) required across the X-ray tube
- The *step-down transformer* required to step-down the mains voltage of 240 volts to the low voltage current required to heat the filament
- A *surrounding lead shield* to minimize leakage
- *Surrounding oil* to facilitate heat removal
- *Aluminium filtration* to remove harmful low-energy (soft) X-rays (see Fig. 3.3)
- The *collimator* – a metal disc or cylinder with central aperture designed to shape and limit the beam size to a rectangle (the same size as an intraoral image receptor) or round with a maximum diameter of 6 cm (see Figs 3.3 and 3.4)
- The *spacer cone* or *beam-indicating device (BID)* – a device for indicating the direction of the beam and setting the ideal distance from the focal spot on the target to the skin. The required *focus to skin distances (fsd)* are:
  - 200 mm for sets operating above 60 kV
  - 100 mm for sets operating below 60 kV

It is the length of *the focal spot to skin distance (fsd)* that is important NOT the physical length of the spacer cone. Various designs are illustrated in Fig. 3.4.

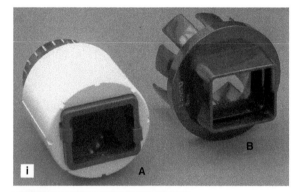

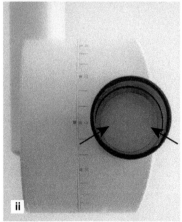

Fig. 3.3 **(i)** Examples of adaptors/collimators designed to change the shape of the beam from circular to rectangular: **A** Sirona Heliodent® DS collimator; **B** Dentsply's Universal collimator. **(ii)** Aluminium filter (arrowed) viewed from down the spacer cone on the Sirona Heliodent® DS.

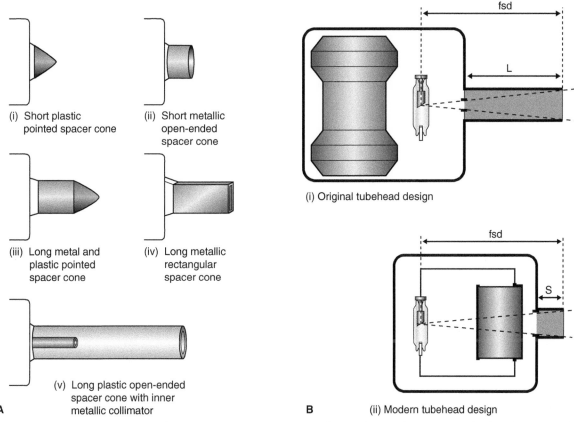

(i) Short plastic pointed spacer cone

(ii) Short metallic open-ended spacer cone

(iii) Long metal and plastic pointed spacer cone

(iv) Long metallic rectangular spacer cone

(v) Long plastic open-ended spacer cone with inner metallic collimator

A

(i) Original tubehead design

(ii) Modern tubehead design

B

Fig. 3.4 A Diagrams showing various designs and shapes of spacer cones or beam-indicating devices. **Note:** The short plastic pointed spacer cone is NOT recommended. **B** Diagrams showing **(i)** the original tubehead design with the X-ray tube at the front of the head, thus requiring a long spacer cone (L) to achieve a near-parallel X-ray beam and the correct *focus to skin distance* (fsd) and **(ii)** the modern tubehead design with the X-ray tube at the back of the head, thus requiring only a short spacer cone (S) to achieve the same *focus to skin distance (fsd)*.

Focal spot size and the principle of line focus

As stated in Chapter 1, the focal spot (the source of the X-rays) should be ideally a *point source* to reduce blurring of the image – the *penumbra effect* – as shown in Fig. 3.5A. However, the heat produced at the target by the bombarding electrons needs to be distributed over as large an area as possible. These two opposite requirements are satisfied by using an angled target and the principle of *line focus*, as shown in Fig. 3.5B.

Main components of the control panel

Examples of three typical control panels are shown in Fig. 3.6. The main components include:

- The *mains on/off* switch and *warning light*

- The *timer*, of which there are three main types:
  - electronic
  - impulse
  - clockwork (inaccurate and no longer used)
- An *exposure time selector* mechanism, usually either:
  - numerical, time selected in seconds
  - anatomical, area of mouth selected and exposure time adjusted automatically
- *Warning lights and audible signals* to indicate when X-rays are being generated
- Other features can include:
  - *Film speed selector*
  - *Patient size selector*
  - *Mains voltage compensator*
  - *Kilovoltage selector*
  - *Milliamperage switch*
  - *Exposure adjustment for digital imaging.*

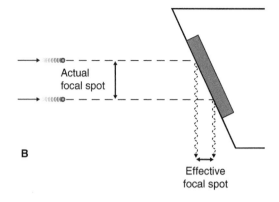

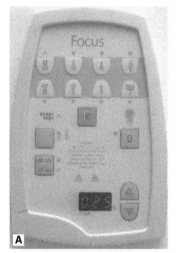

Sharply defined
edge to the image

Point
focal
spot

(i)

Blurring at the
edge of the image
– penumbra effect

Large
focal
spot

A   **(ii)**

Actual
focal spot

B

Effective
focal spot

Fig. 3.5 A Diagrams showing the effect of X-ray beam
source (focal spot) size on image blurring **(i)** a small or
point source, **(ii)** a large source. **B** The principle of line
focus: diagram of the target and focal spot showing how
the angled target face allows a large actual focal spot
but a small *effective* focal spot.

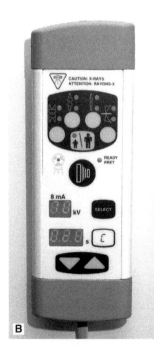

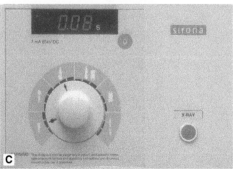

Fig. 3.6 Examples of modern dental X-ray
equipment control panels. **A** Focus® manufactured by
Instrumentarium Imaging. **B** Prostyle Intra®
manufactured by Planmeca. **C** Heliodent® DS
manufactured by Sirona. They are all anatomical
timers suitable for film and digital imaging.

Circuitry and tube voltage

The mains supply to the X-ray machine of 240 volts has two functions:

- To generate the high potential difference (kV) to accelerate the electrons across the X-ray tube via the step-up transformer
- To provide the low-voltage current to heat the tube filament via the step-down transformer.

However, the incoming 240 volts is an alternating current with the typical waveform shown in Fig. 3.7. Half the cycle is positive and the other half is negative. For X-ray production, only the positive half of the cycle can be used to ensure that the electrons from the filament are always drawn towards the target. Thus, the stepped-up high voltage applied across the X-ray tube needs to be *rectified* to eliminate the negative half of the cycle. Four types of rectified circuits are used:

- Half-wave rectified
- Single-phase, full-wave rectified
- Three-phase, full-wave rectified
- Constant potential.

The waveforms resulting from these rectified circuits, together with graphical representation of their subsequent X-ray production, are shown in Fig. 3.8. These changing waveforms mean that equipment is only working at its optimum or peak output at the top of each cycle. The kilovoltage is therefore often described as the *kVpeak* or *kVp*. Thus a 50 kVp half-wave rectified X-ray set only in fact functions at 50 kV for a tiny fraction of the time of any exposure.

Modern designs favour constant potential circuitry, often referred to as *DC units*, which keep

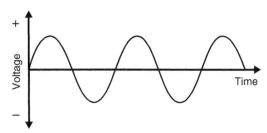

Fig. 3.7 Diagram showing the alternating current waveform.

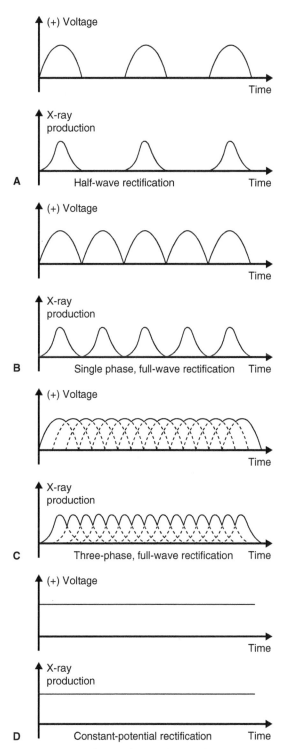

Fig. 3.8 Diagrams showing the waveforms and X-ray production graphs resulting from different forms of rectification.

the kilovoltage at kVpeak throughout any exposure, thus ensuring that:

- X-ray production per unit time is more efficient
- More high-energy, diagnostically useful photons are produced per exposure
- Fewer low energy, harmful photons are produced
- Shorter exposure times are possible.

Other X-ray generating apparatus

The other X-ray generating equipment encountered in dental practices includes:

- Panoramic X-ray machines often combined with cephalometric skull equipment (see Chs 11 and 12)
- Cone beam computed tomography (CBCT) units (see Ch. 13).

The main features and practical components of relevant machines are outlined in later chapters.

Image receptors

In dentistry these include:

- Radiographic film
  - Direct action or packet film
  - Indirect action film used in conjunction with intensifying screens in a cassette
- Digital receptors
  - Solid-state sensors
  - Phosphor plates.

Radiographic film

Radiographic film has traditionally been employed as the image receptor in dentistry and is still widely used. There are two basic types:

- *Direct-action* or *non-screen* film (sometimes referred to as *wrapped* or *packet* film). This type of film is sensitive primarily to X-ray photons.
- *Indirect-action* or *screen* film, so-called because it is used in combination with *intensifying screens* in a *cassette*. This type of film is

sensitive primarily to light photons, which are emitted by the adjacent intensifying screens by the photoelectric effect (see Ch. 2). They respond to shorter exposure of X-rays, enabling a lower dose of radiation to be given to the patient.

Direct-action (non-screen) film
Uses

Direct-action film is used for intraoral radiography where the need for excellent image quality and fine anatomical detail are of importance.

Sizes

Various sizes of film are available, although only three are usually used routinely (see Fig. 3.9).

- 31 × 41 mm ⎫
- 22 × 35 mm ⎬ for periapicals and bitewings
- 57 × 76 mm — for occlusals.

The film packet contents

The contents of a film packet are shown in Fig. 3.10. It is worth noting that:

- The outer packet or wrapper is made of non-absorbent paper or plastic and is sealed to prevent the ingress of saliva.
- The side of the packet that faces towards the X-ray beam has either a pebbled or a smooth surface and is usually white.

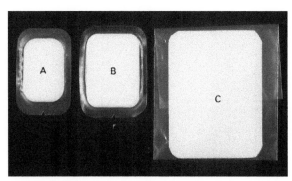

Fig. 3.9 The typical sizes of barrier-wrapped direct-action radiographic film packets available. **A** Small periapical/bitewing film. **B** Large periapical/bitewing film. **C** Occlusal film.

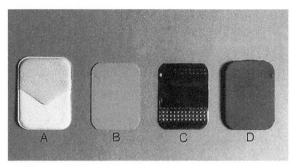

Fig. 3.10 The contents of a film packet. **A** The outer wrapper. **B** The film. **C** The sheet of lead foil. **D** The protective black paper.

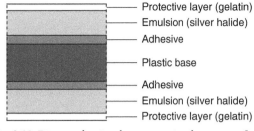

Protective layer (gelatin)
Emulsion (silver halide)
Adhesive
Plastic base
Adhesive
Emulsion (silver halide)
Protective layer (gelatin)

Fig. 3.11 Diagram showing the cross-sectional structure of double emulsion radiographic film.

- The reverse side is usually of two colours so there is little chance of the film being placed the wrong way round in the patient's mouth and different colours represent different film speeds.
- The black paper on either side of the film is there to protect the film from:
  - Light
  - Damage by fingers while being unwrapped
  - Saliva which may leak into the film packet.
- A thin sheet of lead foil is placed behind the film to prevent:
  - Some of the residual radiation that has passed through the film from continuing on into the patient's tissues
  - Scattered secondary radiation, from X-ray photon interactions within the tissues beyond the film, scattering back on to the film and degrading the image.
- The sheet of lead foil contains an embossed pattern so that should the film packet be placed the wrong way round, the pattern will appear on the resultant radiograph. This enables the cause of the resultant pale film to be easily identified (see Ch. 14).

The radiographic film

The cross-sectional structure and components of the radiographic film are shown in Fig. 3.11. It comprises four basic components:

- A *plastic base*, made of clear, transparent cellulose acetate – acts as a support for the emulsion but does not contribute to the final image

- A thin layer of *adhesive* – fixes the emulsion to the base
- The *emulsion* on **both** sides of the base – this consists of silver halide (usually bromide) crystals embedded in a gelatin matrix. The X-ray photons *sensitize* the silver halide crystals that they strike and these sensitized silver halide crystals are later reduced to visible black metallic silver in the developer (see later)
- A *protective layer* of clear gelatin to shield the emulsion from mechanical damage.

Film orientation

The film has an embossed dot on one corner that is used to help orientation. Its position is marked on the back of the packet or can be felt as a raised dot on the front. The side of the film on which the dot is raised is always placed towards the X-ray beam. When the films are mounted, this raised dot is towards the operator and the films are then arranged anatomically and viewed as if the operator were facing the patient.

Film speed

The speed of the film determines how quickly it reacts to X-rays. Thus the faster the film, the less the exposure required for a given film blackening and the lower the radiation dose to the patient. It is determined by the number and size of the silver halide crystals in the emulsion and designated by the letters D, E and F. The larger the crystals, the faster the film, but the poorer the image quality.

In clinical practice, the fastest films consistent with diagnostic results should be used – typically F speed.

Resolution

Resolution, or resolving power, is a measure of the radiograph's ability to differentiate between different structures that are close together. Factors that can affect resolution include penumbra effect (image sharpness), silver halide crystal size and contrast. It is measured in line pairs (lp) per mm. Direct-action film has a resolution of approximately 10 lp per mm.

Indirect-action film
Uses

Film/screen combinations are used as image detectors whenever possible because of the reduced dose of radiation to the patient (particularly when very fine image detail is not essential). The main uses include:

- Extraoral projections, including:
  - Oblique lateral radiographs (Ch. 10)
  - Lateral skull radiographs (Ch. 11)
  - Panoramic radiographs (Ch. 12).

Indirect-action film construction

This type of film is similar in construction to direct-action film described above. However, the following important points should be noted:

- The silver halide emulsion is designed to be sensitive primarily to light rather than X-rays.
- Different emulsions are manufactured which are sensitive to the different colours of light emitted by different types of intensifying screens (see later). These include:
  - *Standard silver halide emulsion* sensitive to BLUE light
  - *Modified silver halide emulsion with ultraviolet sensitizers* sensitive to ULTRAVIOLET light
  - *Orthochromatic emulsion* sensitive to GREEN light
  - *Panchromatic emulsion* sensitive to RED light.
- It is essential that the correct combination of film and intensifying screens is used.
- There is no orientation *dot* embossed in the film so some form of additional identification is

required, e.g. metal letters, **L** or **R**, placed on the outside of the cassette or electronic marking.

- Indirect action film has a resolution of about 5 lp per mm.

Intensifying screens

Intensifying screens consist of *fluorescent phosphors*, which emit light when excited by X-rays, embedded in a plastic matrix. The basic construction and components of an intensifying screen are shown in Fig. 3.12.

Action

Two intensifying screens are used – one in front of the film and the other at the back. The front screen absorbs the low-energy X-ray photons and the back screen absorbs the high-energy photons. The two screens are therefore efficient at stopping the transmitted X-ray beam, which they convert into visible light by the *photoelectric effect* (described in Ch. 2). One X-ray photon will produce many light photons which will affect a relatively large area of film emulsion. Thus, the amount of radiation needed to expose the film is reduced but at the cost of fine detail; *resolution* is decreased. The action of the different screens is shown in Fig. 3.13.

Fluorescent materials

Three main phosphor materials are, or have been, used in intensifying screens:

- Rare earth phosphors including gadolinium and lanthanum

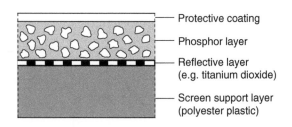

Fig. 3.12 Diagram showing the cross-sectional structure of a typical intensifying screen.

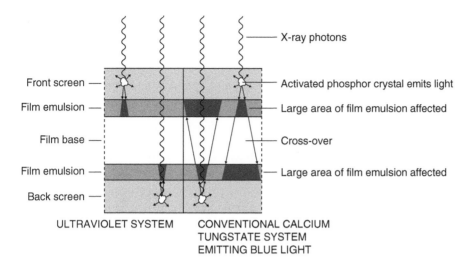

Fig. 3.13 Diagram showing the action of conventional calcium tungstate and ultraviolet systems. Note the small cone of ultraviolet light with no cross-over through the film base, compared to the large cone of blue light and marked cross-over from the calcium tungstate phosphors. These differences result in better resolution and image sharpness with ultraviolet systems.

- Yttrium (a non-rare-earth phosphor but having similar properties)
- Calcium tungstate (CaWO4).

Rare earth and related screens

Modern screens employ these phosphors which produce very fast screen speeds, enabling a substantial reduction in radiation dose to patients, without excessive loss of image detail. The main points can be summarized as follows:

- The rare earth group of elements includes:
  - Lanthanum (Z = 57)
  - Gadolinium (Z = 64)
  - Terbium (Z = 65)
  - Thulium (Z = 69).
- The term *rare earth* is used because it is difficult and expensive to separate these elements from earth and from each other, not because the elements are scarce.
- These phosphors only fluoresce properly when they contain impurities of other phosphors, e.g. gadolinium plus 0.3% terbium. Typical screens include:
  - Terbium-activated gadolinium oxysulphide ($Gd_2O_1S{:}Tb$)
  - Thulium-activated lanthanum oxybromide ($LaOBr{:}Tm$).
- Terbium-activated screens emit GREEN light, while thulium-activated screens emit BLUE light.

- Yttrium (Z = 39), the rare earth related phosphor, in the form of pure yttrium tantalate ($YtaO_4$) emits ULTRAVIOLET light.
- Rare earth and related screens are approximately five times faster than calcium tungstate screens. The amount of radiation required to produce an image is therefore considerably reduced, but they are relatively expensive.
- It is important to use the appropriate films with their correctly matched screens.

Calcium tungstate screens

The original material used, but such screens are now no longer recommended as they are much slower than rare earth screens.

Cassettes

Types

Cassettes are made in a variety of shapes and sizes for different projections. A selection is shown in Fig. 3.14.

Construction

Despite their different shapes, the construction of the cassettes is very similar. They usually consist of a light-tight aluminium or carbon fibre container with the radiographic film sandwiched tightly between two intensifying screens (see Fig. 3.15). Any loss in film/screen

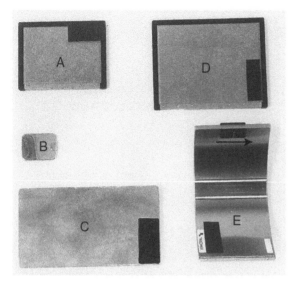

Fig. 3.14 Various cassettes for different radiographic projections. **A** Oblique lateral cassette. **B** Intraoral occlusal cassette. **C** Flat panoramic cassette. **D** Skull cassette. **E** Curved panoramic cassette.

contact will result in degradation of the final image.

Important practical points to note
Film storage

All radiographic film deteriorates with time and manufacturers state expiry dates on film boxes as a guide. However, this does not mean that the film automatically becomes unusable after this date. Storage conditions can have a dramatic effect on the deterioration rate. Ideally films should be stored:

- In a refrigerator in cool, dry conditions
- Away from all sources of ionizing radiation
- Away from chemical fumes including mercury and mercury-containing compounds
- With boxes placed on their edges, to prevent pressure artefacts.

Screen maintenance
Intensifying screens should last for many years if looked after correctly. Maintenance should include:

- Regular cleaning with a proprietary cleaning agent
- Careful handling to avoid scratching or damaging the surface
- Regular checks for loss of film/screen contact.

These aspects are discussed further in Chapter 15.

Digital receptors

There are two types of direct digital image receptors available, namely:

- Solid-state
- Photostimulable phosphor storage plates.

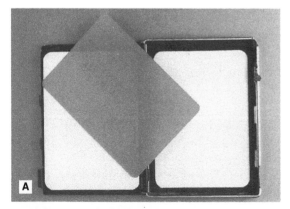

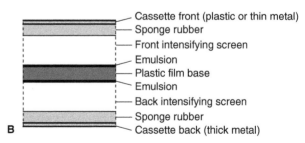

Cassette front (plastic or thin metal)
Sponge rubber
Front intensifying screen
Emulsion
Plastic film base
Emulsion
Back intensifying screen
Sponge rubber
Cassette back (thick metal)

Fig. 3.15 A A standard 18 × 13 cm cassette opened up showing the white intensifying screens and the film. **B** Diagram showing the cross-sectional components in a cassette.

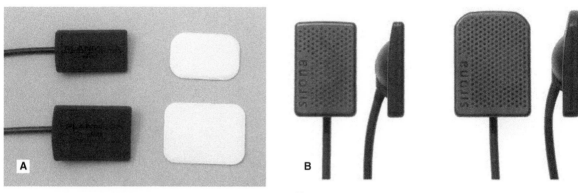

Fig. 3.16 Examples of modern solid-state sensors. **A** Planmeca dixi[2]® and conventional film packets to show their comparative size. **B** Small and large Sirona solid-state sensors showing their thickness.

Uses

Both types of sensors can be used for intraoral (periapical and bitewing) radiography and extraoral radiography, including panoramic and skull radiography. Only phosphor storage plates are available for occlusal and oblique lateral radiography as it is currently too expensive to manufacture sufficiently large solid-state sensors.

Solid-state sensors

Intraoral sensors

The intraoral sensors are small, thin, flat, rigid rectangular boxes usually black in colour and similar in size to intraoral film packets. They vary in thickness from about 5 mm to 7 mm, as shown in Fig. 3.16. Most sensors are cabled to allow data to be transferred directly from the mouth to the computer. Several systems are now available.

For ease of clinical use the sensor cables are usually 1–2 m long and plug into a remote *docking station* which can be conveniently attached to the tubehead supporting arm (see Fig. 3.17). A separate cable then connects the *docking station* to the computer.

A cable-free system is also available. The Schick CDR Wireless™ sensor transmits radiowaves from the mouth to a remote *base station* which is connected by a cable to the computer. This removes the clinical inconvenience of the cable, but additional electronics make the sensor slightly more bulky.

The solid-state sensors are NOT autoclavable. When used clinically they all need to be covered with a protective plastic barrier envelope for infection control purposes (see Ch. 6).

Construction and design

The sensors consist of tiny silicon chip-based pixels and their associated electronics encased in a plastic housing. Underlying technology involves either:

- CCD (charge-coupled devices)
- CMOS (complementary metal oxide semiconductors).

CCD (charge-coupled device)

Individual pixels, consisting of a sandwich of P and N-type silicon, are arranged in rows and columns called an *array* or matrix, above which is a scintillation layer made of similar materials to the rare-earth intensifying screens. The basic design is shown in Fig. 3.18. The X-ray photons that hit the scintillation layer are converted to light. The light interacts via the photoelectric effect with the silicon to create a *charge packet* for each individual pixel, which is concentrated by the electrodes.

The charge pattern formed from the individual pixels in the matrix represents the latent image. The image is read by transferring each row of pixel charges from one row to the next. At the end

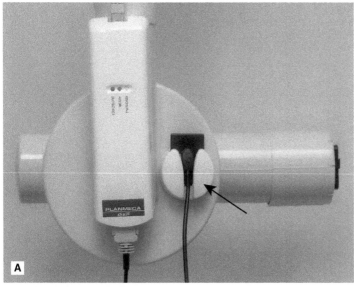

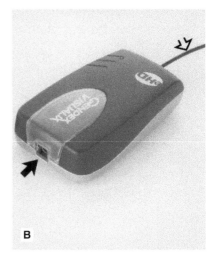

Fig. 3.17 Examples of *docking stations*. **A** Planmeca dixi²® attached to an X-ray tubehead. Note the little holder for conveniently supporting the sensor (arrowed). **B** Gendex Visualix®. The sensor plugs into the arrowed port. The open arrowed cable connects to the computer (kindly provided by Mr R. France.)

of its row, each charge is transferred to a read-out amplifier and transmitted down the cable as an analogue voltage signal to the computer's analogue-to-digital converter, often located in the *docking station*. Each sensor consists of between 1.5 million and 2.5 million pixels and pixel sizes vary from 20 µm microns to 70 µm.

CMOS (complementary metal oxide detectors)

These sensors are similar in construction to CCDs and consist of an array of pixels but they differ from CCDs in the way that the pixel charges are read. Each CMOS pixel is isolated from its neighbour and directly connected to a transistor. The charge packet from each pixel

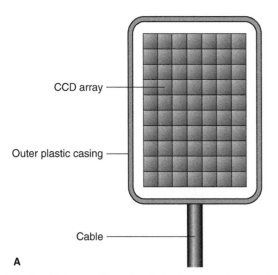

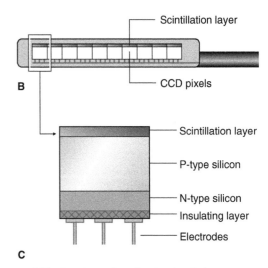

Fig. 3.18 Diagrams illustrating the basic construction of an intraoral CCD sensor. **A** The imaging surface showing the pixel array. **B** Sensor from the side showing the scintillation layer. **C** An individual pixel consisting of a sandwich of N- and P-type silicon.

is transferred to the transistor as a voltage enabling each individual pixel to be assessed separately.

Extraoral sensors

Extraoral sensors contain CCDs in long, thin linear arrays. They are a few pixels wide and many pixels long. The CCD array is incorporated into two different designs of sensor:

- Flat cassette-sized sensors designed to be retro-fitted into existing film-based panoramic equipment to replace conventional cassettes.

- Individually designed sensors as part of completely new solely digital panoramic or skull equipment such as the Schick CDRPanX or the Planmeca dimax$^{3®}$ (see Fig. 3.19).

Although the outward appearances of these sensors is very different, both designs work in a similar fashion. The long narrow pixel array is aligned with a narrow slit-shaped X-ray beam and the equipment scans across the patient. This scanning motion takes several seconds to scan the skull and is discussed in more detail in Chapter 12.

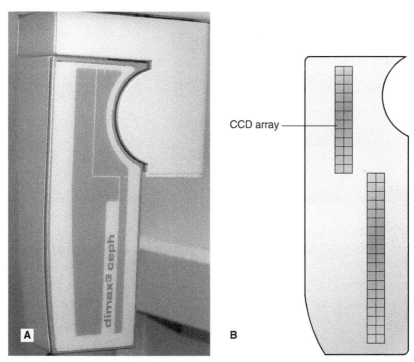

Fig. 3.19 A Specifically designed Planmeca dimax$^{3®}$ sensor for cephalometric radiography (see Ch.12). **B** Diagram showing the basic design with two long thin arrays of CCDs. The lower array is used for panoramic radiography (see Ch.12), both arrays are used for cephalometric radiography (see Ch.11) and the two images obtained are *stitched* together to create one large image.

Photostimulable phosphor storage plates

These digital sensors consist of a range of imaging plates that can be used for both intraoral and extraoral radiography. The plates are not connected to the computer by a cable. Several systems are available and include the DentOptix™ (Gendex) and the Vistascan™ (Durr) and Digora® Optime (intraoral) and PCT (extraoral) (Soredex). A range of intraoral and extraoral plate sizes are available with these systems, identical in size to conventional periapical, occlusal, oblique lateral, panoramic and skull films (see Fig. 3.20). Once cleared (erased), the plates are reusable. Intraoral plates need to be inserted into protective barrier envelopes for control of infection purposes (see Fig. 3.21).

Plate construction and design

The plates typically consist of a layer of barium fluorohalide phosphor on a flexible plastic backing support, as shown in Fig. 3.22.

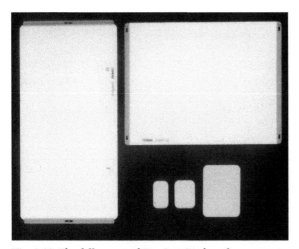

Fig. 3.20 The different sized DenOptix™ plates for panoramic, skull and intraoral radiography.

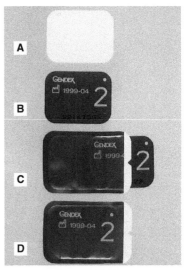

Fig. 3.21 A The white imaging side of a DenOptix™ phosphor plate. **B** The reverse side of the plate. **C** The plate being inserted into the protective barrier envelope – note the reverse side of the plate is visible through the clear side of the envelope. **D** The plate in the envelope ready for clinical use.

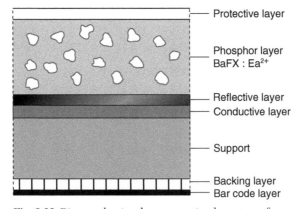

Fig. 3.22 Diagram showing the cross-sectional structure of a typical phosphor imaging plate.

As with using film, image production is not instantaneous with this type of image receptor. Two distinct stages are involved, namely:

- The phosphor layer absorbs and stores the X-ray energy that has not been attenuated by the patient.
- The image plate is then placed in a reader where it is scanned by a laser beam. The stored X-ray energy in the phosphor layer is released as light which is detected by a photomultiplier tube and converted into a voltage which is relayed to the computer and displayed as a digital image. This is described in more detail later in this chapter.

Image processing

Processing is the general term used to describe the sequence of events required to convert the invisible *latent image*, contained in the sensitized film emulsion or in the solid-state or phosphor layer of the digital sensors, into the visible black and white radiographic film or digital image. Two methods are involved, namely:

- Chemical processing
- Computer digital processing.

Chemical processing

It is **crucial** that the stages involved in chemical processing are performed under controlled, standardized conditions with careful attention to detail. Strict quality assurance procedures must be applied (see Ch. 15). Unfortunately, all too often in dental practice poor chemical processing is the cause of radiographic films being of inadequate diagnostic quality, irrespective of how reliable and expensive the X-ray equipment or how accurate the operator's radiographic techniques.

Theory

A detailed knowledge of the chemistry involved in processing is not essential. However, a working knowledge and understanding of the theory of processing is necessary so that processing faults can be identified and corrected. A simplified approach

to the stages involved in converting the green film emulsion into the black/white/grey radiograph is shown in Fig. 3.23 and outlined below:

Stage 1: Development
The **sensitized** silver halide crystals in the emulsion are converted to black metallic silver to produce the *black/grey* parts of the image.

Stage 2: Washing
The film is washed in water to remove residual developer solution.

Stage 3: Fixation
The **unsensitized** silver halide crystals in the emulsion are removed to reveal the *transparent* or *white* parts of the image and the emulsion is hardened.

Stage 4: Washing
The film is washed thoroughly in running water to remove residual fixer solution.

Stage 5: Drying
The resultant *black/white/grey* radiograph is dried.

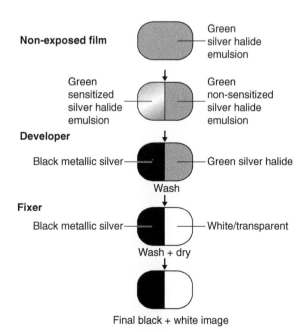

Fig. 3.23 Diagram showing the stages involved in chemical processing, to convert the green film emulsion to the final black and white radiograph. (Courtesy of Mrs J.E. Brown.)

Practical methods

There are three practical chemical processing methods available:

- Manual or wet processing
- Automatic processing
- Using self-developing films.

Manual processing

Manual processing is usually carried out in a *dark-room*, the general requirements of which should include:

- Absolute light-tightness
- Adequate working space
- Adequate ventilation
- Adequate washing facilities
- Adequate film storage facilities
- Safelights – positioned 1.2 m from the work surfaces with 25 W bulbs and filters suitable for the type of film being used (see Ch. 14)
- Processing equipment (see Fig. 3.24):
  - Tanks containing the various solutions
  - Thermometer
  - Immersion heater
  - An accurate timer
  - Film hangers.

Manual processing cycle

1. The exposed film packet is unwrapped and the film clipped on to a hanger.
2. The film is immersed in DEVELOPER and agitated several times in the solution to remove air bubbles and left for about five minutes at 20 °C.
3. The residual developer is rinsed off in water for about 10 seconds.
4. The film is immersed in FIXER for about 8–10 minutes.
5. The film is washed in running water for about 10–20 minutes to remove any residual fixer.
6. The film is allowed to dry in a dust-free atmosphere.

Processing solutions

Two different processing solutions are required, the *developer* and *the fixer*. The typical constituents of these solutions are shown in Tables 3.1 and 3.2.

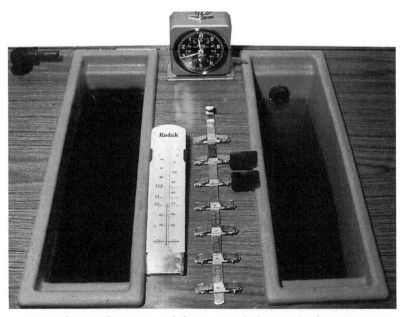

Fig. 3.24 The basic requirements for manual processing including a series of solution tanks, thermometer, timer and film.

Table 3.1 The typical constituents of developer solution and their functions

Constituents	Functions
Phenidone	Helps bring out the image
Hydroquinone	Builds contrast
Sodium sulphite	Preservative – reduces oxidation
Potassium carbonate	Activator – governs the activity of the developing agents
Benzotriazole	Restrainer – prevents fog and controls the activity of the developing agents
Glutaraldehyde	Hardens the emulsion
Fungicide	Prevents fungal growth
Buffer water	Maintains pH (7+) solvent

Table 3.2 The typical constituents of fixer solution and their functions

Constituents	Functions
Ammonium thiosulphate	Removes unsensitized silver halide crystals
Sodium sulphite	Preservative – prevents deterioration of the fixing agent
Aluminium chloride	Hardener
Acetic acid water	Acidifier – maintains pH solvent

Important points to note regarding development

- The alkaline developer solution should be made up to the concentration recommended in the manufacturer's instructions.
- The developer solution is oxidized by air and its effectiveness decreased. Solutions should be used for no more than 10–14 days, irrespective of the number of films processed during that time.
- If the development process is allowed to continue for too long, more silver will be deposited than was intended and the radiograph will be too dark. Conversely, if there is too short a development time the radiograph will be too light.
- Development TIME (in fresh solutions) is dependent on the TEMPERATURE of the solution. The usual value recommended is 5 minutes at 20 °C.
- If the temperature is too high, development is rapid, the film may be too dark and the emulsion may be damaged. If the temperature is too low, development is slowed and a pale film will result.

Important points to note regarding fixing

- Fixer solution should be made up to the concentration recommended by the manufacturer. It is an acid solution so contamination with developer should be avoided.
- Ideally films should be fixed for double the *clearing time*. The clearing time is how long it takes to remove the unsensitized silver halide

crystals. Total fixing time is usually 8–10 minutes.
- Films may be removed from the fixer after 2–4 minutes for *wet* viewing but should be returned to the fixer solution to complete fixing.
- Inadequately fixed films may appear greenish yellow or milky owing to residual emulsion. In time these films may discolour further, becoming brown.

Automatic processing

This term is used when processing is carried out automatically by a machine. There are several automatic processors available which are designed to carry the film through the complete cycle, usually by a system of rollers. Most have a daylight loading facility, eliminating the need for a darkroom (see Fig. 3.25), but in the interests of infection control, saliva-contaminated film packets should be wiped with a disinfecting solution such as 1% hypochlorite, before being placed into the loading facility.

Automatic processing cycle

The cycle is the same as for manual processing except that the rollers squeeze off any excess developing solution before passing the film on to the fixer, eliminating the need for the water wash between these two solutions.

Advantages

The main advantages include:

- Time saving – dry films are produced in about five minutes.
- The need for a darkroom is often eliminated.

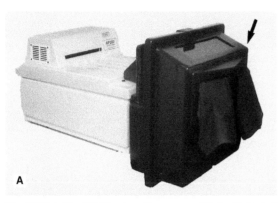
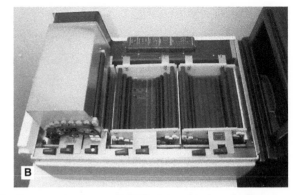

Fig. 3.25 A The AP200 automatic processor fitted with its daylight loading apparatus (arrowed). **B** The internal tanks and roller system of the AP200 processor.

- Controlled, standardized processing conditions are easy to maintain.
- Chemicals can be replenished automatically by some machines.

Disadvantages

The main disadvantages include:

- Strict maintenance and regular cleaning are essential; dirty rollers produce marked films.
- Some models need to be plumbed in.
- Equipment is relatively expensive.
- Smaller machines cannot process large extraoral films.

Self-developing films

Self-developing films are an alternative to manual processing. The X-ray film is presented in a special sachet containing developer and fixer (see Fig. 3.26). Following exposure, the developer tab is pulled, releasing developer solution which is milked down towards the film and massaged around it. After about 15 seconds, the fixer tab is pulled to release the fixer solution which is similarly milked down to the film. After fixing, the used chemicals are discarded and the film is rinsed thoroughly under running water for about 10 minutes.

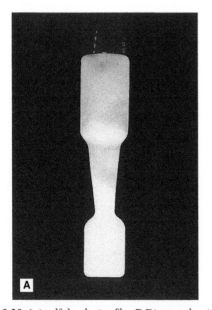
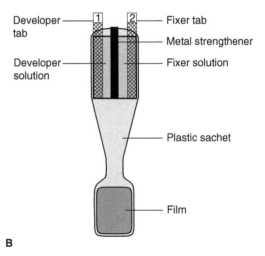

Developer tab
Fixer tab
Metal strengthener
Developer solution
Fixer solution
Plastic sachet
Film

Fig. 3.26 A A self-developing film. **B** Diagram showing the basic internal design.

Advantages

The main advantages include:

- No darkroom or processing facilities are needed.
- Time saving – the final radiograph is ready in about a minute.

Disadvantages

The main disadvantages include:

- Overall image quality is poor.
- The image deteriorates rapidly with time.
- There is no lead foil inside the film packet.
- The film packet is very flexible and easily bent.
- These films are difficult to use in positioning holders.
- The films are relatively expensive.

A rigid, radiopaque plastic backing support tray for the film is manufactured, which helps to reduce the problems of flexibility and lack of lead foil.

Computer digital processing

Digital image

The digital image is captured in pixels (tiny squares), by two different types of sensor – solid-state or photostimulable phosphor plates described earlier. However captured, the digital image is similar to a film-captured image, in that both are two-dimensional representations of a three-dimensional object. In digital imaging, each 2-D pixel represents a 3-D cuboid or *voxel* of the patient. This is shown diagrammatically in Fig. 3.27. The depth of the cuboid is dependent on the thickness of the part of the body being X-rayed. Each pixel measures the total X-ray absorption throughout the whole of each voxel. This 2-D limitation has been overcome with the development of *cone beam computed tomography* (CBCT) (see Ch. 13).

Computer input
Solid-state sensors

As explained earlier, solid-state sensors input the information from each pixel directly (usually down the cable) to the computer's analogue-to-digital converter as an analogue voltage signal.

Phosphor plates

Phosphor plates are **not** directly connected to the computer and therefore an intermediary stage is required when the plate is read. The time taken to read the plate depends on the particular system being used, and the size of the plate, but typically varies between 5 and 100 seconds. Several dental systems are available including Soredex's Digora® Optime (intraoral) and PCT (extraoral), Durr's Vistascan and the Gendex® DenOptix™ (see Fig. 3.28). Although different in design, they all work on the same principle, namely:

- During the radiographic procedure the phosphor layer on the plate absorbs and stores the X-ray energy that has not been attenuated by the patient.
- The plate is then placed in the reader.
- The plate is scanned by a laser beam and the stored X-ray energy is released as light.

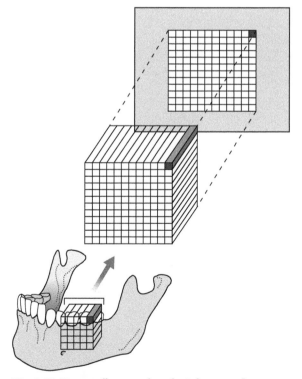

Fig. 3.27 Diagram illustrating how the 3-dimensional jaw is represented as a digital image made up of a grid or matrix of 2-dimensional pixels.

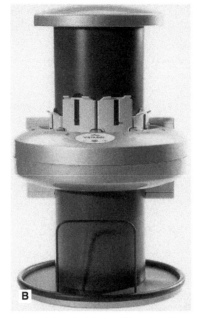

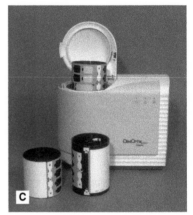

Fig. 3.28 Examples of three phosphor plate readers. **A** Soredex's Digora® Optime (intraoral), **B** Durr's Vistascan and **C** Gendex® DenOptix™.

- The light is detected by a photomultiplier tube and converted into an electrical signal (voltage) and input to the connected computer's analogue-to-digital converter.
- The plate is cleared (erased) ready for reuse.

Computer processing theory

Computers deal with numbers, hence the need for the *analogue* voltage from each pixel to be changed by the analogue-to-digital converter into a discrete *numerical* digital signal. Each pixel has an X and Y coordinate and is allocated a number. Typically using the greyscale there are 256 numbers to select. These range from 0, when the voltage received is at its maximum (no X-ray attenuation in the patient), to 255 when there is no voltage (total X-ray attenuation in the patient). The computer finally allocates an appropriate colour from the greyscale (256 shades of grey from black through to white) to each pixel (0 = black, 255 = white) to create the visual image on the monitor. This concept is illustrated simply in Fig. 3.29 using just eight numbers and eight shades of grey.

The number and size of the pixels, together with the number of shades of grey available, determine the amount of information in an image, the size of the image file and the resolution of the final image (see Fig. 3.30). Pixel sizes vary from 20 μm to 70 μm producing resolution between 7 and 25 line pairs/mm.

Image manipulation

Digital images can be changed by giving the pixels different numbers so altering the shades of grey. Different colours can be used. The coordinates of pixels may be changed or swapped, allowing different parts of the image to be moved around. These variables are the basis for image manipulation and enhancement. Software packages allow several enhancement techniques, some of which are shown in Fig. 3.31. These can include:

- Alteration in contrast
- Alteration in brightness

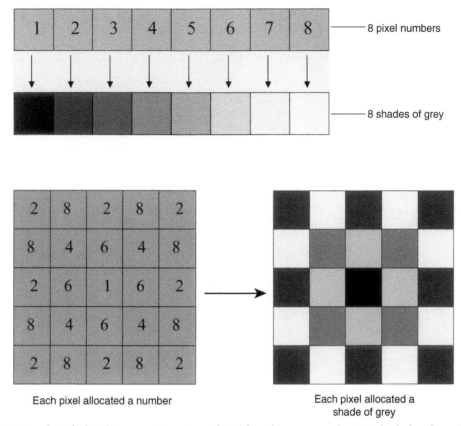

Fig. 3.29 Illustration of simple digital image creation using eight pixel numbers corresponding to eight shades of grey. Each pixel is allocated a number (dependent on the size of the input voltage) and then allocated a shade of grey to create the visual image.

- Inversion (reversed)
- Embossing or pseudo 3-D
- Magnification
- Automated measurement
- Pseudocolourization.

The two most frequently used enhancement functions are altering *brightness* and *contrast*.

Brightness

Brightness can be regarded as equivalent to the *degree of blackening* of a film-captured image. Increasing brightness decreases the degree of blackening and makes the image lighter. This is done by increasing the numerical value of each pixel in the image and allocating it a lighter shade

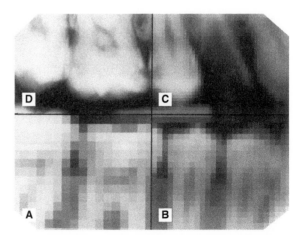

Fig. 3.30 A bitewing radiograph showing the effect on image quality and resolution of different sized pixels gradually reducing from **A** to **D**.

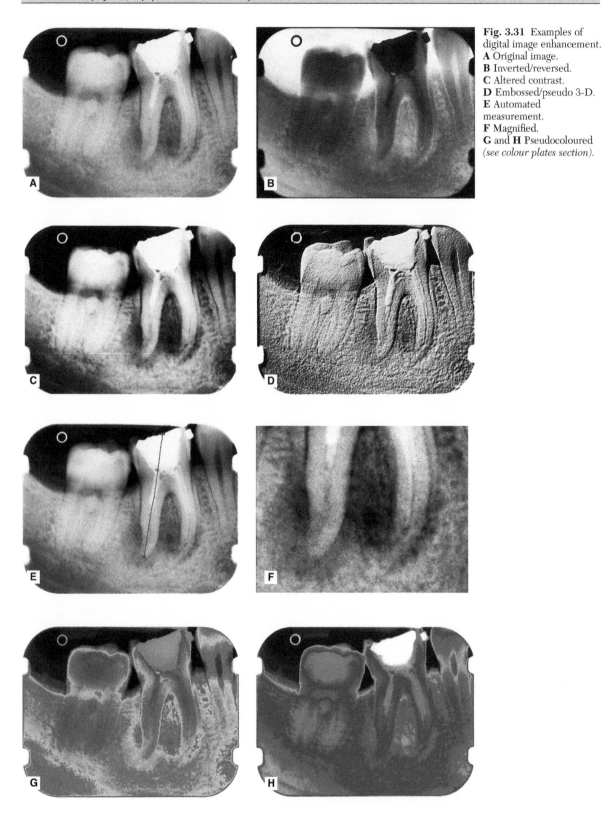

Fig. 3.31 Examples of digital image enhancement.
A Original image.
B Inverted/reversed.
C Altered contrast.
D Embossed/pseudo 3-D.
E Automated measurement.
F Magnified.
G and **H** Pseudocoloured (*see colour plates section*).

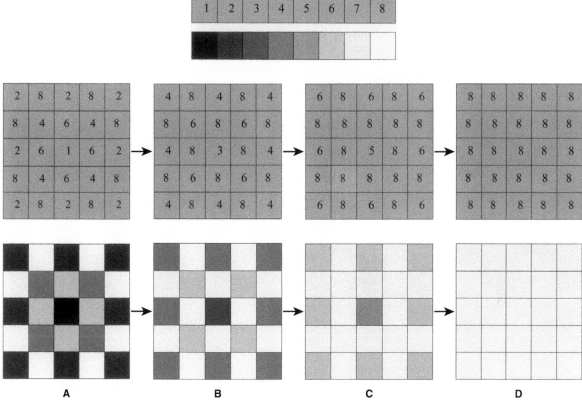

Fig. 3.32 Illustration showing the effect of increasing brightness. **A** The original numbers allocated to the pixels and the original black/white and grey image. **B** Pixel values increased by 2 and the resultant grey/white image. **C** Pixel values increased by 4 and the resultant brighter image. **D** Pixel values increased by 7 (i.e. to extreme end of the brightness scale) and the resultant totally white image.

of grey. Taken to the extreme, every pixel would be allocated the highest number and the image will be totally white. The concept of altering brightness is illustrated in Fig. 3.32, using the same simple model of eight numbers and eight shades of grey. Conversely, decreasing brightness increases the degree of blackening and makes the image darker.

Contrast

Contrast is the visual difference between black and white. Increasing *contrast* increases this difference. This is done by decreasing the pixel numbers in the darker half of the greyscale and increasing the pixel numbers in the lighter half. Taken to the extreme, every pixel would be allocated either the lowest number available or the highest and the image would be black and white only, containing no shades of grey. The concept of altering contrast is illustrated in Fig. 3.33 using the same simple model of eight shades of grey. Conversely, decreasing *contrast* results in a grey image with little visual difference between the pixels.

Note: Despite being able to alter the final image, the computer cannot provide any additional information to that contained in the original image. It should be remembered that, although manipulation and enhancement may make images look aesthetically more pleasing, they also may cause clinical information to be lost and diagnosis compromised.

Hard copy printed images

Hard printed copies of digital images can be obtained on glossy photographic paper by using

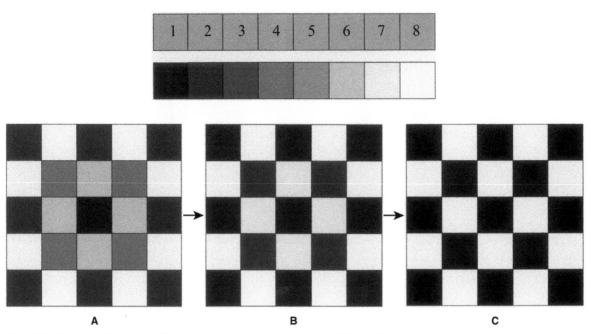

Fig. 3.33 Illustration showing the effect of increasing contrast. **A** The original black/white and grey image. **B** Increased contrast – less visible grey. **C** Complete contrast – the image is only black and white.

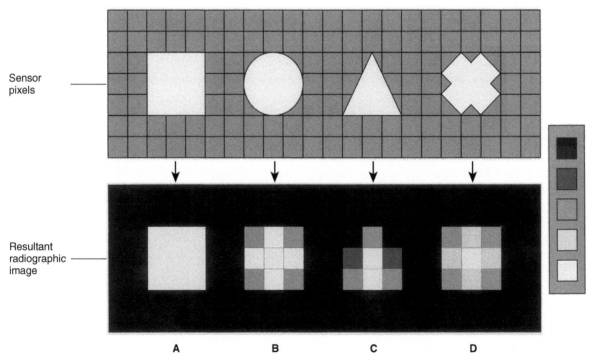

Fig. 3.34 Illustration showing how objects may not be represented accurately on a digital image if pixel size is large, using five shades of grey. **A** The square covers exactly and fills the sensor pixels and is therefore represented exactly radiographically, The outlines of **B** the circle, **C** the triangle and **D** the cross do not exactly cover and fill whole sensor pixels. The number and hence shade of grey allocated to an individual radiographic pixel represents the average of the total X-ray absorption within the whole pixel. Hence, the outlines and shapes of the objects are not represented accurately.

thermal, laser or ink-jet printers. However, image quality is considerably compromised because of the printer's inability to reproduce 256 shades of grey. It is possible to produce excellent quality hard copy images using expensive heat sublimation printers. These print the digital image back onto film and can reproduce all the shades of grey. The quality is comparable to film-captured images.

Advantages

- There is no need for chemical processing, thus avoiding all conventional processing faults (see Ch. 14) and the hazards associated with handling chemical solutions.
- Easy storage and archiving of patient information and incorporation into patient records.
- Easy transfer of images electronically.
- Image enhancement and manipulation.
- Phosphor plates have a wide latitude producing an acceptable image whether underexposed or overexposed.

Disadvantages

- Large pixels result in poor resolution and structures may not be represented accurately, as shown in Figs 3.34 and 3.35.
- Conventional PC screens/monitors reduce or limit image quality. Diagnostic image quality screens/monitors are required for optimal viewing.
- Images need to be backed up to a separate storage area remote from the image-capture computer in case this computer fails.
- Overexposure and overloading of CCD sensors creating the phenomenon of *blooming* (see Ch. 14).
- Loss of image quality and resolution on hard copy printouts when using thermal, laser or ink-jet printers.
- Image enhancement and manipulation:
  - operators need to understand how the image is created and being altered to avoid being misled

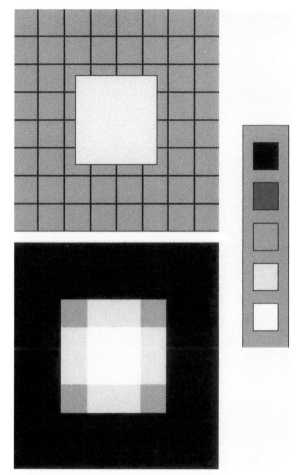

Fig. 3.35 Another illustration showing how an object may not be represented accurately on a digital image if pixel size is large, using five shades of grey. The square from Fig. 3.34 is positioned so that it does not cover *exactly* and fill the sensor pixels. As a result it is now not accurately represented.

  - time-consuming
  - magnification is achieved by enlarging the pixels, but resolution is lost.
- While manufacturers provide safeguards to prevent any tampering with original images within their own software, it is relatively easy to access these images using inexpensive third-party software and then to change them, as shown in Fig. 3.36.

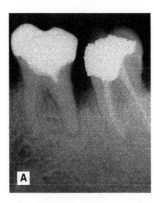 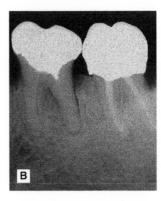

Fig. 3.36 An example of image alteration using third-party software. **A** Original image – note the bony defect between ⌐6 and ⌐7 the lack of contact point and the restoration in ⌐7. **B** After digital manipulation and no clinical treatment.

To access the self assessment questions for this chapter please go to www.whaitesessentialsdentalradiography.com

4 Radiation dose, dosimetry and dose limitation

Several different terms and units have been used in dosimetry over the years. The use of the word *dose* in multiple different descriptors has made this subject even more confusing. However, it is essential that these terms and units are understood to appreciate what is meant by *radiation dose* and to allow meaningful comparisons between different investigations to be made. In addition to explaining the various units and how they are measured/calculated, this chapter also covers the concept of clinical dose limits and dose limitation, as well as summarizing the estimated doses from various sources of ionizing radiation and the magnitude of radiation doses from common dental and medical clinical investigations.

The more important terms in dosimetry include:

- Radiation absorbed dose (D)
- Equivalent dose (H_T)
- Effective dose (E)
- Collective effective dose or collective dose
- Dose limits
- Dose rate

Radiation-absorbed dose (D)

This is a measure of the amount of energy absorbed from the radiation beam per unit mass of tissue and can be measured using a dosimeter.

SI unit: joules/kg (J/kg)
Special name: Gray (Gy)
Subunit names: milligray (mGy) ($\times 10^{-3}$)
microgray (μGy) ($\times 10^{-6}$)

Equivalent dose (H_T)

This is a measure that allows the different radiobiological effectiveness (RBE) of different types of radiation to be taken into account.

For example, alpha particles penetrate only a few millimetres in tissue, lose all their energy and are totally absorbed, whereas X-rays penetrate much further, lose some of their energy and are only partially absorbed. The biological effect of a particular *radiation-absorbed dose* of alpha particles would be considerably more severe than a similar *radiation-absorbed dose* of X-rays.

By introducing a numerical value known as the *radiation weighting factor* (W_R), which represents the biological effects of different radiations on different tissues, the unit of *equivalent dose* (H_T) in a particular tissue provides a common unit allowing comparisons to be made between one type of radiation and another, for example:

X-rays, gamma rays and beta particles	$W_R = 1$
Fast neutrons (10 keV–100 keV) and protons	$W_R = 10$
Alpha particles	$W_R = 20$

Equivalent dose (H_T) = **radiation-absorbed dose (D) × radiation weighting factor (W_R) in a particular tissue**

SI unit: joules/kg (J/kg)
Special name: Sievert (Sv)
Subunit names: millisievert (mSv) ($\times 10^{-3}$)
microsievert (μSv) ($\times 10^{-6}$)

(For X-rays, the *radiation weighting factor* (W_R) = 1, therefore the *equivalent dose* (H_T) in a particular tissue, measured in *Sieverts*, is equal to the *radiation-absorbed dose* (D), measured in *Grays*.)

Effective dose (E)

This measure allows doses from different investigations of different parts of the body to be compared, by converting all doses to an *equivalent whole body dose*. This is necessary because some parts of the body are more sensitive to radiation than others. The International Commission on Radiological Protection (ICRP) has allocated each tissue a numerical value, known as the *tissue weighting factor* (W_T), based on its radiosensitivity, i.e. the risk of the tissue being damaged by radiation – the greater the risk, the higher the *tissue weighting factor*. The sum of the individual *tissue weighting factors* represents the *weighting factor* for the whole body.

The *effective dose* (E) from an individual clinical radiograph, where the x-ray beam is absorbed by different tissues, is calculated as follows:

Effective dose (E) = **Σ Equivalent dose (H_T) in each tissue × relevant tissue weighting factor (W_T)**

Special name: Sievert (Sv)
Subunit name: millisievert (mSv) ($\times 10^{-3}$)
microsievert (μSv) ($\times 10^{-6}$)

The tissue weighting factors recommended by the ICRP in 1990 and revised in 2007 are shown in Table 4.1.

Table 4.1 The tissue weighting factors (W_T) recommended by the ICRP in 1990 and revised in 2007

Tissue	1990 W_T	2007 W_T
Bone marrow	0.12	0.12
Breast	0.05	0.12
Colon	0.12	0.12
Lung	0.12	0.12
Stomach	0.12	0.12
Gonads	0.20	0.08
Bladder	0.05	0.04
Oesophagus	0.05	0.05
Liver	0.05	0.04
Thyroid	0.05	0.04
Bone surface	0.01	0.01
Brain	*	0.01
Kidneys	*	0.01
Salivary glands	—	0.01
Skin	0.01	0.01
Remainder tissues	0.05*	0.12†

*Adrenals, brain, upper large intestine, small intestine, kidney, muscle, pancreas, spleen, thymus and uterus.
†Adrenals, extrathoracic airways, gallbladder, heart wall, kidney, lymphatic nodes, muscle, pancreas, oral mucosa, prostate, small intestine wall, spleen, thymus and uterus/cervix.

The 2007 revised tissue weighting factors include the salivary glands as an individual weighted tissue and the oral mucosa in the remainder tissues. Therefore the *effective dose* for dental radiographic examinations may be considerably higher when calculated using these revised tissue weighting factors.

One way of calculating the *effective dose* is by using a tissue equivalent anthropomorphic phantom with dosimeters placed in the most radiosensitive regions, as shown in Fig. 4.1.

As individual doses are very small from any one examination, a number of radiographic exposures are repeatedly performed (e.g. ten times) using typical exposure factors (time, kV and mA), for that particular examination. The dosemeters are then 'read' to give a measurement of the *radiation-absorbed dose* (D) in the individual tissues. Using this data both the *equivalent dose* (H_T) and the *effective dose* (E) may be calculated as shown in the simplified flow diagram shown in Fig. 4.2.

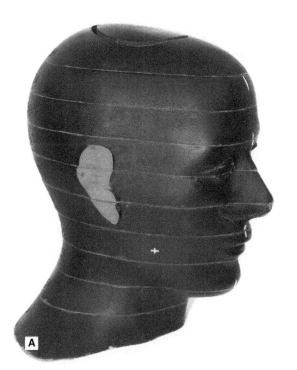
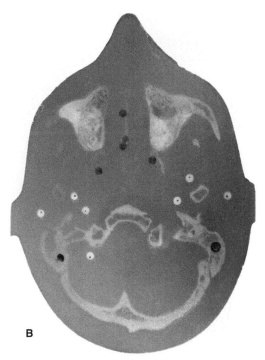

Fig. 4.1 A An example of an anthropomorphic phantom used in dosimetry. **B** One slice of the phantom showing the positions where the individual dosimeters can be placed in specific radiosensitive tissues.

**(1) Radiation-absorbed doses (D)
in 5 radiosensitive tissues**

Tissue	Radiation-absorbed dose (D) (μGy)
Skin	5*
Salivary glands	700
Bone surface	70*
Bone marrow	20*
Thyroid gland	50

*averaged over the total mass of tissue

(2) Equivalent doses (H$_T$) in 5 radiosensitive tissues

Tissue	Equivalent dose (H$_T$) = Radiation-absorbed dose x W$_R$ (μSv)
Skin	5 x 1 = 5
Salivary glands	700 x 1 = 700
Bone surface	70 x 1 = 70
Bone marrow	20 x 1 = 20
Thyroid gland	50 x 1 = 50

(3) Effective doses (E) in 5 radiosensitive tissues

Tissue	Tissue weighting factor (W$_T$)	Equivalent dose (H$_T$) x Tissue weighting factor (W$_T$)
Skin	0.01	5 x 0.01 = 0.05
Salivary glands	0.01	700 x 0.01 = 7
Bone surface	0.01	70 x 0.01 = 0.7
Bone marrow	0.12	20 x 0.12 = 2.4
Thyroid gland	0.04	50 x 0.04 = 2

Overall effective dose for the investigation
= 0.05 + 7 + 0.7 + 2.4 + 2 = **12.15 μSv**

Fig. 4.2 Flow diagram illustrating a very simplified example of how the *effective dose* is calculated for a panoramic radiograph using only five tissues of the anthropomorphic phantom. (1) The *radiation-absorbed doses* for the five tissues. (2) The calculated *equivalent doses* (W$_R$ = 1 for X-rays) for the five tissues. (3) The *effective dose* for the investigation, which is the sum of each equivalent dose (H$_T$) multiplied by the relevant tissue weighting factor (W$_T$), which in this example is 12.15 μSv. For a real dosimetry study **all** the radiosensitive tissues irradiated, with specific weighting factors, would be included in the calculations.

Table 4.2 Typical effective doses for a range of dental and routine medical examinations

X-ray examination	Effective dose (E) (mSv)
Bitewing/periapical radiograph	0.0003–0.022
Panoramic radiograph	0.0027–0.038
Upper standard occlusal	0.008
Lateral cephalometric radiograph	0.0022–0.0056
Skull radiograph (posteroanterior, PA)	0.02
Skull radiograph (lateral)	0.016
Chest (posteroanterior, PA)	0.014
Chest (lateral)	0.038
CT head	1.4
CT chest	6.6
CT abdomen	5.6
CT mandible and maxilla	0.25–1.4
Barium swallow	1.5
Barium enema	2.2
Dento-alveolar cone beam CT (CBCT)	0.01–0.67
Craniofacial cone beam CT (CBCT)	0.03–1.1

Based broadly on the 2011 HPA publication *Frequency and Collective Dose for Medical and Dental X-ray Examinations in the UK* and the 2011 SEDENTEXCT publication *Radiation Protection: Cone Beam CT for Dental and Maxillofacial Radiology* and the 2013 *Selection Criteria for Dental Radiography (3e)*.

When the simple term *dose* is applied loosely, it is the *effective dose (E)* that is usually being described. *Effective dose* can thus be thought of as a broad indication of the risk to health from any exposure to ionizing radiation, irrespective of the type or energy of the radiation or the part of the body being irradiated. A comparison of effective doses from different investigations is shown in Table 4.2.

Collective effective dose or collective dose

This measure is used when considering the total effective dose to a population, from a particular investigation or source of radiation, and is measured in man-sieverts (man-Sv).

Collective dose = **effective dose (E) × population**

For example, in the UK in 2008, the collective dose to the population from all X-ray examinations was calculated by the Health Protection Agency to be 24,700 man-Sv.

Dose limits

In addition to setting *tissue weighting factors* the International Commission for Radiological Protection (ICRP) also sets maximum annual *dose limits* for radiation workers – those people who are exposed to radiation during the course of their work. This exposure carries no benefit only risk. The ICRP divides radiation workers into two subgroups depending on the level of occupational exposure:

- Classified workers
- Non-classified workers.

The *dose limits* for each group are based on the principle that the risk to any worker who receives the full *dose limit* will be such that the worker will be at no greater risk than a worker in another hazardous, but non-radioactive, environment. By way of example, Table 4.3 shows the previous and current annual dose limits in force in the UK.

Table 4.3 The previous annual dose limits and those currently in force in the UK

	Old dose limits	Current dose limits
Classified workers	50 mSv	20 mSv
Non-classified workers	15 mSv	6 mSv
General public	5 mSv	1 mSv

Dose rate

This is a measure of the dose per unit time, e.g. dose/hour, and is sometimes a more convenient, and measurable, figure than the total annual dose limits shown in Table 4.3.

SI unit: microsievert/hour ($\mu Sv\ h^{-1}$)

Estimated annual doses

Everyone is exposed to some form of ionizing radiation from the environment in which we live. Sources include:

- Natural background radiation
  - Cosmic radiation from the earth's atmosphere
  - Gamma radiation from the rocks and soil in the earth's crust
  - Ingestion of radioisotopes, e.g. ^{40}K, in certain foods
  - Inhalation of radon gas and its decay products, ^{222}Rn is a gaseous decay product of uranium that is present naturally in granite. As a gas, radon diffuses readily from rocks through soil and can be trapped in poorly ventilated houses and then breathed into the lungs.
  - Inhalation of thoron gas
- Artificial background radiation
  - Fallout from nuclear explosions
  - Radioactive waste discharged from nuclear establishments
- Medical and dental diagnostic radiation
- Radiation from occupational exposure.

The Radiation Protection Division of the Health Protection Agency has estimated the annual doses from these various sources in the UK, as illustrated in Table 4.4. As shown, an individual's average dose from natural background radiation is estimated at about **2.23 mSv** per year (84%) with an additional **0.423 mSv** (16%) from artificial sources (*total average dose approximately 2.7 mSv*) including dental radiography. In the USA natural background radiation is estimated at approximately **3.2 mSv** per year with an additional **3.0 mSv** from artificial sources (*total average dose 6.2 mSv*). These figures are useful to remember when considering the magnitude of the doses associated with various diagnostic procedures as shown previously in Table 4.2.

Table 4.4 Health Protection Agency estimated average annual doses to the UK population from various sources of ionizing radiation in 2005

Radiation source	Average annual dose (μSv)	Approximate %
Natural sources		
Cosmic radiation	330	
External exposure from earth's crust	350	
Internal radiation from certain foodstuffs	250	
Exposure to radon/thoron and their decay products	1,300	
Total from natural sources	2,230	84
Artificial sources		
Fallout	6	
Radioactive waste	1	
Medical and dental diagnostic radiation	410	
Occupational exposure	6	
Total from artificial sources	423	16
Total from all sources	~2.7 mSv	100

Dose limitation

As mentioned previously, the International Commission on Radiological Protection (ICRP) regularly publishes data not only on radiation dose but also on general recommendations on dose limits and dose limitation based on the following general principles:

- No practice shall be adopted unless its introduction produces a positive net benefit (*Justification*)
- All exposures shall be kept as **low as reasonably practicable** (ALARP), taking economic and social factors into account (*Optimization*)
- The dose equivalent to individuals shall not exceed the limits recommended by the ICRP (*Limitation*).

For the purposes of dose limitation, the ICRP has divided the population into three groups:

- Patients
- Radiation workers (classified and non-classified)
- General public.

Patients

Radiograhic investigations involving patients are divided into four subgroups:

- Examinations directly associated with illness
- Systematic examinations (periodic health checks)
- Examinations for occupational, medico-legal or insurance purposes
- Examinations for medical research.

Examinations directly associated with illness

- There are no set dose limits
- The decision to carry out such an investigation should be based on:
  - A correct assessment of the indications
  - The expected yield
  - The way in which the results are likely to influence the diagnosis and subsequent treatment

  - The clinician having an adequate knowledge of the physical properties and biological effects of ionizing radiation (i.e., *adequately trained*).
- The number, type and frequency of the radiographs requested or taken (selection criteria) are the responsibility of the clinician. Evidence-based selection criteria recommendations have been published in different countries in recent years to provide guidance in this clinical area of radiation protection. In the UK, the booklet *Selection Criteria for Dental Radiography* is published and regularly updated by the Faculty of General Dental Practice of the Royal College of Surgeons of England (3rd Edition published in 2013). National selection criteria documentation should be regarded as essential reading for all dentists and from an integral part of the *justification* process. An example of these radiation protection recommendations in practice are shown in Chapter 5.

Systematic examinations (periodic health checks)

- There are no set dose limits.
- There should be a high probability of obtaining useful information – hence the usefulness of selection criteria.
- The information obtained should be important to the patient's health.

Examinations for occupational, medico-legal or insurance purposes

- There are no set dose limits.
- The benefit is primarily to a third party.
- The patient should at least benefit indirectly.
- In the UK the 2001 *Guidance Notes* emphasize that the need for, and the usefulness of, these examinations should be critically assessed when deciding whether they are justified. They also recommend that these types of examinations should be requested only by medical/dental practitioners and that the patient's consent should be obtained.

Examinations for medical research

- There are no set dose limits.
- All research projects should be approved on the advice of an appropriate expert group or Ethics Committee and subject to Local Rules and regulations.
- All volunteers should have a full understanding of the risks involved and give their consent.

Radiation workers

As described earlier, the ICRP further divides workers who are exposed to radiation during the course of their work into two subgroups depending on the level of occupational exposure:

- Classified workers
- Non-classified workers.

The ICRP maximum dose limits for each group as shown in Table 4.3 is based on the principle that the risk to any worker who receives the full dose limit will be such that the worker will be at no greater risk than a worker in another hazardous, but non-radioactive environment.

The main features of each group of radiation workers are summarized below:

Classified workers

- Receive high levels of exposure to radiation at work (if *Local Rules* are observed this is highly unlikely in dental practice).
- Require compulsory personal monitoring.
- Require compulsory annual health checks.

Non-classified workers (most dental staff, including dental care professionals)

- Receive low levels of exposure to radiation at work (as in the dental surgery).
- The annual dose limits are 3/10 of the classified workers' limits. Provided the *Local Rules* are observed, all dental staff should receive an annual effective dose of considerably less than the limit of 6 mSv. Hence, the regulations in the UK suggest the setting of '*Dose Constraints*'. These represent the upper level of individual dose that should not be exceeded in

a well-managed practice, and for dental radiography the following recommendations are made:

1 mSv	for employees directly involved with the radiography (operators)
0.3 mSv	for employees not directly involved with the radiography and for members of the general public.

In addition to above dose limits, the legal person must ensure that the dose to the fetus of any pregnant member of staff is unlikely to exceed 1 mSv during the declared term of the pregnancy.

- Personal monitoring (see Chapter 5) is not compulsory in the UK, although it is recommended if the risk assessment indicates that individual doses could exceed 1 mSv per year. The 2001 *Guidance Notes* state that in practice this should be considered for those staff whose weekly workload exceeds 100 intraoral or 50 panoramic images, or a pro-rata combination of each type of examination.
- Annual health checks are not required.

The radiation dose to dental care professionals can come from:

- The primary beam, if they stand in its path
- Scattered radiation from the patient
- Radiation leakage from the tubehead.

The main practical radiation protection measures to limit the dose that workers are exposed to are described in Chapter 5.

General public

This group includes everyone who is not receiving a radiation dose either as a patient or as a radiation worker, but who may be exposed inadvertently, for example, someone in a dental surgery waiting room, in other rooms in the building or passers-by. The annual dose limits for this group have been lowered to 1 mSv, as shown in Table 4.3 although the suggested dose constraint is 0.3 mSv (see earlier). The general public is at risk from the primary beam and the main practical radiation protection measures to limit the dose are described in Chapter 5.

The biological effects associated with X-rays, risk and practical radiation protection

Radiation-induced tissue damage

The action of radiation on cells and the resultant damage are classified as:

- Direct action or damage as a result of ionization of macromolecules
- Indirect action or damage as a result of the free radicals produced by the ionization of water.

Direct action or damage

The X-ray photons, or high-energy ejected electrons, interact directly with, and ionize, vital biologic macromolecules such as DNA, RNA, proteins and enzymes, as shown in Fig. 5.1A. This ionization results in the breakage of the macromolecule's chemical bonds, causing them to become abnormal structures, which may in turn lead to inappropriate chemical reactions. Rupture of one of the chemical bonds in a DNA macromolecule may sever one of the side chains of the ladder-like structure. This type of injury to DNA is called a *point mutation*. The subsequent chromosomal effects from direct damage could include:

- Inability to pass on information
- Abnormal replication
- Cell death
- Only temporary damage – the DNA being repaired successfully before further cell division.

If the radiation directly affects somatic cells, the effects on the DNA (and hence the chromosomes) could result in a radiation-induced malignancy. If the damage is to reproductive stem cells, the result could be a radiation-induced congenital abnormality.

What actually happens in the cell depends on several factors, including:

- The type and number of nucleic acid bonds that are broken
- The intensity and type of radiation
- The time between exposures
- The ability of the cell to repair the damage
- The stage of the cell's reproductive cycle when irradiated.

Indirect action or damage

This process, which is shown in Fig. 5.1B, involves the ionization of the water molecule producing both ions and *free radicals* which can combine to damage the vital biologic macromolecules such as DNA. The sequence of events involved is summarized in Fig. 5.2. The free radicals can recombine to form hydrogen peroxide, a cellular poison, and a hydroperoxyl radical, another toxic substance. Both of these substances are highly reactive and produce biological damage. By themselves, free radicals may transfer excess energy to other molecules, thereby breaking their chemical bonds and having an even greater effect. As about 80% of the body consists of water, the vast majority of the interactions with ionizing radiation are indirect.

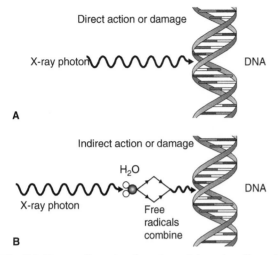

A

B

Fig. 5.1 Diagram illustrating the action and damaging effects of radiation on cells. **A** *Direct action or damage* – the X-ray photon interacts directly with the DNA. **B** *Indirect action or damage* – the X-ray photon ionizes water to produce free radicals which damage the DNA.

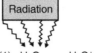

(1) $H_2O \longrightarrow H_2O^+ + e^-$

(2) The positive ion immediately breaks up:
$H_2O^+ \longrightarrow H^+ + OH$

(3) The electron (e^-) attaches to a neutral water molecule:
$H_2O + e^- \longrightarrow H_2O^-$

(4) The resulting negatively charged molecule dissociates:
$H_2O^- \longrightarrow H + OH^-$

(5) The electrically neutral H and OH are the free radicals. They are unstable and highly reactive and can combine together or with oxygen (O_2), e.g. :
$OH + OH \longrightarrow H_2O_2$ (hydrogen peroxide)
$H + O_2 \longrightarrow HO_2$ (hydroperoxyl radical)

This radical and hydrogen peroxide destructively unite and damage DNA and macromolecules

Fig. 5.2 A diagrammatic summary of the sequence of events following ionization of water molecules leading to *indirect damage* to the cell.

Classification of the biological effects

Whatever the actual mechanism for the DNA and cellular damage, the biological effects of ionizing radiation are classified into two main categories:

- *Tissue reactions* (*deterministic* effects)
- *Stochastic* effects.

Tissue reactions (deterministic effects)

These are the non-cancer damaging effects, to the body of the person exposed, that will **definitely** result from a specific high dose of radiation. The severity of the effect is proportional to the dose received, and in most cases a *threshold* dose exists below which there will be no effect. They were previously referred to as deterministic effects, but are now referred to as tissue reactions by the International Commission on Radiological Protection (ICRP) because it now recognizes that some of these effects are not determined solely at the time of irradiation but can be modified after radiation exposure. They are further subdivided into:

- Early tissue reactions – appearing shortly after exposure, e.g. skin erythema or mucositis

- Late tissue reactions – appearing months to years after exposure, e.g. osteoradionecrosis.

Stochastic effects

Stochastic effects are those that **may** develop. Their development is random and depends on the laws of chance or probability. These damaging effects **may** be induced when the body is exposed to **any** dose of radiation. Experimentally it has not been possible to establish a *safe dose* – i.e. a dose below which stochastic effects do not develop. It is therefore assumed that there is *no threshold dose*, and that every exposure to ionizing radiation carries with it the **possibility** of inducing a stochastic effect. The lower the radiation dose, the lower the probability of cell damage. However, the severity of the damage is **not related** to the size of the inducing dose. This is the underlying philosophy behind present radiation protection recommendations described later. Stochastic effects are further subdivided into:

- Cancer induction
- Heritable effects (genetic effects).

Cancer induction

If a somatic (body) cell is irradiated a radiation-induced malignancy cancer may develop. Quantifying the risk is complex and controversial. Data from groups exposed to high doses of radiation have been analysed and the results used to provide an estimate of the risk from the low doses of radiation encountered in diagnostic radiology. The high-dose groups studied include:

- The survivors of the atomic explosions at Hiroshima and Nagasaki
- Patients receiving radiotherapy
- Radiation workers – people exposed to radiation in the course of their work
- The survivors of the nuclear disaster at Chernobyl.

The problem of quantifying the risk is compounded because cancer is a common disease, so in any group of individuals studied there is likely to be some incidence of cancer. In the groups listed above, that have been exposed to high doses of radiation, the incidence of cancer is likely to be increased and is referred to as the *excess cancer incidence*. From the data collected, it has been possible to construct *dose – response curves* (Fig. 5.3), showing the relationship between excess cancers and radiation dose. The graphs can be extrapolated to zero (the controversy on risk assessment revolves around exactly how this extrapolation should be done), and a risk factor for induction of cancer by low doses of radiation can be calculated.

After reviewing all the available evidence, the International Commission on Radiological Protection suggest there is a 1 in 20,000 chance of developing a fatal cancer for every 1 mSv of effective dose. Using this estimate, a broad estimate of risk from various X-ray examinations may be calculated and these are shown in Table 5.1.

Table 5.1 A broad estimate of the risk of a standard 30-year-old adult patient developing a fatal radiation-induced malignancy from a variety of dental and medical X-ray examinations

X-ray examination	Estimated risk of fatal cancer
Bitewing/periapical radiograph (70 kV, round collimation, D-speed film)	1 in 1,000,000
Bitewing/periapical radiograph (70 kV, rectangular collimation, F-speed film)	1 in 10,000,000
Panoramic radiograph (average)	1 in 1,000,000
Upper standard occlusal	1 in 2,500,000
Lateral cephalometric radiograph	1 in 5,000,000
Skull radiograph (PA)	1 in 1,000,000
Skull radiograph (lateral)	1 in 1,250,000
Chest (PA)	1 in 1,430,000
Chest (lateral)	1 in 540,000
CT head	1 in 14,300
CT chest	1 in 3000
CT abdomen	1 in 3500
CT mandible and maxilla	1 in 80,000 to 1 in 14,300
Barium swallow	1 in 13,300
Barium enema	1 in 9100
Dento-alveolar cone beam CT	1 in 2,000,000 to 1 in 30,000
Craniofacial cone beam CT	1 in 670,000 to 1 in 18,200

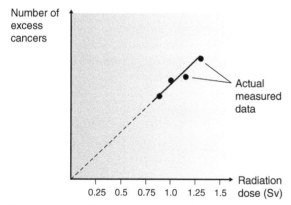

Fig. 5.3 A typical dose – response curve, showing excess cancer incidence plotted against radiation dose and a linear extrapolation of the data to zero.

Table 5.2 The multiplication factor for risk for different age groups based on the 2004 *European Guidelines on Radiation Protection in Dental Radiology*

Age group (yr)	Multiplication factor for risk
<10	×3
10–20	×2
20–30	×1.5
30–50	×0.5
50–80	×0.3
80+	Negligible risk

Risk is age-dependent, being highest for the young and lowest for the elderly. The risks shown in Table 5.1 are for a 30-year-old adult. The 2004 *European Guidelines on Radiation* recommend that these should be modified by the multiplication factors shown in Table 5.2, which represent averages for the two sexes. In fact, at all ages, risks for females are slightly higher and risks for males slightly lower.

This epidemiological information is being updated continually and recent reports suggest that the risk from low-dose radiation may be considerably greater than thought previously. However, the present figures at least provide an idea of the comparative order of magnitude of the risk involved from different investigations. Dental radiology employs low doses of radiation and hence the risk of stochastic cancer-induction is very small. However, the total number of intraoral and extraoral dental radiographs taken is very high – estimated at around 20 million per year in the UK alone. It is thought that diagnostic radiology (medical and dental) is responsible for about 700 cases of cancer per year in the UK of which about 10 cases are attributable to dental radiology – hence the need for the practical radiation measures outlined later.

Heritable effects (genetic effects)

Mutations result from any sudden change to a gene or chromosome. They can be caused by external factors, such as radiation or may occur spontaneously.

Radiation to the reproductive organs **may** damage the DNA of the sperm or egg cells. This **may** result in a congenital abnormality in the offspring of the person irradiated. However, there is no certainty that these effects will happen, so all genetic effects are described as stochastic.

A cause-and-effect relationship is difficult, if not impossible, to prove. Although ionizing radiation has the potential to cause genetic damage, there are no human data that show convincing evidence of a direct link with radiation. Risk estimates have been based mainly on experiments with mice. It is estimated that a dose to the gonads of 0.5–1.0 Sv would double the spontaneous mutation rate. Once again it is assumed that there is *no threshold dose*.

Effects on the unborn child

The developing fetus is particularly sensitive to the effects of radiation, especially during the period of organogenesis (3–7 weeks after conception). The major problems are:

- Congenital abnormalities or death associated with large doses of radiation
- Mental retardation and reduction in Intelligence Quotient (IQ)
- Cancer induction.

As a result, there is a maximum permissible dose allowable to the abdomen of a woman who is pregnant. The implications for radiation protection for pregnant women during dental radiography are described later.

Summary of the harmful effects important in dental radiology

In dentistry, the size of the doses used routinely are relatively small (see Ch. 4) and well below the threshold doses required to produce *tissue reactions* (deterministic effects). However, the *stochastic effects* can develop with **any** dose of ionizing radiation. Dental radiology does not usually involve irradiating the reproductive organs, thus in dentistry the heritable effects are of limited importance and the main concern is that of cancer induction.

Practical radiation protection

As a result of these damaging effects ionizing radiation is the subject of considerable safety legislation designed to minimize the risks to radiation workers and to patients. As described in Chapter 4, the International Commission on Radiological Protection (ICRP) regularly publishes general radiation protection recommendations based on the general principles of justification, optimization and limitation. Their main aims of radiation protection are to:

- Prevent the detrimental tissue reaction (deterministic effects) by having rules and guidelines based on scientific evidence to ensure known threshold doses are not exceeded.
- Limit the probability of stochastic effects to acceptable levels by determining the level of risk involved.

Their recommendations to try to achieve these aims are usually incorporated eventually into national legislation and guidelines, although the precise details may vary from one country to another. A summary of the current UK legislation and recommendations and guidelines can be found www.whaitesessentialsdentalradiography.com. This section summarizes generic practical radiation protection measures and good practice appropriate for patients, the general public and dental staff.

Practical radiation protection of patients

The main radiation dose to patients comes from:

- Being irradiated in the first place which is totally dependent of the decision and clinical judgement of their dentist
- The main beam of the X-ray equipment.

The main practical radiation protection measures can therefore be considered under three headings:

- Clinical judgement
- Equipment
- Radiographic technique and the technical skill of the staff undertaking the radiography.

Clinical judgement

- All dentists must have received adequate training in dental radiology and should undertake continuing education and training after qualification to keep their knowledge and skills up to date, particularly in relation to the clinical applications of new technology, e.g. cone beam CT (CBCT) (see Ch. 13). This seems reasonable as it is the dentist who decides on the acceptability of the risk to which the patient is being subjected.
- Before an exposure can take place, it must be clinically justified by a dentist (i.e. assessed to ensure that it will lead to a change in the patient's management and prognosis). Every exposure should be justified on the grounds of:
  - The availability and/or findings of previous radiographs
  - The specific objectives of the exposure in relation to the history and following clinical examination of the patient
  - The total potential diagnostic benefit to the patient
  - The radiation risk associated with the radiographic examination
  - The efficacy, benefits and risks of alternative techniques having the same objective, but involving no or less exposure to ionizing radiation.
- To assist with the justification process dentists should make use of published evidence-based selection criteria. For example, in 2013 the Faculty of General Dental Practice (UK) of the Royal College of Surgeons of England published the 3rd Edition of their booklet *Selection Criteria for Dental Radiography*. Their recommendations are graded on the quality of the evidence available using the following scale:
  - **A** = based on evidence from at least one study with *in vitro* validation as part of the body of literature of overall good quality and consistency
  - **B** = based on evidence from well conducted clinical trials but with no specific *in vitro* validation studies
  - **C** = based on evidence from expert committee reports or opinions and/or clinical experience of respected authorities and indicates an absence of directly applicable studies of good quality
  - **NSR** = based on evidence from high-quality, non-systematic literature review.

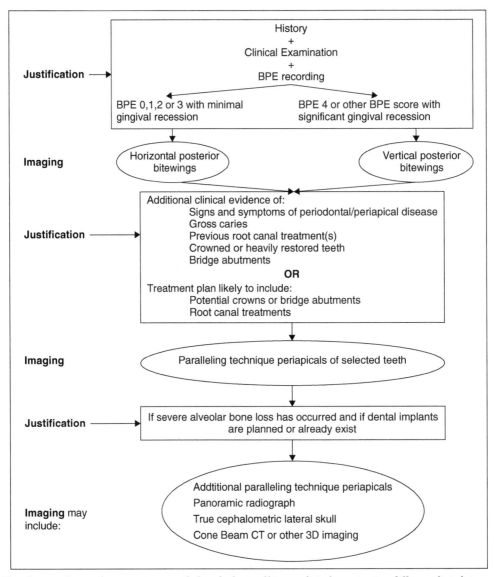

Fig. 5.4 Flow diagram showing how imaging is *justified* on the basic of history, clinical examination, different clinical signs and symptoms of disease and possible treatment plans – based broadly on the imaging strategy for a dentate or partially dentate adult patient from the Faculty of General Dental Practice (UK)'s 2013 *Selection Criteria for Dental Radiography* (3rd Edn).

A variety of their recommendations are included later in Chapter 17, 18 and 19. A flow diagram showing how imaging is *justified* on the basis of history, clinical examination, different clinical signs and symptoms of disease and possible treatment plans – based broadly on the recommendations in the 2013 *Selection Criteria* booklet is shown in Figure 5.4.

Equipment

• All dental X-ray generating equipment should:

– Be installed correctly and tested by a medical physicist for safety and output before being used on a patient
– Be checked regularly by a medical physicist, for example every 1–3 years
– Function within agreed parameters – typically 60–70 kV, 7–12 mA
– Contain adequate filtration (inherent and added) – typically 1.5 mm of aluminium for sets operating below 70 kV and 2.5 mm for sets operating about 70 kV (see Ch. 3)

- Have the main beam collimated to cover the rectangular image receptor (film packet or digital sensor) being used (see Ch. 3) and should not exceed 40×50 mm
- Have a focus to skin distance (fsd) of at least 100 mm if operating below 60 kV and at least 200 mm if operating above 60 kV
- Have an exposure switch (timer) that only functions when continuous pressure is maintained and that terminates if pressure is released
- Be provided with film speed controls and finely adjustable exposure time setting
- Be assessed as to the actual dose delivered to enable comparison with national Diagnostic Reference Levels (DRLs) – if available.
- All panoramic X-ray generating equipment should:
  - Be installed correctly and tested by a medical physicist for safety and output before being used on a patient
  - Be checked regularly by a medical physicist, for example every 1–3 years
  - Function within agreed parameters – typically 60–90–kV
  - Contain adequate filtration (inherent and added)
  - Have the beam collimated to 125 mm or 150 mm (height) × 5 mm (width) at the image receptor
  - Have an exposure switch (timer) that only functions when continuous pressure is maintained and that terminates if pressure is released
  - Be provided with adequate patient-positioning aids incorporating light beam markers (see Ch. 12)
  - Ideally be provided with facilities for field-limitation techniques (see Ch. 12).
- All image receptors should:
  - Be the fastest available (F speed film, rare earth screens or digital sensors) that will produce satisfactory diagnostic images.

Radiographic technique

- All dentists and dental care professionals involved in X-raying patients should:
  - Have received adequate training and should undertake continuing education and training

after qualification to keep their knowledge and skills up to date
  - Undertake radiography accurately to avoid retakes, for example by using image receptor holders and beam-aiming devices for intraoral radiography described in Chapters 7 and 18 or by using patient positioning aids during panoramic radiography described in Chapter 12
  - Use the minimum number of projections
  - Optimize all exposure settings to ensure that all doses are kept as low as reasonably practicable (ALARP) consistent with the intended purpose
  - Ensure all image processing (chemical or computer) (see Chapter 3) is carried to the highest standards so that images do not have to be retaken
  - Consider the use of lead protection.

Confusion and controversy still surround the use of lead protection for patients in different countries. In the UK current guidance suggests that patient protection is best achieved by implementation of the practical dose reduction measures outlined above in relation to clinical judgement, equipment and radiographic technique, and not by lead protection. The latest UK *Guidance Notes* state:

- There is no justification for the routine use of lead aprons for patients undergoing intraoral or panoramic radiography.
- Thyroid collars, as shown in Fig. 5.5, should be used in those few cases where the thyroid may be in the primary beam. (In the authors' opinion, this can include maxillary occlusal radiography and CBCT, and thyroid protection is therefore shown in Chs 11 and 16.)
- Lead aprons do not protect against radiation scattered internally within the body.
- Protective aprons, having a lead equivalence of not less than 0.25 mm, should be provided for any adult who provides assistance by supporting a patient during radiography.
- When a lead apron is provided, it must be correctly stored (e.g. over a suitable hanger) and not folded. Its condition must be routinely checked including a visual inspection at annual intervals.

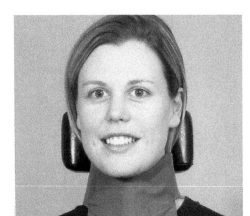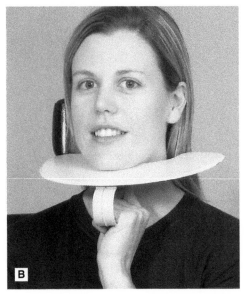

Fig. 5.5 Examples of thyroid lead protection. **A** Lead collar (0.5 mm Pb equivalent). **B** Hand-held neck shield (0.5 mm Pb equivalent).

Specific radiation protection requirements for female patients of childbearing age

The developing fetus is most susceptible to the dangers of ionizing radiation during the period of organogenesis (3–7 weeks) – often before the woman knows that she is pregnant. Legislation usually prohibits the carrying out of a medical exposure of a female of childbearing age without an enquiry as to whether she is pregnant or likely to be pregnant **if** the primary beam is likely to irradiate the pelvic area. This is highly unlikely in dental radiography. If a patient is known to be pregnant then the patient should be reassured that the risk to the foetus is negligible during dental radiography and all routine radiation protection measures employed. Alternatively, because of the emotive nature of radiography during pregnancy, the patient could be given the option to delay the radiography until after the baby is born – if clinical treatment would not be compromised.

Practical radiation protection of the general public

This group includes everyone who is not receiving a radiation dose either as a patient or as a radiation worker, but who may be exposed inadvertently, for example, someone in a dental surgery waiting room, in other rooms in the building or passers-by. The general public are at risk from the primary beam, so specific consideration should be given to:

- The siting of X-ray equipment to ensure that the primary beam is not aimed directly into occupied rooms or corridors
- The thickness/material of partitioning walls
- Advice from a medical physicist on the siting of all X-ray equipment, surgery design and the placement of radiation warning signs, as shown in Fig. 5.6.

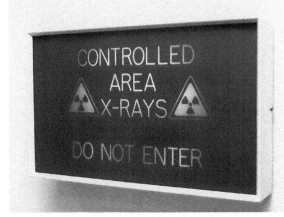

Fig. 5.6 An example of a controlled area warning sign. The words DO NOT ENTER are illuminated when the exposure button is pressed.

Practical radiation protection of radiation workers

The radiation dose to dentists and their staff can come from:

- The primary beam, if they stand in its path
- Scattered radiation from the patient if they stand too close
- Radiation leakage from the tubehead.

The main protective measures to limit the dose that workers might receive are therefore based mainly on a combination of common sense and the knowledge that ionizing radiation is attenuated by distance and obeys the inverse square law (see Fig. 5.7).

- The main practical radiation protection measures include:
  - Ensuring all radiation workers (dental staff) know the risks to their own health created by exposure to X-rays and the safety precautions they need to take including:
  - Always standing outside the so-called controlled area – approximately 1.5 m from the X-ray machine and the patient (or behind appropriate lead screens/barriers) and never in the path of the main beam, as shown in Fig. 5.8
  - Never holding an image receptor in a patient's mouth
  - Never holding the X-ray tubehead during an exposure
  - Always using the X-ray equipment safely and in accordance with current guidance and good practice.

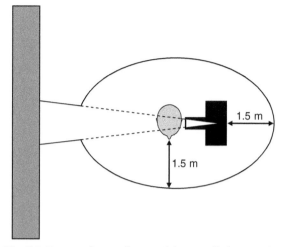

Fig. 5.8 Diagram showing the size of the controlled area, 1.5 m in any direction from the patient and tubehead and anywhere in the line of the main beam until it is attenuated by a solid wall.

Monitoring

Dental staff are almost always designated as non-classified workers by the International Commission on Radiological Protection (ICRP). As explained in Chapter 4, the ICRP sets annual dose limits for different categories of radiation workers and for non-classified workers the current limit is 6 mSv per year. In the UK, the Health Protection Agency regards an annual limit of 1 mSv as more appropriate for dental staff working in general dental practice. The amount of radiation received by individuals can be monitored and measured using a variety of different monitoring devices and can include:

- Film badges
- Thermoluminescent dosimeters (TLD)
  - Badge
  - Extremity monitor
- Optically stimulated luminescence dosimeters (OSLD)
- Personal electronic dosimeters (PED).

These devices do not protect against radiation. They merely provide data as to the amount of radiation that has been received over a period of time. More immediate information that the wearer is being irradiated can be provided by personal electronic dosimeters including sophisticated systems such as the recently developed Unfors Alert dosimeter. A selection of various dosimeters is shown in Fig. 5.9.

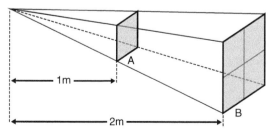

Fig. 5.7 Diagrammatic representation of the inverse square law. Doubling the distance from the source means that the area of B is four times the area of A, thus the radiation per unit area at B is one-quarter that at A.

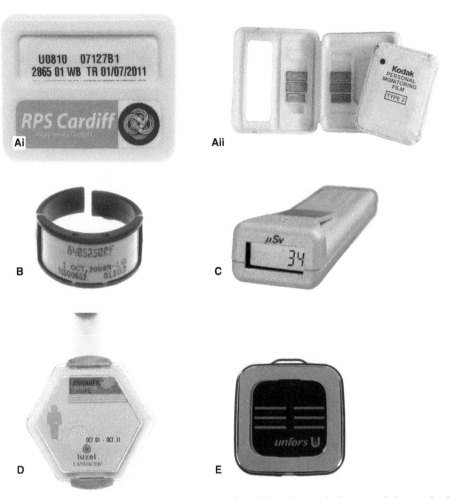

Fig. 5.9 A selection of monitoring devices. **A(i)** Personal monitoring plastic film badge, **(ii)** badge opened showing the different metal filters and the film. **B** Personal TLD extremity (finger) monitor. **C** Personal electronic dosimeter. **D** Personal OSLD badge. **E** Unfors Alert dosimeter.

Film badges

The main features of film badges are:

- They consist of a plastic frame (usually blue or white) containing a variety of different metal filters and a small radiographic film which reacts to radiation
- They are worn on the outside of the clothes, usually at the level of the reproductive organs, for 1–3 months before being processed
- They are the most common form of personal monitoring device currently in use.

Advantages

- Provide a permanent record of dose received.
- May be checked and reassessed at a later date.
- Can measure the type and energy of radiation encountered.
- Simple, robust and relatively inexpensive.

Disadvantages

- No immediate indication of exposure – all information is retrospective.
- Processing is required which may lead to errors.
- The badges are prone to filter loss.

Thermoluminescent dosimeters (TLDs)
The main features of TLDs are:

- They are used for personal monitoring of the whole body and/or the extremities, as well as measuring the skin dose from particular investigations.
- They contain materials such as lithium fluoride (LiF) which absorb radiation and then release the energy in the form of light when heated.
- The intensity of the emitted light is proportional to the radiation energy absorbed originally.
- Personal monitors consist of a yellow or orange plastic holder, worn like the film badge for 1–3 months.

Advantages
- The lithium fluoride is re-usable.
- Read-out measurements are easily automated and rapidly produced.
- Suitable for a wide variety of dose measurements.

Disadvantages
- Read-out is destructive, giving no permanent record, results cannot be checked or reassessed.
- Only limited information provided on the type and energy of the radiation.
- Dose gradients are not detectable.
- Relatively expensive.

Optically stimulated luminescent dosimeters (OLSDs)
The main features of OSLDs are:

- They are used for personal monitoring of the whole body.
- They consist of a badge containing an aluminium oxide detector and metal and plastic filters.
- The detector is read by exposing it to a light source, which releases the stored radiation energy in the aluminium oxide as blue light (luminescence).
- The radiation exposure can be calculated from the amount and intensity of blue light released.

Advantages
- Quick non-destructive readout.
- Multiple readouts possible so radiation doses can be verified if required.

- Good sensitivity and respond to a wide range of energies.
- Relatively robust.

Disadvantages
- No immediate indication of exposure – all information is retrospective.

Personal electronic dosimeters (PEDs)
The main features of PEDs are:

- They are battery operated devices normally worn in the operator's pocket for personal monitoring of the whole body.
- They are usually based on an energy-activated silicon diode (a solid-state detector) to measure radiation dose.
- Some also measure the dose rate and have an audible alarm to indicate radiation as it is received.

Advantages
- Direct digital read-out gives immediate information.
- Once purchased, no ongoing running costs
- Relatively robust.

Disadvantages
- Initial cost can be expensive.
- Only sophisticated devices give a permanent record of exposure.
- No indication given of the type or energy of the radiation.
- Not very sensitive to low-energy radiation, and so may not be reliable in the energy range encountered in dental radiography.

Footnote

All dental staff should be fully aware of the biological effects associated with X-rays, the risks involved for both patients and themselves and hence the practical radiation protection measures that are required. Although monitoring of dental workers is not usually a mandatory requirement, it seems sensible for all staff to be monitored at least for a short period of time for their own peace of mind.

To access the self assessment questions for this chapter please go to www.whaitesessentialsdentalradiography.com

Radiography

PART CONTENTS

6

Dental radiography – general patient considerations including control of infection

This short chapter is designed as a preface to the radiography section. It summarizes the general guidelines relating to patient care, pertinent to all aspects of dental radiography, thus avoiding unnecessary repetition in subsequent chapters. Measures aimed at the control of infection during radiography are also discussed.

General guidelines on patient care

- For intraoral radiography the patient should be positioned comfortably in the dental chair, ideally with the occlusal plane horizontal and parallel to the floor. For most projections the head should be supported against the chair to minimize unwanted movement. This upright positioning is assumed in subsequent chapters when describing radiographic techniques. However, some operators elect to X-ray their patients in the supine position along with most other dental surgery procedures. All techniques need to be modified accordingly, but it can sometimes be more difficult to assess angulations and achieve accurate alignment of image receptor and tubehead with the patient lying down.
- For extraoral views the patient should be reassured about the large, possibly frightening or unfriendly looking equipment, before being positioned within the machine. This is of particular importance with children.
- The procedure should be explained to the patients in terms they can understand, including warning them not to move during the investigation.
- Spectacles, dentures or orthodontic appliances should be removed. Jewellery, including earrings, may also need to be removed for certain projections.

- A protective lead thyroid collar, if deemed appropriate for the investigation being carried out, should be placed on the patient (see Ch. 5).
- The exposure factors on the control panel should be selected before positioning the intraoral image receptor and X-ray tubehead, in order to reduce the time of any discomfort associated with the investigation.
- Intraoral image receptors should be positioned carefully to avoid trauma to the soft tissues taking particular care where tissues curve, e.g. the anterior hard palate, lingual to the mandibular incisor teeth and distolingual to the mandibular molars.
- The radiographic investigation should be carried out as accurately and as quickly as possible, to avoid having to retake the radiograph and to lessen patient discomfort.
- The patient should always be watched throughout the exposure to check that he/she has obeyed instructions and has not moved.

Specific requirements when X-raying children and patients with disabilities

These two groups of patients can present particular problems during radiography, including:

- Difficulty in obtaining cooperation
- Anatomical difficulties, such as:
  - large tongue (macroglossia)
  - small mouth (microstomia)
  - tight oral musculature
  - limited neck movement
  - narrow dental arches
  - shallow palate
  - obesity

73

- Neurological disabilities, such as:
  - communication and learning difficulties
  - tremor
  - palsy

As a result of these difficulties, the following additional guidelines should be considered:

- Only radiographic investigations appropriate to the limitations imposed by the patient's age, cooperation or disability should be attempted.
- Select intraoral image receptors of appropriate size, modifying standard techniques as necessary.
- Utilize assistant(s) to help hold the image receptor and/or steady and reassure the patient. This can be accomplished by using an accompanying relative, rather than repeatedly using a member of staff.

Note: Radiation protection regulations usually require that during an exposure a designated *controlled area* or exclusion zone must exist around the X-ray set and theoretically only the patient is allowed in this area (see Ch. 5). Therefore, if assistance is needed and this requirement cannot be fulfilled, a *radiation protection adviser* (RPA) or a medical physics expert must advise on the appropriate protective measures for the assistant.

- Perform any necessary radiography under general anaesthesia, if an uncooperative patient is having their dental treatment in this manner (see Fig. 6.1). Radiographs taken are usually restricted to oblique laterals and periapicals, although bitewings can be taken.
- Avoid panoramic radiography because of the need for the patient to remain still for approximately 18 seconds (see Ch. 12). Oblique lateral radiographs should be regarded as the extraoral views of choice.
- Use the paralleling technique, if possible, for periapical radiography because with this technique the relative positions of the image receptor, teeth and X-ray beam are maintained, irrespective of the position of the patient's head (see Ch. 7).

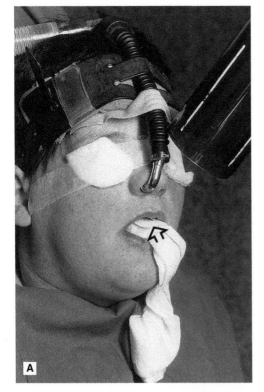

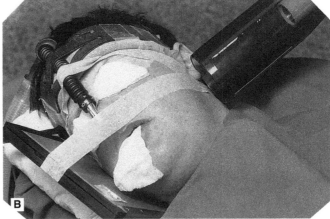

Fig. 6.1 Patient positioning for radiography under general anaesthesia. **A** Periapical radiography of upper incisor teeth. Note the film packet (arrowed) supported in the desired position by a gauze pack. **B** Oblique lateral radiography. Note the tape used to stabilize the cassette and maintain the correct patient position. (Kindly provided by Mr P. Erridge.)

Control of infection

In the UK, the Health and Safety at Work, etc. Act of 1974 states that every person working in hospitals or general practice (referred to as *health care workers* or HCWs) has a legal duty to ensure that all necessary steps are taken to prevent cross-infection to protect themselves, their colleagues and the patients. In addition, The Management of Health and Safety Regulations 1992 requires that a risk assessment is carried out for all procedures to reduce the possibility of harm to staff and patients. Effective infection control measures are therefore required in dental radiography even though most investigations are regarded as *non-invasive* or *non-exposure prone procedures*, because they do not involve breaches of the mucosa or skin. The main risk of cross-infection is from one patient to another from salivary contamination of work areas and equipment. HCWs themselves are not at great risk during radiography but there are no grounds for complacency.

Main infections of concern

- *Infective hepatitis caused by hepatitis B (HBV) or hepatitis C (HCV) viruses.* The WHO estimates that of the 2 billion people that have been infected with HBV, more than 350 million have chronic (lifelong) infections. In the developing world, 8–10% of people in the general population become chronically infected. HBV is thought to be 50–100 times more infectious than HIV. The WHO estimates that 3% of the world's population has been infected with HCV.
- *Human immunodeficiency virus (HIV disease and AIDS caused by HIV).*
- *Tuberculosis (TB).* The incidence of all forms of TB is rising.
- *Cold sores caused by herpes simplex virus (HSV).* HCWs are at risk of getting herpetic whitlow, a painful finger infection, although this has reduced since the adoption of the use of gloves.
- *Rubella (German measles).*
- *Syphilis.*
- *Diphtheria.*
- *Mumps.*
- *Influenza.*
- *Transmissible spongiform encephalopathies (TSEs), e.g. Creutzfeldt – Jakob disease (CJD).*

A thorough medical history should therefore be obtained from all patients. However, the medical history and examination may not identify asymptomatic carriers of infectious diseases.

It is therefore safer for HCWs to accept that ALL patients may be an infection risk – age or class is no barrier – and universal precautions should be adopted. This means that the same infection control measures should be used for all patients, the only exception being for patients known to have or suspected of having TSEs and the small number of patients in the defined risk groups for TSEs.

Important point to note

If dental clinicians are requesting other HCWs to take their radiographs, either in hospitals or general dental practice, it is their responsibility to ensure that these workers are made aware of any known medical problems or risks, e.g. epilepsy or current infections.

Infection control measures

As mentioned previously, in dental radiography the main concerns arise from salivary contamination of work areas and equipment. Suitable precautions include:

- Training of all staff in infection control procedures and monitoring their compliance.
- All clinical staff should be vaccinated against hepatitis B, have their response to this vaccine checked and maintain this vaccination.
- Open wounds on the hands should be covered with waterproof dressings.
- Protective non-sterile, non-powdered medical gloves should be worn for all radiographic procedures and changed after every patient.
- Eye protection – either safety glasses or visors (see Fig. 6.2) should be worn but masks are not usually necessary for radiography.

- All required image receptors and holders should be placed on disposable trays to avoid contamination of work surfaces.
- To prevent salivary contamination of film packets, they can be placed in small barrier envelopes or preferably purchased pre-packed in such envelopes, before use (see Fig. 6.3). After being used in the mouth, the film packet can be emptied out of the barrier envelope onto a clean surface and then handled safely.
- Digital radiography sensors must also be placed inside appropriate barrier envelopes (see Fig. 6.4).
- Film packets must only be introduced into daylight-loading processors using clean hands or washed gloves. Powdered gloves may cause artefacts on the films.
- Contaminated disposable trays, barrier envelopes and film packaging should be discarded directly into suitable clinical waste disposal bags.

- All image receptor holders/bite blocks/bite pegs should be decontaminated and sterilized in an autoclave as set out in national guidance, for example in the UK the Department of Health's document HTM 01-05 *Decontamination in Primary Care Dental Practices* updated in 2013.
- X-ray equipment, including the tubehead, control panel, timer switch and cassettes which have been touched during the radiographic procedure should be wiped after each patient with a suitable surface disinfectant, e.g. Mikrozid®.
- Alternatively, all pieces of equipment can be covered, for example with cling film or dedicated barrier *sleeves*, which can be replaced after every patient (see Fig. 6.5).
- Soiled gloves and cleaning swabs should be placed in suitable disposal bags and sealed for incineration.

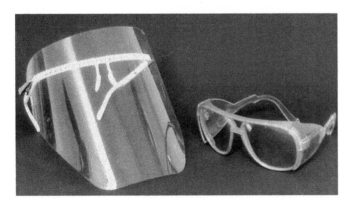

Fig. 6.2 Plastic safety glasses and Vista-Tec visor (Polydentia SA) suitable for eye protection during dental radiography.

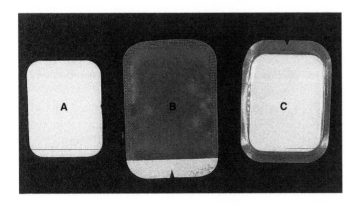

Fig. 6.3 A 31 × 41 mm periapical film packet. **B** Plastic barrier envelope to take the periapical film. **C** Prepacked periapical film packet inside its barrier envelope.

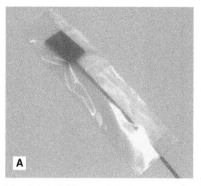
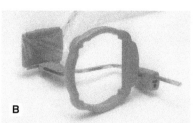
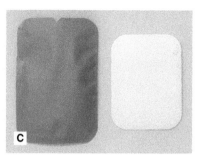

Fig. 6.4 **A** Solid-state digital sensor inside a barrier envelope. **B** Barrier wrapped solid-state sensor inserted into a sensor holder. **C** Barrier envelope for the 31 × 41 mm digital photostimulable phosphor plate shown.

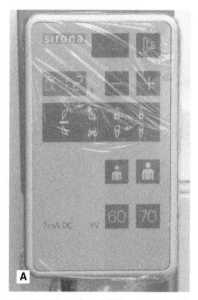
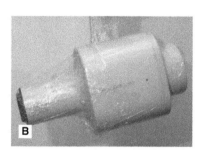
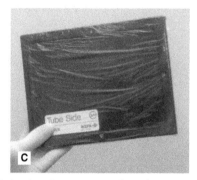

Fig. 6.5 Examples of different pieces of equipment barrier-wrapped in cling film and ready for clinical use: **A** a control panel including the exposure button; **B** an X-ray tubehead and **C** a cassette for extraoral use.

Important point to note

- When X-raying known or suspected TSE patients, extraoral radiographic techniques, that avoid salivary contamination, should be chosen whenever possible (preferably using a technique that does not involve any form of intraoral positioning device) and films should be processed immediately and not left on work surfaces.

Footnote

The importance of effective control of infection measures during dental radiography cannot be overemphasized. All dental care professionals should remember that they have a duty of care to do no harm to their patients. Inadequate infection control measures may put other/subsequent patients at risk from infection, whether transmitted directly or indirectly.

To access the self assessment questions for this chapter please go to www.whaitesessentialsdentalradiography.com

7 Periapical radiography

Periapical radiography describes intraoral techniques designed to show individual teeth and the tissues *around the apices*. Each film usually shows two to four teeth and provides detailed information about the teeth and the surrounding alveolar bone.

Main indications

The main clinical indications for periapical radiography include:

- Detection of apical infection/inflammation
- Assessment of the periodontal status
- After trauma to the teeth and associated alveolar bone
- Assessment of the presence and position of unerupted teeth
- Assessment of root morphology before extractions
- During endodontics
- Preoperative assessment and postoperative appraisal of apical surgery
- Detailed evaluation of apical cysts and other lesions within the alveolar bone
- Evaluation of implants postoperatively.

Ideal positioning requirements

The ideal requirements for the position of the image receptor and the X-ray beam, relative to a tooth, are shown in Fig. 7.1. They include:

- The tooth under investigation and the image receptor should be in contact or, if not feasible, as close together as possible.

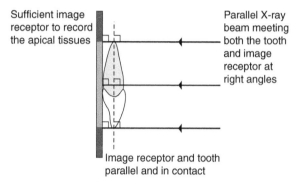

Fig. 7.1 Diagram illustrating the ideal geometrical relationship between image receptor, tooth and X-ray beam.

- The tooth and the image receptor should be parallel to one another.
- The image receptor should be positioned with its long axis vertically for incisors and canines, and horizontally for premolars and molars with sufficient receptor beyond the apices to record the apical tissues.
- The X-ray tubehead should be positioned so that the beam meets the tooth and the image receptor at right angles in both the vertical and the horizontal planes.
- The positioning should be reproducible.

Radiographic techniques

The anatomy of the oral cavity does not always allow all these ideal positioning requirements to be satisfied. In an attempt to overcome the problems, two techniques for periapical radiography have been developed:

- The paralleling technique
- The bisected angle technique.

Paralleling technique

Theory

1. The image receptor is placed in a holder and positioned in the mouth **parallel** to the long axis of the tooth under investigation.
2. The X-ray tubehead is then aimed at right angles (vertically and horizontally) to both the tooth and the image receptor.
3. By using a film or sensor holder with fixed image receptor and X-ray tubehead positions, the technique is reproducible.

This positioning has the potential to satisfy four of the five ideal requirements mentioned earlier. However, the anatomy of the palate and the shape of the arches mean that the tooth and the image receptor cannot be both parallel and in contact. As shown in Fig. 7.2, the image receptor has to be positioned some distance from the tooth.

To prevent the magnification of the image that this separation would cause, a parallel, non-diverging, X-ray beam is required (see Fig. 7.3). As explained in Chapter 3, this is achieved usually by having a **long** *focal spot to skin distance (fsd)*, ideally of 200 mm.

Film packet/sensor holders

A variety of holders has been developed for this technique. The choice of holder is a matter of personal preference and dependent on the type of image receptor – film packet or digital sensor (solid-state or phosphor plate) – being used. The different holders vary in cost and design, as shown in Fig. 7.4 but essentially consist of three basic components:

- A mechanism for holding the image receptor parallel to the teeth that also prevents bending of the receptor
- A bite block or platform
- An X-ray beam-aiming device. This may or may not provide additional collimation of the beam.

The different components of the various holders usually need to be assembled together before the holder can be used clinically. The holder design used depends upon whether the tooth under investigation is:

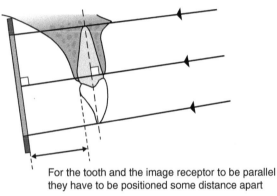

For the tooth and the image receptor to be parallel they have to be positioned some distance apart

Fig. 7.2 Diagram showing the position the image receptor has to occupy in the mouth to be parallel to the long axis of the tooth, because of the slope of the palate.

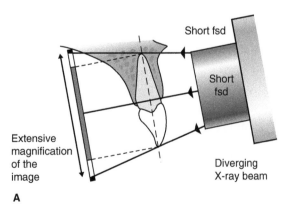

A

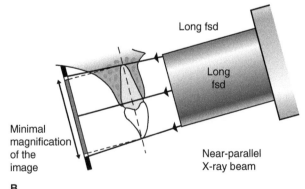

B

Fig. 7.3 Diagrams showing the magnification of the image that results from using **A** a short focal spot to skin distance (fsd) and a diverging X-ray beam and **B** a long focal spot to skin distance (fsd) and a near-parallel X-ray beam.

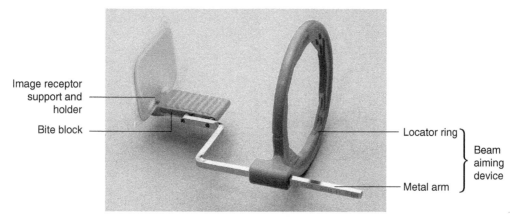

Fig. 7.4 Posterior Rinn XCP image receptor holder showing the three basic components common to most holders.

- Anterior or posterior
- In the mandible or maxilla
- On the right- or the left-hand side of the jaw.

These variables mean that assembling the holder can be confusing, but it must be done correctly. To facilitate this assembly some manufacturers now colour-code the various components. Once assembled correctly the entire image receptor should be visible when viewed through the beam-aiming device, as shown in Fig. 7.5. A selection of different holders is shown in Fig. 7.6.

Typically, the **same** anterior holder can be used for **right** and **left** maxillary **and** mandibular *incisors* and *canines* utilizing a small image receptor (22 × 35 mm) with its long axis vertical. Four images in the maxilla and three images in the mandible are usually required to cover the right and left incisors and canines, as shown in Fig. 7.7.

Typically **different** holders are required for the **right** and **left** *premolar and molar* maxillary and mandibular posterior teeth. The different designs allow the holders to hook around the

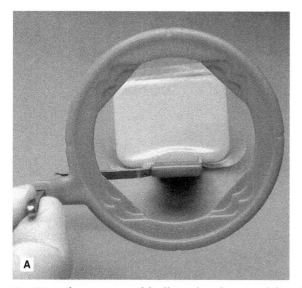
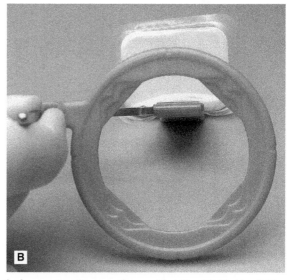

Fig. 7.5 A The appearance of the film packet when viewed through the locator ring of a correctly assembled Rinn XCP holder. **B** The appearance when the image receptor holder has been assembled incorrectly.

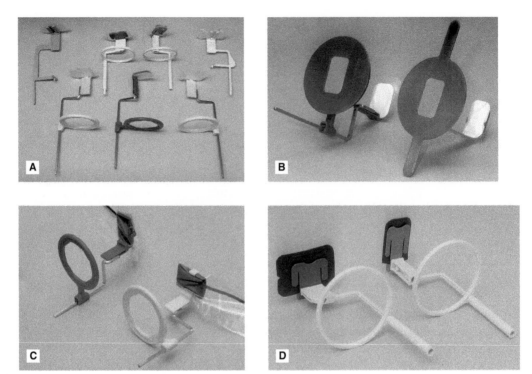

Fig. 7.6 A A selection of film packet and digital phosphor plate holders designed for the paralleling technique. Note how some manufacturers use colour coding to identify holders for different parts of the mouth. **B** Holders incorporating additional rectangular collimation – the Masel Precision all-in-one metal holder and the Rinn XCP holder with the metal collimator attached to the locator ring. **C** Blue anterior and yellow posterior Rinn XCP-DS solid-state digital sensor holders. **D** Green/yellow anterior and red/yellow posterior Hawe – Neos holders suitable for film packets and digital phosphor plates (shown here). *(See colour plates section)*

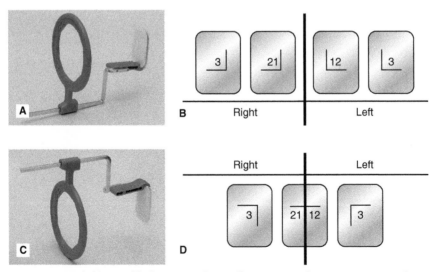

Fig. 7.7 A The anterior Rinn XCP holder suitable for imaging the maxillary incisors and canines. **B** Diagram showing the four small image receptors required to image the right and left maxillary incisors and canines. **C** The same anterior Rinn XCP holder suitable for imaging the mandibular incisors and canines. **D** Diagram showing the three small image receptors required to image the right and left mandibular incisors and canines. *(See colour plates section)*

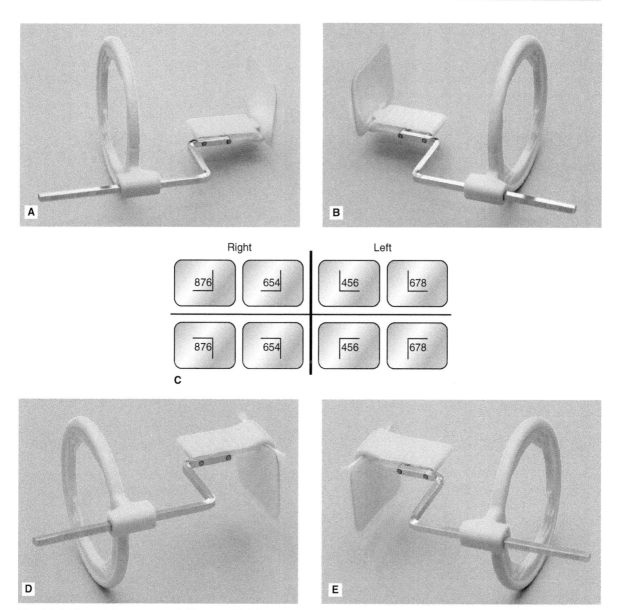

Fig. 7.8 A The posterior Rinn XCP holder assembled for imaging the RIGHT maxillary premolars and molars. **B** The posterior Rinn XCP holder assembled for imaging the LEFT maxillary premolars and molars. **C** Diagram showing the two large image receptors required to image the right and left premolars and molars in each quadrant. **D** The posterior Rinn XCP holder assembled for imaging the RIGHT mandibular premolars and molars. **E** The posterior Rinn XCP holder assembled for imaging the LEFT mandibular premolars and molars. (*See colour plates section*)

cheek and corner of the mouth. A large image receptor (31 × 41 mm) is ideally utilized with its long axis horizontal. Two images are usually required to cover the premolar and molar teeth in each quadrant, as shown is Fig. 7.8.

Positioning techniques

The radiographic techniques for the permanent dentition can be summarized as follows:

1. The patient is positioned with the head supported and with the occlusal plane horizontal.
2. The holder and image receptor are placed in the mouth as follows:
   a. *Maxillary incisors and canines* – the image receptor is positioned sufficiently posteriorly to enable its height to be accommodated in the vault of the palate
   b. *Mandibular incisors and canines* – the image receptor is positioned in the floor of the mouth, approximately in line with the lower canines or first premolars
   c. *Maxillary premolars and molars* – the image receptor is placed in the midline of the palate, again to accommodate its height in the vault of the palate
   d. *Mandibular premolars and molars* – the image receptor is placed in the lingual sulcus next to the appropriate teeth.
3. The holder is rotated so that the teeth under investigation are touching the bite block.
4. A cottonwool roll is placed on the reverse side of the bite block. This often helps to keep the tooth and image receptor parallel and may make the holder less uncomfortable.
5. The patient is requested to bite **gently** together, to stabilize the holder in position.
6. The locator ring is moved down the indicator rod until it is just in contact with the patient's face. This ensures the correct focal spot to film distance (fsd).
7. The spacer cone is aligned with the locator ring. This automatically sets the vertical and horizontal angles and centres the X-ray beam on the image receptor.
8. The exposure is made.

Positioning clinically using film packets and digital phosphor plates is shown in Figs 7.9–7.16 for the following different areas of the mouth:

Maxillary central incisor (Fig. 7.9)

Maxillary canine (Fig. 7.10)

Maxillary premolars (Fig. 7.11)

Maxillary molars (Fig. 7.12)

Mandibular incisors (Fig. 7.13)

Mandibular canine (Fig. 7.14)

Mandibular premolars (Fig. 7.15)

Mandibular molars (Fig. 7.16)

Note:

1. *Full mouth survey* is the terminology used to describe the full collection of 15 periapical radiographs (seven anterior and eight posterior) showing the full dentition.
2. When using film packets and digital phosphor plates the end of the receptor with the orientation dot should be placed opposite the crowns of the teeth to avoid subsequent superimposition of the dot over an apex.

Positioning using solid-state digital sensors

Clinical positioning of holders for the paralleling technique when using solid-state digital sensors can be more difficult because of the bulk and absolute rigidity of the sensor. Those systems employing cables also require extra care with regard to the position of the cable to avoid damaging it. Once the holder is inserted into the mouth, the positioning of the tubehead is the same as described previously when using other types of image receptors and is shown in Fig. 7.17 for different parts of the mouth.

Maxillary incisors

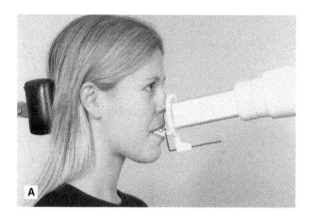

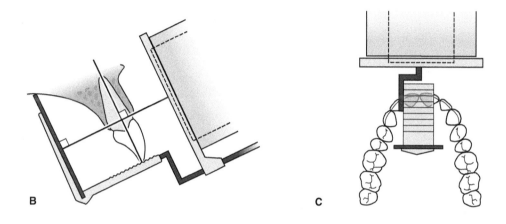

B   C

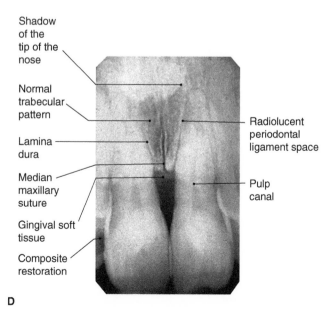

Shadow of the tip of the nose

Normal trabecular pattern

Lamina dura

Median maxillary suture

Gingival soft tissue

Composite restoration

Radiolucent periodontal ligament space

Pulp canal

D

Fig. 7.9 A Patient positioning (maxillary central incisor). **B** Diagram of the positioning. **C** Plan view of the positioning. **D** Resultant radiograph with the main anatomical features indicated.

Maxillary canine

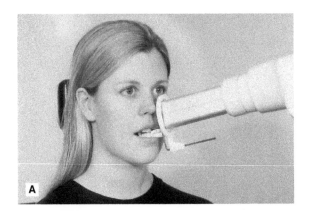

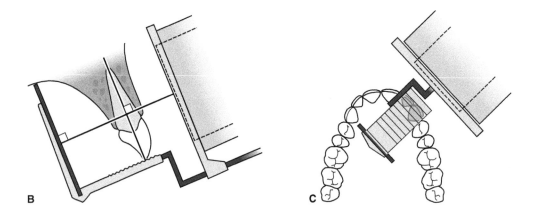

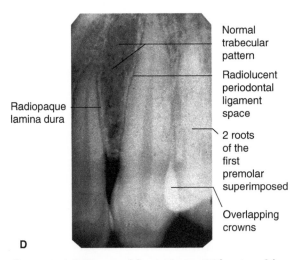

Fig. 7.10 A Patient positioning (maxillary canine). **B** Diagram of the positioning. **C** Plan view of the positioning. **D** Resultant radiograph with the main anatomical features indicated.

Maxillary premolars

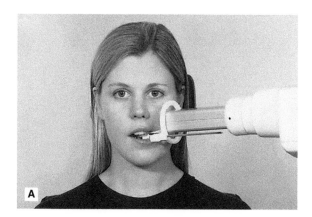

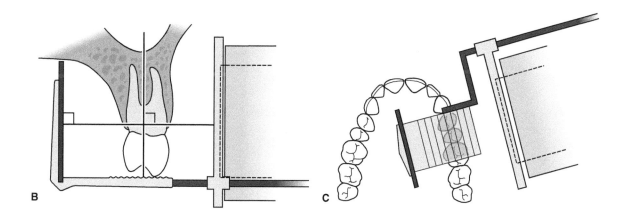

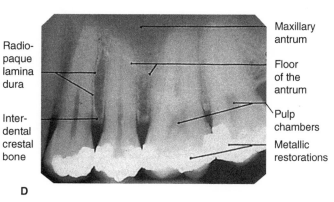

Radio-
paque
lamina
dura

Inter-
dental
crestal
bone

Maxillary
antrum

Floor
of the
antrum

Pulp
chambers

Metallic
restorations

Fig. 7.11 A Patient positioning (maxillary premolars). **B** Diagram of the positioning. **C** Plan view of the positioning. **D** Resultant radiograph with the main anatomical features indicated.

Maxillary molars

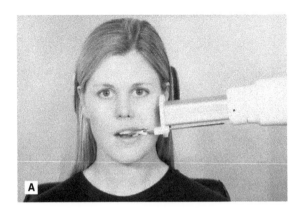

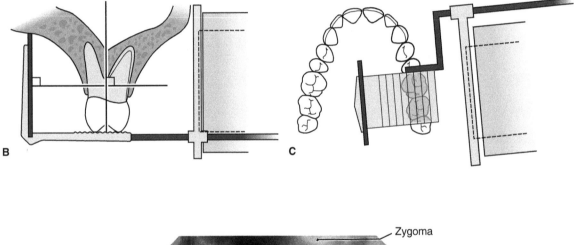

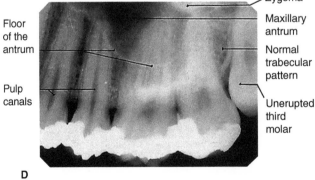

Fig. 7.12 A Patient positioning (maxillary molars). **B** Diagram of the positioning. **C** Plan view of the positioning. **D** Resultant radiograph with the main anatomical features indicated.

Mandibular incisors

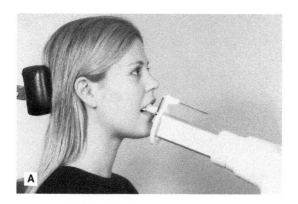

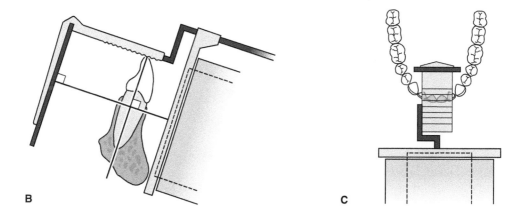

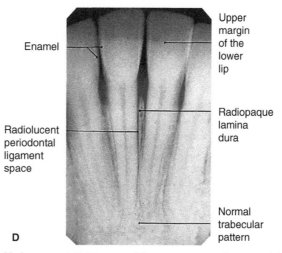

Fig. 7.13 A Patient positioning (mandibular incisors). **B** Diagram of the positioning. **C** Plan view of the positioning. **D** Resultant radiograph with the main anatomical features indicated.

Mandibular canine

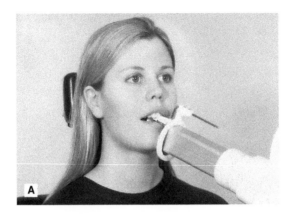

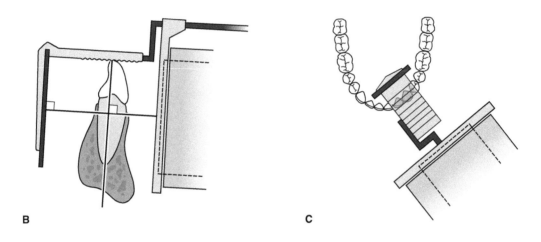

B   C

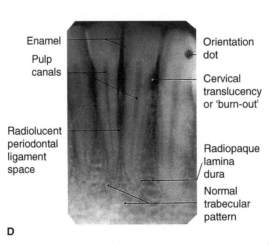

Enamel

Pulp canals

Radiolucent periodontal ligament space

Orientation dot

Cervical translucency or 'burn-out'

Radiopaque lamina dura

Normal trabecular pattern

D

Fig. 7.14 A Patient positioning (mandibular lateral and canine). **B** Diagram of the positioning. **C** Plan view of the positioning. **D** Resultant radiograph with the main anatomical features indicated.

Mandibular premolars

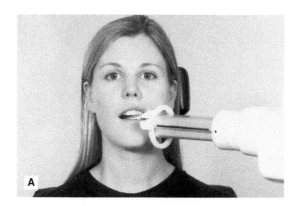

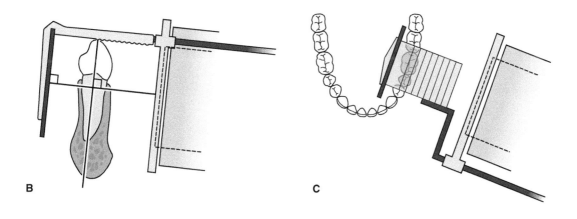

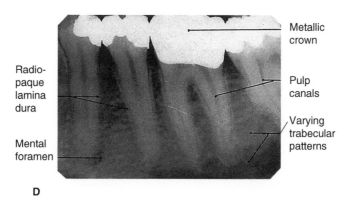

Fig. 7.15 A Patient positioning (mandibular premolars). **B** Diagram of the positioning. **C** Plan view of the positioning. **D** Resultant radiograph with the main anatomical features indicated.

Mandibular molars

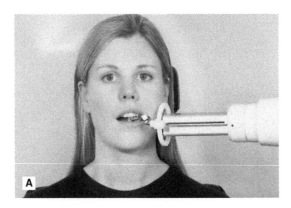

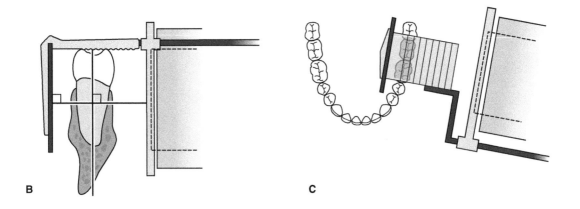

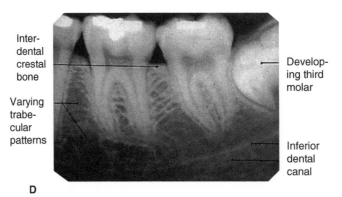

Fig. 7.16 A Patient positioning (mandibular molars). **B** Diagram of the positioning. **C** Plan view of the positioning. **D** Resultant radiograph with the main anatomical features indicated.

Solid-state digital sensor positioning

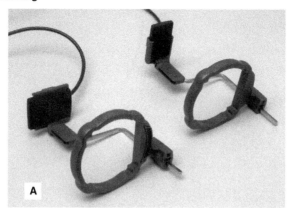

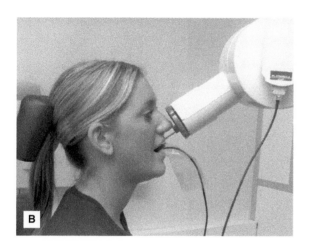

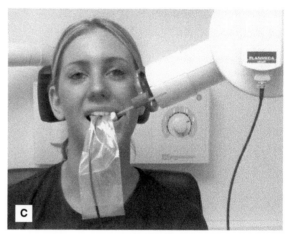

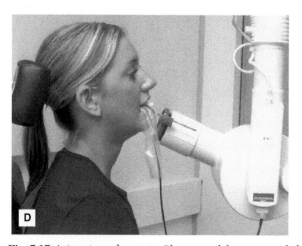

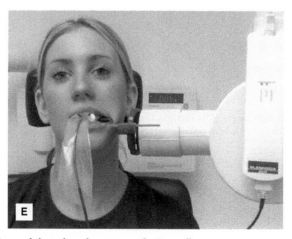

Fig. 7.17 A Anterior and posterior Planmeca solid-state sensor holders and their clinical positioning for **B** maxillary incisors. **C** Maxillary molars. **D** Mandibular incisors. **E** Mandibular molars.

Bisected angle technique

Theory

The theoretical basis of the bisected angle technique is shown in Fig. 7.18 and can be summarized as follows:

1. The image receptor is placed as close to the tooth under investigation as possible without bending the receptor.
2. The angle formed between the long axis of the tooth and the long axis of the image receptor is assessed and mentally bisected.
3. The X-ray tubehead is positioned at right angles to this bisecting line with the central ray of the X-ray beam aimed through the tooth apex.
4. Using the geometrical principle of similar triangles, the actual length of the tooth in the mouth will be equal to the length of the image of the tooth on the image.

Vertical angulation of the X-ray tubehead

The angle formed by continuing the line of the central ray until it meets the occlusal plane determines the *vertical angulation* of the X-ray beam to the occlusal plane (see Fig. 7.18).

Note: These vertical angles are often quoted but inevitably they are only approximate. Patient differences including head position, and individual tooth position and inclination mean that each positioning should be assessed independently. The vertical angulations suggested below in Figs 7.23–7.30 should be taken as a general guide only.

Horizontal angulation of the X-ray tubehead

In the horizontal plane, the central ray should be aimed through the interproximal contact areas, to avoid overlapping the teeth. The *horizontal angulation* is therefore determined by the shape of the arch and the position of the teeth (see Fig. 7.19).

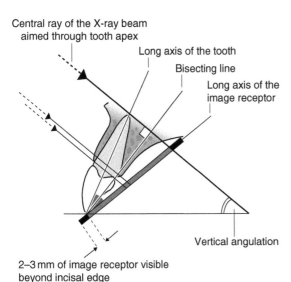

Central ray of the X-ray beam aimed through tooth apex

Long axis of the tooth

Bisecting line

Long axis of the image receptor

Vertical angulation

2–3 mm of image receptor visible beyond incisal edge

Fig. 7.18 Theoretical basis of the bisected angle technique. The angle between the long axes of the tooth and image receptor is bisected and X-ray beam aimed at right angles to this line, through the apex of the tooth. With this geometrical arrangement, the length of the tooth in the mouth is equal to the length of the image of the tooth on the image receptor, but, as shown, the periodontal bone levels will not be represented accurately.

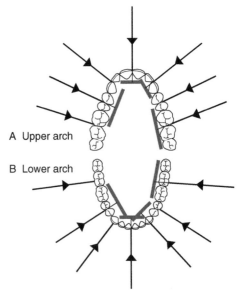

A Upper arch

B Lower arch

Fig. 7.19 Diagram of **A** the upper arch and **B** the lower arch. The various horizontal angulations of the X-ray beam are shown.

Positioning techniques

The bisected angle technique can be performed either by using an image receptor holder to support the image receptor in the patient's mouth or by asking the patient to support the image receptor **gently** using either an index finger or thumb. Both techniques are described.

It is, however, good practice that the image receptor should be held by the patient only when it cannot otherwise be kept in position.

Using film packet/digital sensor holders

Various holders are available, a selection of which are shown in Fig. 7.20. The Rinn Bisected Angle Instruments (BAI) closely resemble the paralleling technique holders and consist of the same three basic components – image receptor holding mechanism, bite block and an X-ray beam-aiming device – but the image receptor is not held parallel to the teeth. The more simple holders and the disposable bite blocks hold the image receptor in the desired position but the X-ray tubehead then has to be aligned independently. In summary:

1. The image receptor is pushed securely into the chosen holder. Either a large or small size of image receptor is used so that the particular tooth being examined is in the middle of the receptor, as shown in Fig. 7.21. When using a film packet, the white surface faces the X-ray tubehead and the film orientation dot is opposite the crown.
2. The X-ray tubehead is positioned using the beam-aiming device if available OR the operator has to assess the *vertical* and *horizontal* *angulations* and then position the tubehead without a guide.
3. The exposure is made.

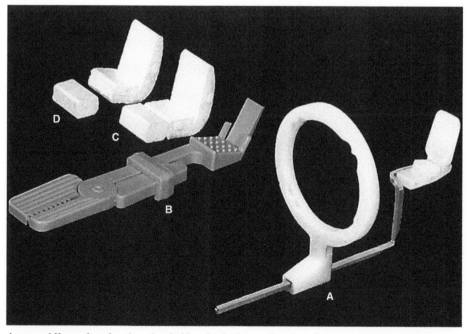

Fig. 7.20 A selection of film packet/phosphor plate holders for the bisected angle technique. **A** The Rinn bisected angle instrument (BAI). **B** The Emmenix® film holder. **C** The Rinn Greene Stabe® bite block. **D** The Rinn Greene Stabe® bite block reduced in size for easier positioning and for use in children.

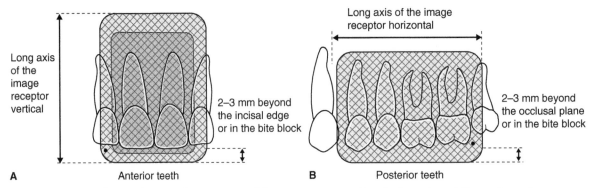

A   Anterior teeth   **B**   Posterior teeth

Fig. 7.21 Diagrams showing the general requirements of the image receptor position for **A** anterior and **B** posterior teeth.

Using the patient's finger

1. The appropriate-sized image receptor is positioned and orientated in the mouth as shown in Fig. 7.21 with about 2 mm extending beyond the incisal or occlusal edges, to ensure that all of the tooth will appear on the image. The patient is then asked to gently support the image receptor using either an index finger or thumb.

2. The operator then assesses the *vertical* and *horizontal angulations* and positions the tubehead without a guide. The effects of incorrect tubehead position are shown in Fig. 7.22.
3. The exposure is made.

The specific positioning for different areas of the mouth, using both simple holders and the patient's finger to support the image receptor, is shown in Figs 7.23–7.30.

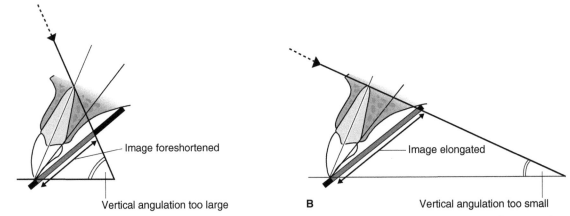

A   Vertical angulation too large   **B**   Vertical angulation too small

Fig. 7.22 Diagrams showing the effects of incorrect vertical tubehead positioning. **A** Foreshortening of the image. **B** Elongation of the image.

Maxillary central incisors

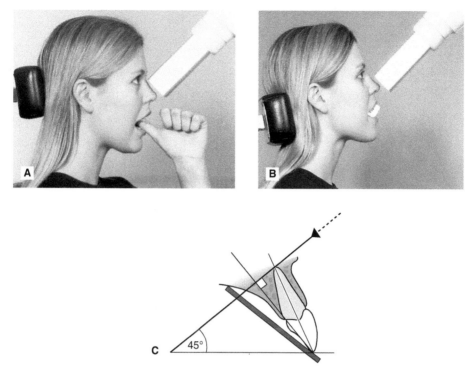

Fig. 7.23 Patient positioning with the patient **A** supporting the image receptor with the ball of the left thumb and **B** using the Rinn Greene Stabe® bite block. **C** Diagram of the relative positions of image receptor, tooth and X-ray beam.

Maxillary canine

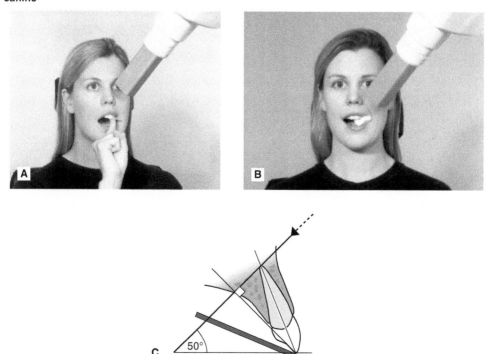

Fig. 7.24 Patient positioning with the patient **A** supporting the image receptor with the ball of the right index finger and **B** using the Rinn Greene Stabe® bite block. **C** Diagram of the relative positions of image receptor, tooth and X-ray beam.

Maxillary premolars

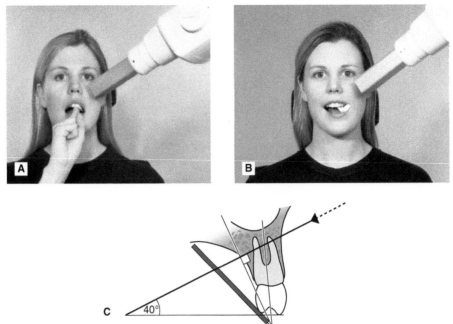

Fig. 7.25 Patient positioning with the patient **A** supporting the image receptor and **B** using the Rinn Greene Stabe® bite block. **C** Diagram of the relative positions of image receptor, tooth and X-ray beam.

Maxillary molars

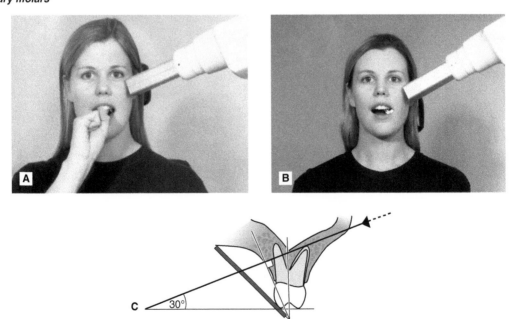

Fig. 7.26 Patient positioning with the patient **A** supporting the image receptor and **B** using the Rinn Greene Stabe® bite block. **C** Diagram of the relative positions of image receptor, tooth and X-ray beam.

Mandibular incisors

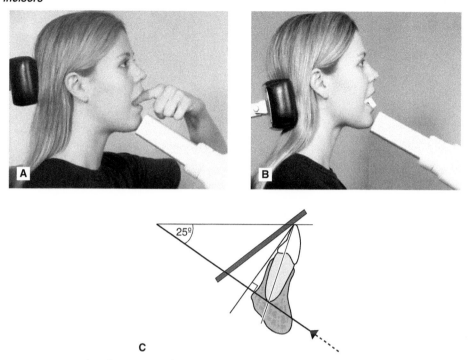

Fig. 7.27 Patient positioning with **A** the patient's index finger on the upper edge of the image receptor, supporting and depressing it into the floor of the mouth and **B** using the Rinn Greene Stabe® bite block. **C** Diagram of the relative positions of image receptor, tooth and X-ray beam.

Mandibular canine

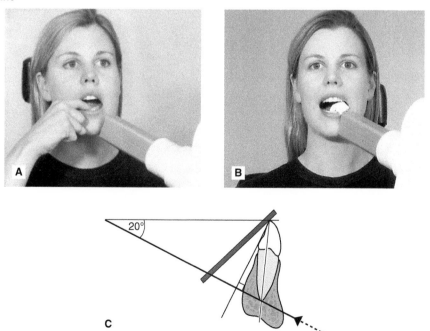

Fig. 7.28 Patient positioning with the patient **A** supporting and depressing the upper edge of the image receptor and **B** using the Rinn Greene Stabe® bite block. **C** Diagram of the relative positions of image receptor, tooth and X-ray beam.

Mandibular premolars

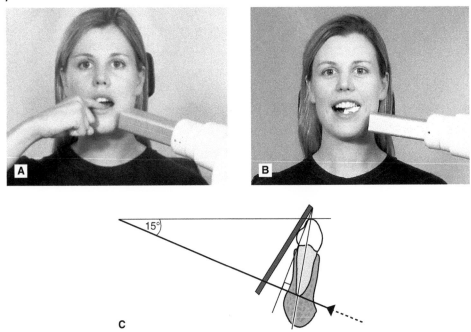

Fig. 7.29 Patient positioning with the patient **A** supporting the image receptor and **B** using the Rinn Greene Stabe® bite block. **C** Diagram of the relative positions of image receptor, tooth and X-ray beam.

Mandibular molars

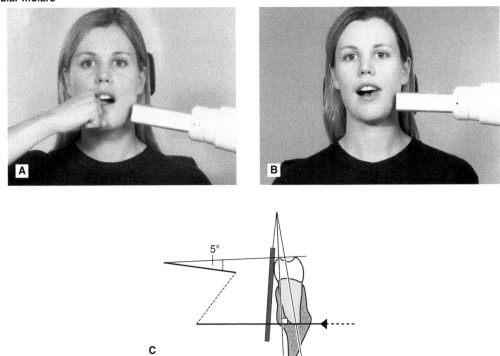

Fig. 7.30 Patient positioning with the patient **A** supporting the image receptor and **B** using the Rinn Greene Stabe® bite block. **C** Diagram of the relative positions of image receptor, tooth and X-ray beam.

Comparison of the paralleling and bisected angle techniques

The advantages and disadvantages of the two techniques can be summarized as follows.

Advantages of the paralleling technique

- Geometrically accurate images are produced with little magnification.
- The shadow of the zygomatic buttress appears **above** the apices of the molar teeth.
- The periodontal bone levels are well represented.
- The periapical tissues are accurately shown with minimal foreshortening or elongation.
- The crowns of the teeth are well shown enabling the detection of approximal caries.
- The horizontal and vertical angulations of the X-ray tubehead are automatically determined by the positioning devices if placed correctly.
- The X-ray beam is aimed accurately at the centre of the image receptor – all areas of the image receptor are irradiated and there is no *coning off or cone cutting*.
- Reproducible radiographs are possible at different visits and with different operators.
- The relative positions of the image receptor, teeth and X-ray beam are always maintained, irrespective of the position of the patient's head. This is useful for some patients with disabilities.

Disadvantages of the paralleling technique

- Positioning of the image receptor can be very uncomfortable for the patient, particularly for posterior teeth, often causing gagging.
- Positioning the holders within the mouth can be difficult for inexperienced operators.
- The anatomy of the mouth sometimes makes the technique impossible, e.g. a shallow, flat palate.
- The apices of the teeth can sometimes appear very near the edge of the image receptor.
- Positioning the holders in the lower third molar regions can be very difficult.

- The technique cannot be performed satisfactorily using a short focal spot to skin distance (i.e. a short spacer cone) because of the resultant magnification.
- The holders need to be autoclavable or disposable.

Advantages of the bisected angle technique

- Positioning of the image receptor is reasonably comfortable for the patient in all areas of the mouth.
- Positioning is relatively simple and quick.
- If all angulations are assessed correctly, the image of the tooth will be the same length as the tooth itself and should be *adequate* (but not ideal) for most diagnostic purposes.

Disadvantages of the bisected angle technique

- The many variables involved in the technique often result in the image being badly distorted.
- Incorrect vertical angulation will result in foreshortening or elongation of the image.
- The periodontal bone levels are poorly shown.
- The shadow of the zygomatic buttress frequently overlies the roots of the upper molars.
- The horizontal and vertical angles have to be assessed for every patient and considerable skill is required.
- It is not possible to obtain reproducible views.
- *Coning off or cone cutting* may result if the central ray is not aimed at the centre of the image receptor, particularly if using rectangular collimation.
- Incorrect horizontal angulation will result in overlapping of the crowns and roots.
- The crowns of the teeth are often distorted, thus preventing the detection of approximal caries.
- The buccal roots of the maxillary premolars and molars are foreshortened.

A visual comparison between the two techniques, showing how dramatic the variation in image quality and reproducibility can be, is shown in Figs 7.31 and 7.32.

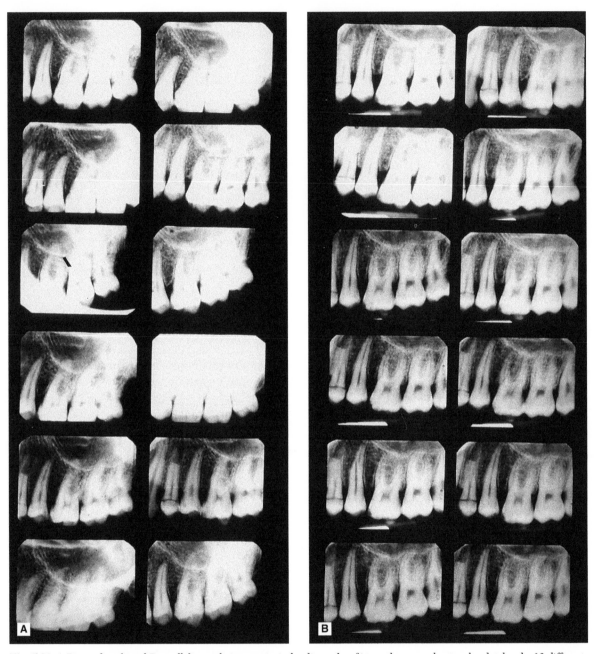

Fig. 7.31 A Bisected angle and **B** paralleling technique periapical radiographs of |6 on the *same* phantom head, taken by 12 *different* experienced operators. The obvious reproducibility and accurate imaging show why the paralleling technique should be regarded as the technique of choice.

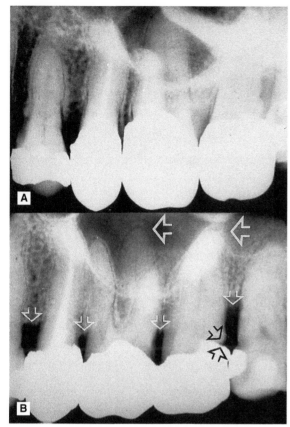

Fig. 7.32 A Bisected angle and **B** paralleling technique periapicals of the ⌊45678 taken on the *same* patient, by the *same* operator, on the *same* day. Note the difference in the periodontal bone levels (small white open arrows), the restoration in ⌊7 (black open arrows) and the apical tissues ⌊67 (large white open arrows).

Conclusion

The diagnostic advantages of the accurate, reproducible images produced by the paralleling technique using film holders and beam-aiming devices ensure that this technique should be regarded as the technique of choice for periapical radiography. It is good practice that, whenever practicable, techniques using image receptor holders with beam-aiming devices should be adopted.

Positioning difficulties often encountered in periapical radiography

Placing the image receptor intraorally, in the *textbook-described* positions, is not always possible clinically. The radiographic techniques described

earlier often need to be modified. The main difficulties encountered involve:

- Mandibular third molars
- Gagging
- Endodontics
- Edentulous alveolar ridges
- Children
- Patients with disabilities (see Ch. 6).

Problems posed by mandibular third molars

The main difficulty is placement of the image receptor sufficiently posteriorly to record the entire third mandibular molar (particularly when it is horizontally impacted) **and** the surrounding tissues, including the inferior dental canal (see Fig. 7.33).

Possible solutions

These include:

- Using specially designed or adapted holders as shown in Fig. 7.34 to hold and position the image receptor in the mouth, as follows:

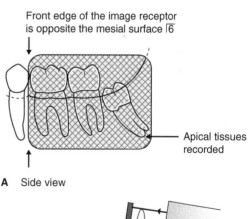

Front edge of the image receptor is opposite the mesial surface ⌊6

Apical tissues recorded

A Side view

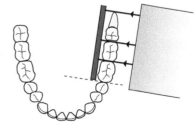

B Plan view

Fig. 7.33 Diagrams showing the ideal image receptor position for mandibular third molars to ensure the tooth and apical tissues are recorded.

1. The holder is clipped securely on to the top edge of the image receptor.
2. With the mouth open, the image receptor is positioned gently in the lingual sulcus as far posteriorly as possible.
3. The patient is asked to close the mouth (so relaxing the tissues of the floor of the mouth) and at the same time the image receptor is eased further back into the mouth, if required, until its front edge is opposite the mesial surface of the mandibular first molar.
4. The patient is asked to bite on the holder and to support it in position.
5. The X-ray tubehead is positioned at right angles to the third molar and the image receptor and centred 1 cm up from the lower border of the mandible, on a vertical line dropped from the outer corner of the eye (see Fig. 7.34).

- Taking two radiographs of the third molar using two different horizontal tubehead angulations, as follows:
  1. The image receptor is positioned as posteriorly as possible (using the technique described with the holders).
  2. The X-ray tubehead is aimed with the *ideal* horizontal angulation so the X-ray beam passes between the second and third molars. (With horizontally impacted third molars, the apex may not be recorded using this positioning, as shown in Fig. 7.35.)

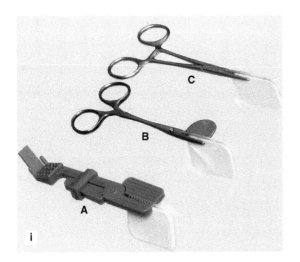

i

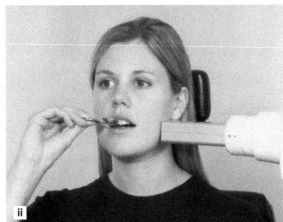

ii

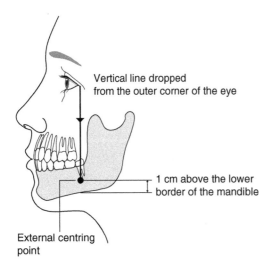

Vertical line dropped from the outer corner of the eye

1 cm above the lower border of the mandible

External centring point

(iii)

Fig. 7.34 (i) A selection of film packet/phosphor plate holders for mandibular third molars: **A** Emmenix® film holder; **B** Worth film holder; **C** a conventional pair of artery forceps. (ii) Patient positioning – having closed the mouth, the patient is stabilizing the image receptor holder with a hand. (iii) Diagram indicating the external centring point for the X-ray beam.

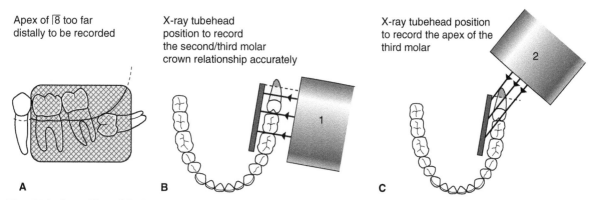

Fig. 7.35 The problem of the horizontal third molar. **A** Side view showing the often achievable image receptor position. **B** Plan view showing X-ray tubehead position 1. **C** Plan view showing X-ray tubehead position 2.

3. A *second* image receptor is placed in the same position as before, but the X-ray tubehead is positioned further posteriorly aiming forwards to project the apex of the third molar on to the film. (With this positioning, the crowns of the second and third molars will be overlapped, as shown in Fig. 7.35.)

Note: The vertical angulation of the X-ray tubehead is the same for both projections.

Problems of gagging

The gag reflex is particularly strong in some patients. This makes the placement of the image receptor in the desired position particularly difficult, especially in the upper and lower molar regions.

Possible solutions

These include:

- Patient sucking a local anaesthetic lozenge before attempting to position the image receptor.
- Asking the patient to concentrate on breathing deeply while the image receptor is in the mouth.

- Placing the image receptor flat in the mouth (in the occlusal plane) so it does not touch the palate, and applying the principles of the bisected angle technique – the long axes of the tooth and image receptor are assessed and the X-ray tubehead's position modified accordingly, as shown in Fig. 7.36.

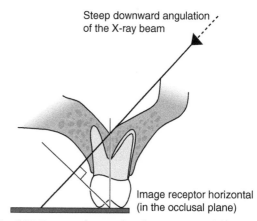

Fig. 7.36 Diagram showing the relative position of the X-ray beam to the maxillary molar and the image receptor when it is placed in the occlusal plane. **Note**: The length of the image of the tooth on the radiograph should again equal the length of the tooth in the mouth. However, there will be considerable distortion of the surrounding tissues.

Problems encountered during endodontics

The main difficulties involve:

- Image receptor placement and stabilization when endodontic instruments, rubber dam and rubber dam clamps are in position
- Identification and separation of root canals
- Assessing root canal lengths from foreshortened or elongated radiographs.

Possible solutions

These include:

- The problem of image receptor placement and stabilization can be solved by:
  - Using a simple image receptor holder such as the Rinn Eezee-Grip®, as shown in Fig. 7.37. This is positioned in the mouth and then held in place by the patient.
  - Using one of the special endodontic image receptor holders that have been developed. These incorporate a modified bite platform area, to accommodate the handles of the endodontic instruments, while still allowing the image receptor and the tooth to be parallel (see Fig. 7.38).

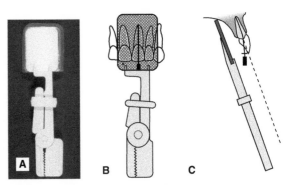

Fig. 7.37 A The Rinn Eezee – Grip® film/phosphor plate holder. **B** and **C** Diagrams showing its use in endodontics. (**Note:** Rubber dam not shown.)

- The problem of identifying and separating the root canals can be solved by taking at least two radiographs, using different horizontal X-ray tubehead positions, as shown in Fig. 7.39.
- The problems of assessing root canal length can be solved by:
  - Taking an accurate paralleling technique periapical preoperatively and measuring the lengths of the root(s) directly from the radiograph before beginning the endodontic treatment. The amount of distortion on subsequent images can then be assessed.

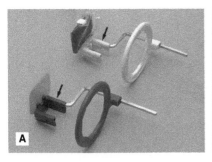
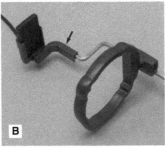
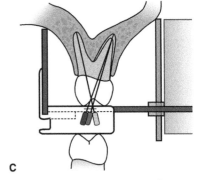

Fig. 7.38 Specially designed image receptor holders and beam-aiming devices for use during endodontics. **A** Rinn Endoray® suitable for film packets and digital phosphor plates (green) and solid-state digital sensors (white). **B** Anterior Planmeca solid-state digital sensor holder. Note the modified designs of the biteblocks (arrowed) to accommodate the handles of the endodontic instruments. Colour coding of holders by some manufacturers is now used to facilitate clinical use. **C** Diagram of the Rinn Endoray® in place. (*See colour plates section*)

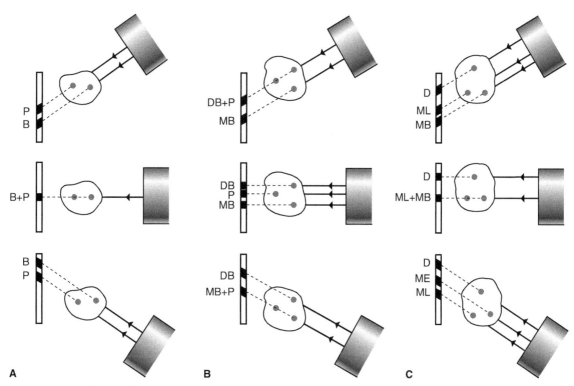

A   **B**   **C**

Fig. 7.39 Diagrams showing the effect of different horizontal X-ray tubehead positions on root separation for **A** maxillary premolars, **B** maxillary first molars and **C** mandibular first molars. (The images of the canals are designated: P = palatal, B = buccal, MB = mesiobuccal, DB = distobuccal, ML = mesiolingual and D = distal.)

– Calculating mathematically the actual length of a root canal from a distorted bisected angle technique periapical taken with the diagnostic instrument within the root canal at the clinically assessed apical *stop*.

The calculation is done as follows (see Fig. 7.40):

1. Measure:
   a. The *radiographic tooth length*
   b. The *radiographic instrument length*
   c. The *actual instrument length*
2. Substitute the measurements into the formula:

$$\text{Actual tooth length} = \frac{\text{Radiographic tooth length} \times \text{Actual instrument length}}{\text{Radiographic instrument length}}$$

3. Calculate the *actual tooth length* and adjust the working length of the instrument as necessary.

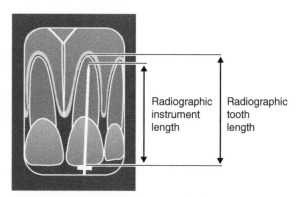

Fig. 7.40 Diagram showing the required radiographic measurements in endodontics to calculate the actual tooth length.

Problems of the edentulous ridge

The main difficulty in the edentulous and partially dentate patient is again image receptor placement.

Possible solutions

These include:

- In edentulous patients, the lack of height in the palate, or loss of lingual sulcus depth, contraindicates the paralleling technique and all periapical radiographs should be taken using a modified bisected angle technique. The long axes of the image receptor and the alveolar ridge are assessed and the X-ray tubehead position adjusted accordingly, as shown in Fig. 7.41.
- In partially dentate patients, the paralleling technique can usually be used. If the edentulous area causes the image receptor holder to be displaced, the deficiency can be built up by using cottonwool rolls, as shown in Fig. 7.42.

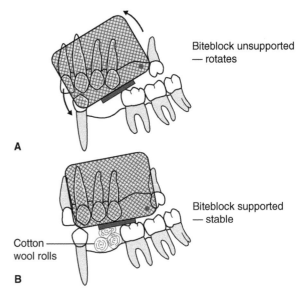

Fig. 7.42 Diagrams showing **A** the effect on the position of the image receptor and holder created by an edentulous area, and **B** how the problem can be solved using cottonwool rolls to rebuild the edentulous area, thus supporting the bite block.

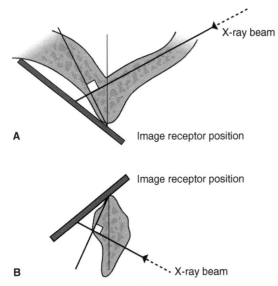

Fig. 7.41 Diagrams showing the relative position of the image receptor and X-ray beam. **A** For the molar region of an edentulous maxillary ridge. **B** For the molar region of an edentulous mandibular ridge.

Problems encountered in children

Once again the main technical problem (as opposed to management problems) encountered in children is the size of their mouths and the difficulty in placing the image receptor intraorally. The paralleling technique is not possible in very small children, but can often be used (and is recommended) anteriorly, for investigating traumatized permanent incisors. The reproducibility afforded by this technique is invaluable for future comparative purposes.

A modified bisected angle technique is possible in most children, with the image receptor placed flat in the mouth (in the occlusal plane) and the position of the X-ray tubehead adjusted accordingly, as shown in Fig. 7.43.

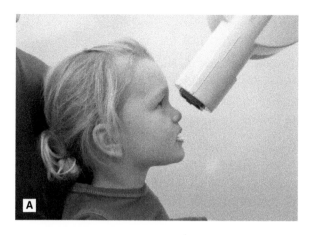

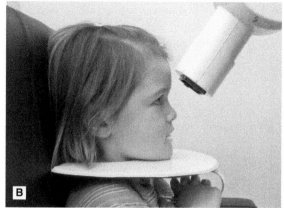

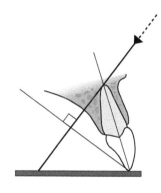

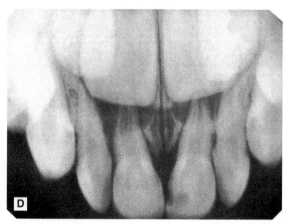

Fig. 7.43 Positioning for a child's maxillary incisors, **A** in 3-year-old and **B** in a 6-year-old, showing the use of a thyroid shield. **C** Diagram showing the relative positions of the image receptor, in the occlusal plane, and the X-ray beam. **D** An example of the resultant radiograph.

Assessment of image quality

Assessment of the quality of **all** radiographic images should be regarded as a routine part of any quality assurance (QA) programme (see Ch. 14). Essentially image quality assessment involves three separate stages, namely:

- Comparison of the image against ideal quality criteria
- Subjective rating of image quality using published standards
- Detailed assessment of rejected films to determine the sources of error.

Ideal quality criteria

Irrespective of the type of image receptor or technique being used, typical quality criteria for a periapical radiograph include:

- The image should have acceptable definition with no distortion or blurring.
- The image should include the correct anatomical area together with the apices of the tooth/ teeth under investigation with at least 3–4 mm of surrounding bone.
- There should be no overlap of the approximal surfaces of the teeth.

- The desired density and contrast for film-captured images will depend on the clinical reasons for taking the radiograph, e.g.
  - to assess *caries, restorations and the periapical tissues* films should be well exposed and show good contrast to allow differentiation between enamel and dentine and between the periodontal ligament space, the lamina dura and trabecular bone.
  - to assess the *periodontal status* films should be underexposed to avoid burnout of the thin alveolar crestal bone (see Ch. 19).
- The images should be free of *coning off or cone cutting* and other film handling errors.
- The images should be comparable with previous periapical images both geometrically and in density and contrast.

Subjective rating of image quality

A simple three-point subjective rating scale for all intraoral and extraoral film-captured radiographs was published in the UK in 2001 in the *Guidance Notes for Dental Practitioners on the Safe Use of X-ray Equipment*. A summary is shown in Table 7.1, and is repeated in Chapters 8 and 12. Image quality is discussed in detail, together with the errors associated with exposure factors and chemical processing, in Chapter 14. Patient preparation and positioning errors in periapical radiography are described below.

Assessment of rejected films and determination of errors

Patient preparation and positioning (radiographic technique) errors (Fig. 7.44)

These can include:

- Failure to remove dentures or orthodontic appliances
- Failure to position the image receptor correctly to capture the area of interest, thereby failing to image the apices and periapical tissues
- Failure to position the image receptor correctly causing it to bend (if flexible) creating geometrical distortion
- Failure to orientate the image receptor correctly and using it back-to-front
- Failure to align the X-ray tubehead correctly in the horizontal plane, either
  - Too far anteriorly or posteriorly (*coning off or cone cutting*)
  - Not aimed through the contact areas at right angles to the teeth and the image receptor causing overlapping of the contact areas
- Failure to align the X-ray tubehead correctly in the vertical plane, either
  - Too far superiorly or inferiorly (*coning off or cone cutting*)
  - Too steep an angle causing foreshortening and geometrical distortion
  - Too shallow an angle causing elongation and geometrical distortion
- Failure to instruct the patient to remain still during the exposure with subsequent movement resulting in blurring
- Failure to set correct exposure settings (see Ch. 14)
- Careless inadvertent use of the image receptor twice.

Note: Many of these technique errors can be avoided by using the paralleling technique.

Table 7.1 Subjective quality rating criteria for film-captured images published in the 2001 *Guidance Notes for Dental Practitioners on the Safe Use of X-ray Equipment*

Rating	Quality	Basis
1	Excellent	No errors of patient preparation, exposure, positioning, processing or film handling
2	Diagnostically acceptable	Some errors of patient preparation, exposure, positioning, processing or film handling, but which do not detract from the diagnostic utility of the radiograph
3	Unacceptable	Errors of patient preparation, exposure, positioning, processing or film handling, which render the radiograph diagnostically unacceptable

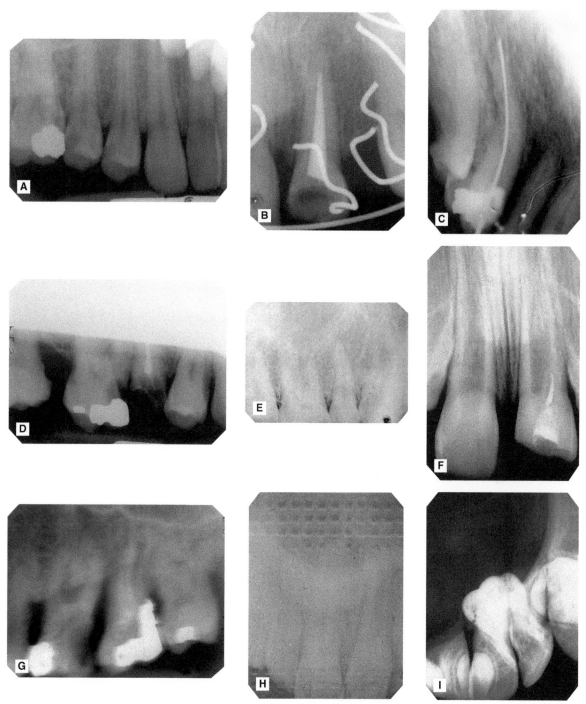

Fig. 7.44 A selection of patient preparation and positioning (radiographic technique) errors. **A** Image receptor not positioned sufficiently apically to cover the area of interest – apices and periapical tissues not shown. **B** Failure to remove an orthodontic appliance. **C** Image receptor positioned incorrectly and bent during exposure – image geometrically distorted. **D** Failure to align the X-ray tubehead correctly in the vertical plane – coning off of the superior part of the image. **E** X-ray tubehead positioned at too steep an angle in the vertical plane – foreshortening and geometrical distortion of the image. **F** X-ray tubehead positioned at too shallow an angle in the vertical plane – elongation and geometrical distortion of the image. **G** Failure to instruct the patient to remain still – image blurred as a result of movement. **H** Image receptor (film packet) incorrectly placed back to front – pattern of the lead foil is evident. **I** Image receptor (film packet) inadvertently used twice – double exposure.

To access the self assessment questions for this chapter please go to www.whaitesessentialsdentalradiography.com

8 Bitewing radiography

Bitewing radiographs take their name from the original technique which required the patient to *bite* on a small *wing* attached to an intraoral film packet (see Fig. 8.1). Modern film holders, as shown later, have eliminated the need for the wing (now termed a *tab*), and digital image receptors (solid-state or phosphor plate) can be used instead of film, but the terminology and clinical indications have remained the same. An individual image is designed to show the crowns of the premolar and molar teeth on one side of the jaws.

Main indications

The main clinical indications include:

- Detection of dental caries
- Monitoring the progression of dental caries
- Assessment of existing restorations
- Assessment of the periodontal status.

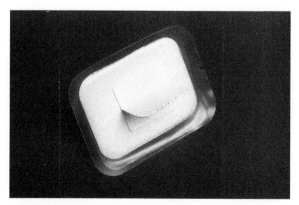

Fig. 8.1 An intraoral barrier-wrapped film packet with a *wing* or *tab* attached.

Ideal technique requirements

These include:

- An appropriate image receptor holder with beam-aiming device should be used and is recommended in the UK in the 2001 *Guidance Notes for Dental Practitioners on the Safe Use of X-ray Equipment.*
- The image receptor should be positioned centrally within the holder with the upper and lower edges of the image receptor parallel to the bite platform.
- The image receptor should be positioned with its long axis horizontally for a *horizontal bitewing* or vertically for a *vertical bitewing* (Fig. 8.2).
- The posterior teeth and the image receptor should be in contact or as close together as possible.
- The posterior teeth and the image receptor should be parallel – the shape of the dental arch may necessitate two separate image receptor positions to achieve this requirement for the premolars and the molars (Fig. 8.3).
- The beam-aiming device should ensure that in the horizontal plane the X-ray tubehead is aimed so that the beam meets the teeth and the image receptor at right angles, and passes directly through **all** the contact areas (Fig. 8.3).
- The beam-aiming device should ensure that in the vertical plane the X-ray tubehead is aimed downwards (approximately 5°–8° to the horizontal) to compensate for the upwardly rising curve of Monson (Fig. 8.4).
- The positioning should be reproducible.

It is sometimes not possible to use an image receptor holder (with beam-aiming device) and achieve these ideal technical requirements –

113

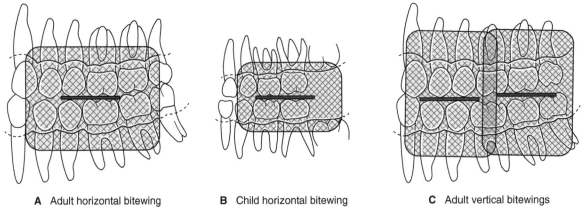

A Adult horizontal bitewing   **B** Child horizontal bitewing   **C** Adult vertical bitewings

Fig. 8.2 Diagrams showing the ideal image receptor position for different types of bitewings.

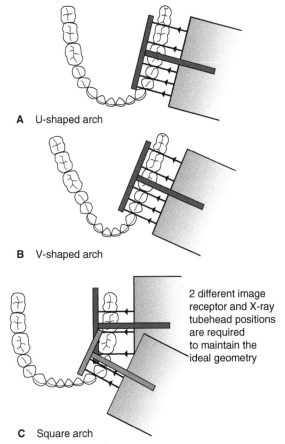

A U-shaped arch

B V-shaped arch

2 different image
receptor and X-ray
tubehead positions
are required
to maintain the
ideal geometry

C Square arch

Fig. 8.3 Diagrams showing the ideal image receptor and X-ray tubehead positions (determined by the beam-aiming device) for different arch shapes.

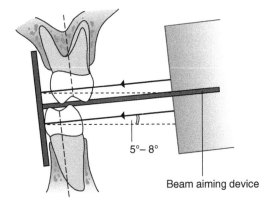

5°– 8°

Beam aiming device

Fig. 8.4 Diagram showing the ideal image receptor position and the approximate 5°–8° downward vertical angulation of the X-ray beam (determined by the beam-aiming device) compensating for the curve of Monson.

particularly in children. Dental care professionals therefore still need to be aware of the original technique of using a tab attached to the film packet or phosphor plate and aligning the X-ray tubehead by eye.

Positioning techniques

Using image receptor holders with beam-aiming devices

Several image receptor holders with different beam-aiming devices have been produced for use with film packets or digital phosphor plates and

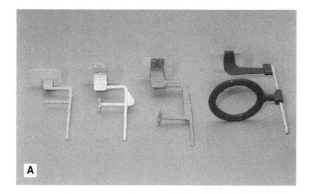

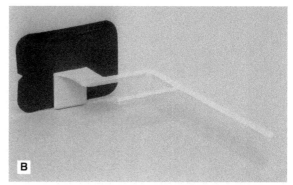

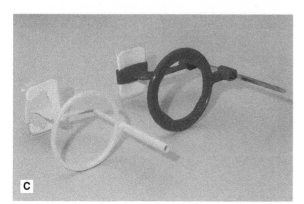

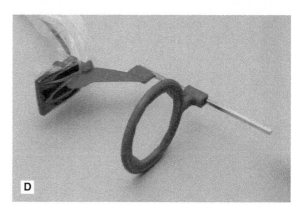

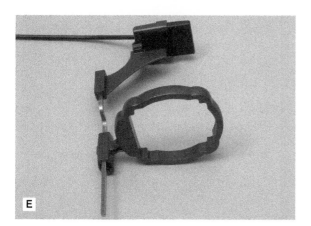

Fig. 8.5 Bitewing image receptor holders with beam-aiming devices. **A** A selection of horizontal bitewing holders set-up using a film packet as the image receptor – note the red colour coding for the Rinn XCP System. **B** The Hawe–Neos Kwikbite horizontal holder set-up using a digital phosphor plate. **C** Vertical bitewing holders – the red Rinn XCP holder and the yellow Hawe–Neos Parobite holder set-up using film packets. **D** The red Rinn XCP-DS horizontal bitewing solid-state digital sensor holder. **E** The Planmeca horizontal bitewing holder designed specifically for use with their dixi2 solid-state digital sensors. (*See colour plates section*)

with digital solid-state sensors, held either horizontally or vertically. A selection of different holders is shown in Fig. 8.5. As in periapical radiography, the choice of holder is a matter of personal preference and dependent upon the type of image receptors being employed. The various holders vary in cost and design but essentially consist of the same three basic components that make up periapical holders (see Ch. 7), namely:

- A mechanism for holding the image receptor parallel to the teeth
- A bite platform that replaces the original wing
- An X-ray beam-aiming device.

The radiographic technique can be summarized as follows:

1. The desired holder is selected together with an appropriate-sized image receptor – typically a

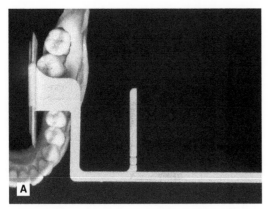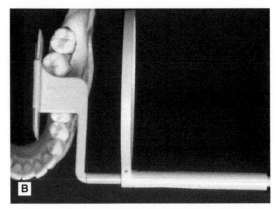

Fig. 8.6 A Position of the simple Hawe–Neos Kwikbite holder in relation to the teeth. **B** Position of the Hawe–Neos Kwikbite holder (with circular beam-aiming device) in relation to the teeth.

31 × 41 mm film packet or phosphor plate or the equivalent sized solid-state sensor.

2. The patient is positioned with the head supported and with the occlusal plane horizontal.

3. The holder is inserted carefully into the lingual sulcus opposite the posterior teeth.

4. The anterior edge of the image receptor should be positioned opposite the distal aspect of the lower canine – in this position the image receptor extends usually just beyond the mesial aspect of the lower third molar (see Fig. 8.6).

5. The patient is asked to close the teeth firmly together onto the bite platform. (Note: Extra care needs to be taken of solid-state sensor cables.)

6. The X-ray tubehead is aligned accurately using the beam-aiming device to achieve optimal horizontal and vertical angulations (see Fig. 8.7).

7. The exposure is made.

8. If required, the procedure is repeated for the premolar teeth with a new image receptor and X-ray tubehead position.

Advantages

- Relatively simple and straightforward.
- Image receptor is held firmly in position and cannot be displaced by the tongue.
- Position of X-ray tubehead is determined by the beam-aiming device so assisting the operator in ensuring that the X-ray beam is always at right angles to the image receptor.
- Avoids *coning off* or *cone cutting* of the anterior part of the image receptor.
- Holders are autoclavable or disposable.

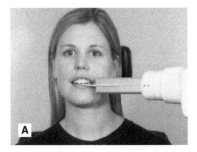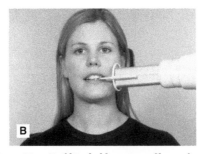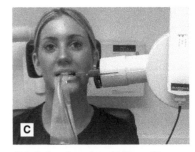

Fig. 8.7 Clinical positioning for **A** simple Hawe–Neos Kwikbite holder using a film packet or digital phosphor plate, **B** Hawe–Neos holder (with circular beam-aiming device) using a film packet or digital phosphor plate and **C** Planmeca holder using a solid-state digital sensor.

Disadvantages

- Position of the holder in the mouth is operator-dependent, therefore images are not 100% reproducible, so not absolutely ideal for monitoring progression of caries.
- Positioning of the film holder and image receptor can be uncomfortable for the patient, particularly when using solid-state digital sensors.
- Some holders are relatively expensive.
- Holders not usually suitable for children.

Using a tab attached to the image receptor

The traditional bitewing technique is particularly suitable when using film packets or digital phosphor plates as the image receptor. Although, as explained below, the technique is very operator-dependent and not recommended for adults, it is still widely used for children.

The radiographic technique can be summarized as follows:

1. The appropriate sized barrier-wrapped film packet or phosphor plate is selected and the tab attached, orientated appropriately for *horizontal* or *vertical* projections, as shown in Fig. 8.8A:
   - Large film packets/phosphor plates (31 × 41 mm) for adults
   - Small film packets/phosphor plates (22 × 35 mm) for children under 12 years. Once the second permanent molars have erupted the adult size is required
   - Occasionally a long film packet/phosphor plate (53 × 26 mm) is used for adults.
2. The patient is positioned with the head supported and with the occlusal plane horizontal.
3. The shape of the dental arch and the number of films required are assessed.
4. The operator holds the tab between thumb and forefinger and inserts the image receptor into the lingual sulcus opposite the posterior teeth.
5. The anterior edge of the image receptor should again be positioned opposite the distal

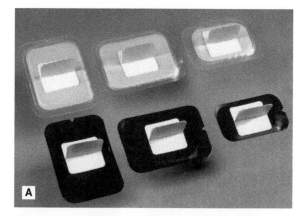

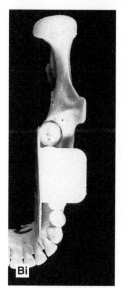

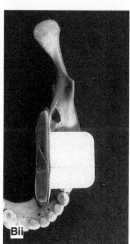

Fig. 8.8 A Film packets and phosphor plates with tabs attached suitable for adult *vertical* bitewings, adult *horizontal* bitewings and child's *horizontal* bitewings. **B** The ideal bitewing and film packet position in relation to the teeth for (**i**) an adult and (**ii**) a child.

aspect of the lower canine – in this position, the posterior edge of the film packet extends usually just beyond the mesial aspect of the lower third molar (see Fig. 8.8B).

6. The tab is placed on to the occlusal surfaces of the lower teeth.
7. The patient is asked to close the teeth firmly together on the tab.
8. As the patient closes the teeth, the operator pulls the tab firmly between the teeth to ensure that the image receptor and teeth are in contact.

9. The operator releases the tab.
10. The operator assesses the horizontal and vertical angulations and positions the X-ray tubehead so that the X-ray beam is aimed directly through the contact areas, at right angles to the teeth and the image receptor, with an approximately 5°–8° downward vertical angulation (see Fig. 8.9A and B).
11. The exposure is made.
12. If required, the procedure is repeated for the premolar teeth with a new image receptor and X-ray tubehead position.

Note: When positioning the X-ray tubehead, after the patient has closed the mouth, the film can no longer be seen. To ensure that the anterior part of the image receptor is exposed and to avoid *coning off* and *cone cutting*, a simple guide to remember is that the front edge of the open-ended spacer cone should be positioned adjacent to the corner of the mouth.

Advantages

- Simple.
- Inexpensive.
- The tabs are disposable, so no extra cross-infection control procedures required.
- Can be used easily in children.

Disadvantages

- Arbitrary, operator-dependent assessment of horizontal and vertical angulations of the X-ray tubehead.
- Images not accurately reproducible, so not ideal for monitoring the progression of caries.
- *Coning off or cone cutting* of anterior part of image receptor is common.
- Not compatible with using solid-state digital sensors.
- The tongue can easily displace the image receptor.

Resultant radiographs

Whichever radiographic technique is used, the resultant radiographic images and the anatomical structures they show are very similar – it is their accuracy that varies. Examples are shown in Figs 8.10–8.12.

Assessment of image quality

As described in Chapter 7, image quality assessment essentially involves three separate stages, namely:

- Comparison of the image against ideal quality criteria
- Subjective rating of image quality using published standards
- Detailed assessment of rejected films to determine the source of error.

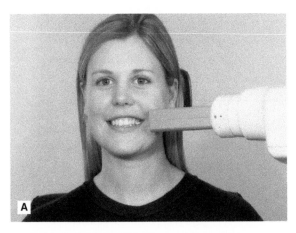
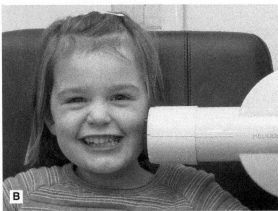

Fig. 8.9 A Adult patient and X-ray tubehead positioning for a left bitewing. **B** Positioning for a child.

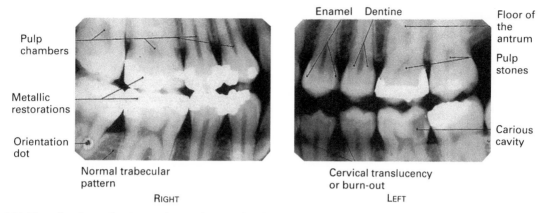

Pulp chambers

Metallic restorations

Orientation dot

Normal trabecular pattern

Enamel   Dentine

Floor of the antrum

Pulp stones

Carious cavity

Cervical translucency or burn-out

RIGHT   LEFT

Fig. 8.10 Examples of typical RIGHT and LEFT horizontal adult bitewing radiographs, suitable for the assessment of caries and restorations, with the main radiographic features indicated.

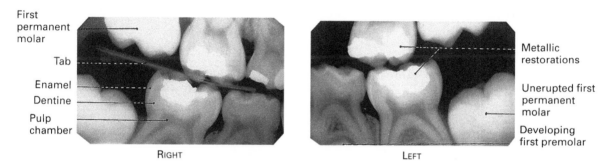

First permanent molar

Tab

Enamel

Dentine

Pulp chamber

Metallic restorations

Unerupted first permanent molar

Developing first premolar

RIGHT   LEFT

Fig. 8.11 Examples of typical RIGHT and LEFT bitewing radiographs of a child, with the main radiographic features indicated.

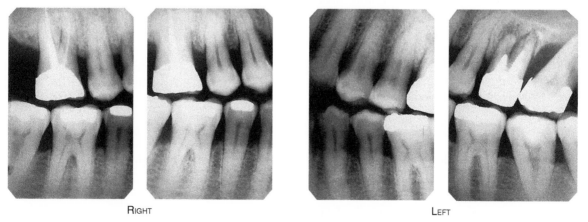

RIGHT   LEFT

Fig. 8.12 Example of typical RIGHT and LEFT vertical adult bitewing radiographs. Note that two films are used on each side to image both the premolars and molars.

Ideal quality criteria

Irrespective of the type of image receptor being used, typical quality criteria for a bitewing radiograph include:

- The image should have acceptable definition with no distortion or blurring.
- The image should include from the mesial surface of the first premolar to the distal surface of the second molar – if the third molars are erupted then the 7/8 contact should be included.
- The occlusal plane/bite platform should be in the middle of the image so that the crowns and coronal parts of the roots of the maxillary teeth are shown in the upper half of the image and the crowns and coronal parts of the roots of the mandibular teeth are shown in the lower half of the image, and the buccal and lingual cusps should be superimposed.
- The maxillary and mandibular alveolar crests should be shown.
- There should be no overlap of the approximal surfaces of the teeth.
- The desired density and contrast for film-captured images will depend on the clinical reasons for taking the radiograph, e.g.
  - To assess *caries and restorations* films should be well exposed and show good contrast to allow differentiation between enamel and dentine and to allow the enamel–dentine junction (EDJ) to be seen
  - To assess the *periodontal status* films should be underexposed to avoid *burn-out* of the thin alveolar crestal bone (see Ch. 19).
- The image should be free of *coning off or cone cutting* and other film handling errors.
- The image should be comparable with previous bitewing images both geometrically and in density and contrast.

Subjective rating of image quality

The simple three-point subjective rating scale published in the 2001 *Guidance Notes* was introduced in Chapter 7 and is discussed in detail, together with the errors associated with exposure factors and chemical processing, in Chapter 14. A summary is shown again in Table 8.1. Patient

Table 8.1 Subjective quality rating criteria for film-captured images published in the 2001 *Guidance Notes for Dental Practitioners on the Safe Use of X-ray Equipment*

Rating	Quality	Basis
1	Excellent	No errors of patient preparation, exposure, positioning, processing or film handling
2	Diagnostically acceptable	Some errors of patient preparation, exposure, positioning, processing or film handling, but which do not detract from the diagnostic utility of the radiograph
3	Unacceptable	Errors of patient preparation, exposure, positioning, processing or film handling, which render the radiograph diagnostically unacceptable

preparation and positioning errors in bitewing radiography are described below.

Assessment of rejected films and determination of errors

Patient preparation and positioning (radiographic technique) errors (Fig. 8.13)

These can include:

- Positioning the image receptor too far posteriorly in the mouth thereby failing to image the premolar teeth
- Failure to insert the image receptor correctly into the lingual sulcus between the tongue and posterior teeth allowing the tongue to displace the image receptor
- Failure to align the X-ray tubehead correctly in the horizontal plane, either
  - Too far posteriorly (coning off or cone cutting)
  - Too far anteriorly – rarely (coning off or cone cutting)
  - Not aimed through the contact areas at right angles to the line of the arch and the image receptor causing overlapping of the contact areas
- Failure to align the X-ray tubehead correctly in the vertical plane thereby not superimposing the buccal and lingual cusps

- Failure to set correct exposure settings
- Failure to instruct the patient to remain still during the exposure with subsequent movement resulting in blurring.

Note: Many of these positioning errors can be avoided by using image receptor holders with beam-aiming devices but are relatively common when not using a holder and aligning and positioning the X-ray tubehead without a guide.

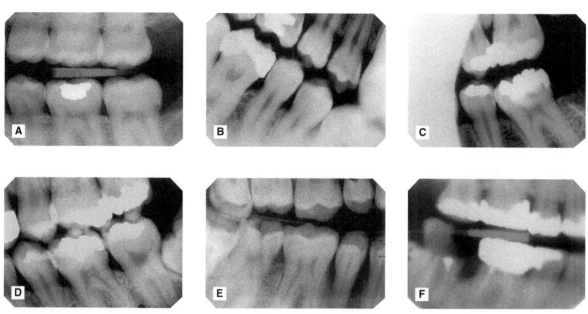

Fig. 8.13 A selection of bitewings showing patient preparation and positioning errors.
A Image receptor positioned too far posteriorly – the edentulous area distal to the lower second is imaged but not the premolar teeth.
B Image receptor displaced by tongue – occlusal plane not horizontal.
C Failure to align the X-ray tubehead correctly in the horizontal plane – *coning off* of the anterior part of the image.
D Failure to align the X-ray tubehead correctly in the horizontal plane – overlapping of the contact areas.
E Failure to align the X-ray tubehead correctly in the vertical plane – buccal and lingual cusps not superimposed and distortion of the teeth.
F Failure to instruct the patient to remain still – image blurred as a result of movement.

To access the self assessment questions for this chapter please go to www.whaitesessentialsdentalradiography.com

9 Occlusal radiography

Occlusal radiography is defined as those intraoral radiographic techniques taken using a dental X-ray set where the image receptor (film packet or digital phosphor plate – 5.7 × 7.6 cm) is placed in the occlusal plane. Suitable sized solid-state digital sensors are not currently available.

Terminology and classification

The terminology used in occlusal radiography is very confusing. The British Standards Glossary of Dental Terms (BS 4492: 1983) is inadequate in defining the various occlusal projections and in differentiating between them. The result is that there is still little uniformity in terminology among different publications and teaching institutions.

The terminology used here is based broadly on the British Standards terms, but they have been modified in an attempt to make them more explicit, straightforward and practical.

Maxillary occlusal projections

- *Upper standard (or anterior) occlusal* (standard occlusal)
- *Upper oblique occlusal* (oblique occlusal)
- *Vertex occlusal* (vertex occlusal) – no longer used.

Mandibular occlusal projections

- *Lower 90° occlusal* (true occlusal)
- *Lower 45° (or anterior) occlusal* (standard occlusal)
- *Lower oblique occlusal* (oblique occlusal).

Upper standard (or anterior) occlusal

This projection shows the anterior part of the maxilla and the upper anterior teeth.

Main clinical indications

The main clinical indications include:

- Periapical assessment of the upper anterior teeth, especially in children but also in adults unable to tolerate periapical holders
- Detecting the presence of unerupted canines, supernumeraries and odontomes
- As the midline view, when using the parallax method for determining the bucco/palatal position of unerupted canines
- Evaluation of the size and extent of lesions such as cysts or tumours in the anterior maxilla
- Assessment of fractures of the anterior teeth and alveolar bone.

Technique and positioning

The technique can be summarized as follows:

1. The patient is seated with the head supported and with the occlusal plane horizontal and parallel to the floor and is asked to support a protective thyroid shield.
2. The image receptor, suitably barrier wrapped, is placed flat into the mouth on to the occlusal surfaces of the lower teeth. The patient is asked to bite together gently. The image receptor is placed centrally in the mouth with its long axis crossways in adults and anteroposteriorly in children.
3. The X-ray tubehead is positioned above the patient in the midline, aiming downwards through the bridge of the nose at an angle of 65°–70° to the image receptor (see Fig. 9.1).

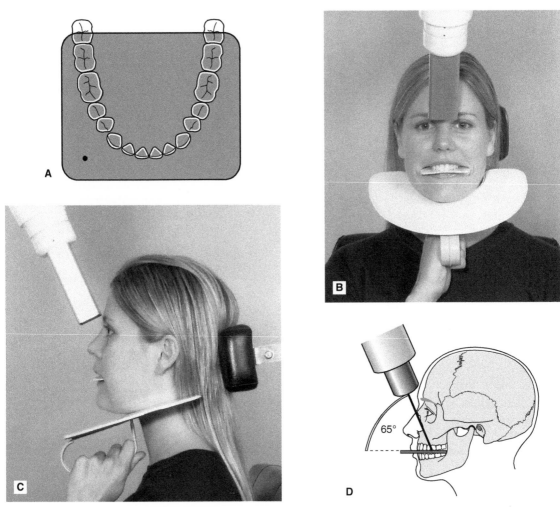

Fig. 9.1 A Diagram showing the position of the image receptor in relation to the lower arch. **B** Positioning from the front; note the use of the protective thyroid shield. **C** Positioning from the side. **D** Diagram showing the positioning from the side. The resultant radiograph is shown in Fig. 9.2.

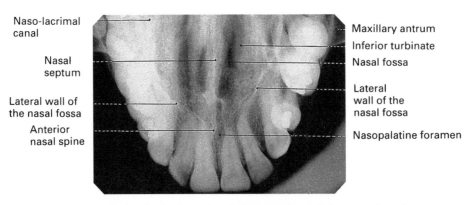

Fig. 9.2 An example of an upper standard occlusal radiograph with the main anatomical features indicated.

Upper oblique occlusal

This projection shows the posterior part of the maxilla and the upper posterior teeth on one side.

Main clinical indications

- Periapical assessment of the upper posterior teeth, especially in adults unable to tolerate periapical image receptors
- Evaluation of the size and extent of lesions such as cysts, tumours or osteodystrophies affecting the posterior maxilla
- Assessment of the condition of the antral floor
- As an aid to determining the position of roots displaced inadvertently into the antrum during attempted extraction of upper posterior teeth
- Assessment of fractures of the posterior teeth and associated alveolar bone including the tuberosity.

Technique and positioning

1. The patient is seated with the head supported and with the occlusal plane horizontal and parallel to the floor.
2. The image receptor, suitably barrier wrapped, is inserted into the mouth onto the occlusal surfaces of the lower teeth, with its long axis anteroposteriorly. It is placed to the side of the mouth under investigation, and the patient is asked to bite together gently.
3. The X-ray tubehead is positioned to the side of the patient's face, aiming downwards through the cheek at an angle of 65°–70° to the image receptor, centring on the region of interest (see Fig. 9.3).

Note: If the X-ray tubehead is positioned too far posteriorly, the shadow cast by the body of the zygoma will obscure the posterior teeth.

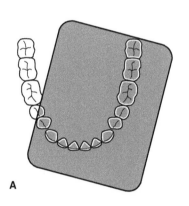
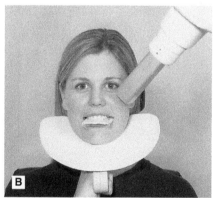
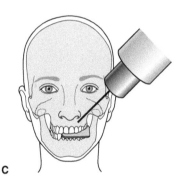

A

B

C

Fig. 9.3 A Diagram showing the position of the image receptor in relation to the lower arch for a LEFT upper oblique occlusal. **B** Positioning for the LEFT upper oblique occlusal from the front; note the use of the protective thyroid shield. **C** Diagram showing the positioning from the front. The resultant radiograph is shown in Fig. 9.4.

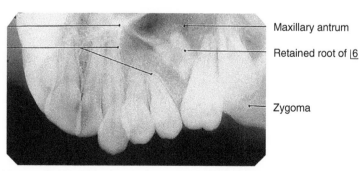

Floor of the nasal fossa

Anterior wall and floor of the antrum

Maxillary antrum

Retained root of |6

Zygoma

Fig. 9.4 An example of an upper left oblique occlusal radiograph with the main anatomical features indicated.

Lower 90° occlusal

This projection shows a plan view of the tooth-bearing portion of the mandible and the floor of the mouth. A minor variation of the technique is also used to show unilateral lesions.

Main clinical indications

- Detection of the presence and position of radiopaque calculi in the submandibular salivary ducts
- Assessment of the buccolingual position of unerupted mandibular teeth
- Evaluation of the buccolingual expansion of the body of the mandible by cysts/tumours
- Assessment of fracture displacement of the anterior mandible in the horizontal plane
- Assessment of mandibular width prior to implant placement.

Technique and positioning

1. The image receptor, suitably barrier wrapped and facing downwards, is placed centrally into the mouth, on to the occlusal surfaces of the lower teeth, with its long axis crossways. The patient is asked to bite together gently.
2. The patient *then* leans forwards and *then* tips the head backwards as far as is comfortable, where it is supported.
3. The X-ray tubehead, with circular collimator fitted, is placed below the patient's chin, in the midline, centring on an imaginary line joining the first molars, at an angle of 90° to the image receptor (see Fig. 9.5).

Variation of technique
To show a particular part of the mandible, the image receptor is placed in the mouth with its long axis anteroposteriorly over the area of interest. The X-ray tubehead, still aimed at 90° to the image receptor, is centred below the body of the mandible in that area.

Note: The lower 90° occlusal is mounted as if the examiner were looking into the patient's mouth. The radiographic film is therefore mounted with the embossed dot pointing *away* from the examiner.

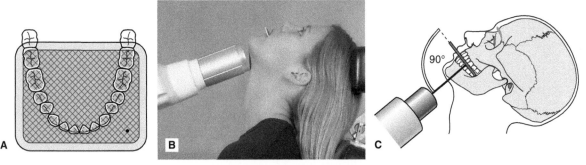

Fig. 9.5 A Diagram showing the position of the image receptor (facing downwards) in relation to the lower arch. **B** Positioning for the lower 90° occlusal from the side. **C** Diagram showing the positioning from the side. The resultant radiograph is shown in Fig. 9.6.

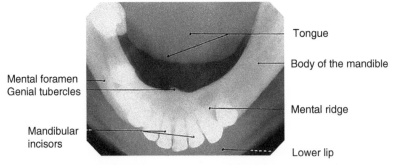

Fig. 9.6 An example of a lower 90° occlusal radiograph with the main anatomical features indicated.

Lower 45° (or anterior) occlusal

This projection is taken to show the lower anterior teeth and the anterior part of the mandible. The resultant radiograph resembles a large bisected angle technique periapical of this region.

Main clinical indications

- Periapical assessment of the lower incisor teeth, especially useful in adults and children unable to tolerate periapical image receptors
- Evaluation of the size and extent of lesions such as cysts or tumours affecting the anterior part of the mandible

- Assessment of fracture displacement of the anterior mandible in the vertical plane.

Technique and positioning

1. The patient is seated with the head supported and with the occlusal plane horizontal and parallel to the floor.
2. The image receptor, suitably barrier wrapped and facing downwards, is placed centrally into the mouth, on to the occlusal surfaces of the lower teeth, with its long axis anteroposteriorly, and the patient is asked to bite gently together.
3. The X-ray tubehead is positioned in the midline, centring through the chin point, at an angle of 45° to the image receptor (see Fig. 9.7).

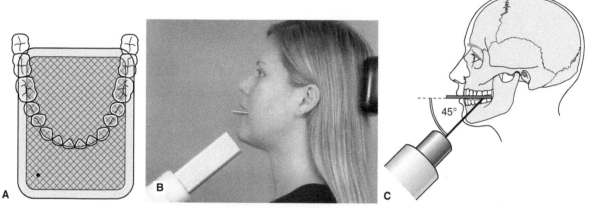

Fig. 9.7 A Diagram showing the position of the image receptor (facing downwards) in relation to the lower arch. **B** Positioning for the lower 45° occlusal from the side. **C** Diagram showing the positioning from the side. The resultant radiograph is shown in Fig. 9.8.

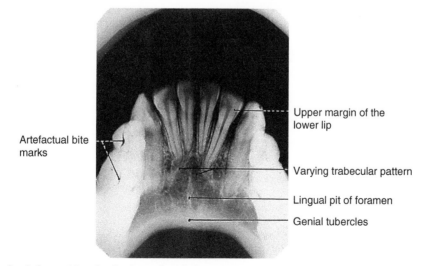

Fig. 9.8 An example of a lower 45° occlusal radiograph with the main anatomical features indicated.

Lower oblique occlusal

This projection is designed to allow the image of the submandibular salivary gland, on the side of interest, to be projected on to the film. However, because the X-ray beam is oblique, all the anatomical tissues shown are distorted.

Main indications

The main clinical indications include:

- Detection of radiopaque calculi in a submandibular salivary gland
- Assessment of the buccolingual position of unerupted lower wisdom teeth
- Evaluation of the extent and expansion of cysts, tumours or osteodystrophies in the posterior part of the body and angle of the mandible.

Technique and positioning

The technique can be summarized as follows:

1. The image receptor, suitably barrier wrapped and facing downwards, is inserted into the mouth, onto the occlusal surfaces of the lower teeth, over to the side under investigation, with its long axis anteroposteriorly. The patient is asked to bite together gently.
2. The patient's head is supported, then rotated away from the side under investigation and the chin is raised. This rotated positioning allows the subsequent positioning of the X-ray tubehead.
3. The X-ray tubehead with circular collimator is aimed upwards and forwards towards the image receptor, from below and behind the angle of the mandible and parallel to the lingual surface of the mandible (see Fig. 9.9).

Note: The lower oblique occlusal radiographic film is also mounted with the embossed dot pointing *away* from the examiner.

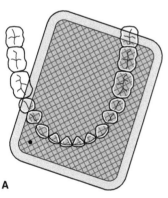

A

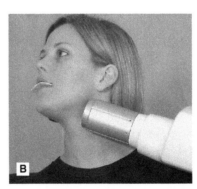

B

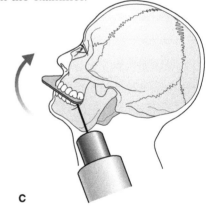

C

Fig. 9.9 A Diagram showing the position of the image receptor (facing downwards) in relation to the lower arch for the LEFT lower oblique occlusal. **B** Positioning for the LEFT lower oblique occlusal from the side. **C** Diagram showing the positioning from the side and indicating that the patient's chin is raised and that the head is rotated AWAY from the side under investigation. The resultant radiograph is shown in Fig. 9.10.

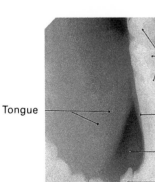

Buccal plate of the mandible

Mandibular molars

Tongue

Lingual plate of the mandible

Floor of the mouth

Mandibular incisors

Fig. 9.10 An example of a lower oblique occlusal radiograph with the main anatomical features indicated.

To access the self assessment questions for this chapter please go to www.whaitesessentialsdentalradiography.com

10 Oblique lateral radiography

Introduction

Oblique lateral radiographs are extraoral views of the jaws that can be taken using a dental X-ray set (see Fig. 10.1). Before the development of panoramic equipment they were the routine extraoral radiographs used both in hospitals and in general practice. In recent years, their popularity has waned, but the limitations of panoramic radiographs (see Ch. 12) have ensured that oblique lateral radiographs still have an important role.

Terminology

Lateral radiographs of the head and jaws are divided into:

- True laterals
- Oblique laterals
- Bimolars (two oblique laterals on one film).

The differentiating adjectives *true* and *oblique* are used to indicate the relationship of the film, patient and X-ray beam, as shown in Fig. 10.2.

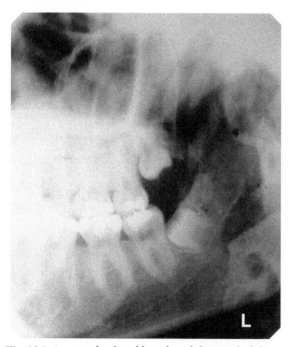

Fig. 10.1 An example of an oblique lateral showing the left molars.

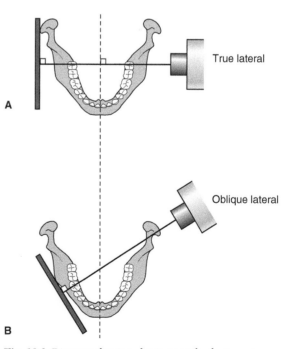

Fig. 10.2 Diagrams showing what is meant by the terms *true* and *oblique* lateral.

True lateral positioning

The image receptor and the sagittal plane of the patient's head are parallel and the X-ray beam is perpendicular to both of them. This is the positioning for the *true lateral skull radiograph* taken in a cephalostat unit described in Chapter 11.

Oblique lateral positioning

The image receptor and the sagittal plane of the patient's head are **not** parallel. The X-ray beam is aimed perpendicular to the image receptor but is *oblique* to the sagittal plane of the patient. As a result, a variety of different *oblique lateral* projections is possible with different head and X-ray beam positions.

Main indications

The main clinical indications for oblique lateral radiographs include:

- Assessment of the presence and/or position of unerupted teeth
- Detection of fractures of the mandible
- Evaluation of lesions or conditions affecting the jaws including cysts, tumours, giant cell lesions, and osteodystrophies
- As an alternative when intraoral views are unobtainable because of severe gagging or if the patient is unable to open the mouth or is unconscious (see Ch. 6, Fig. 6.1)

- As specific views of the salivary glands or temporomandibular joints.

Equipment required

This includes (see Fig. 10.3):

- A dental X-ray set
- An extraoral cassette containing film and intensifying screens or a digital phosphor plate (usually 13 × 18 cm)
- A lead shield to cover half the cassette when taking bimolar views.

Specially constructed angle boards, as shown in Fig. 10.3, can be used to facilitate positioning, but are not considered necessary by the authors.

Basic technique principles

As stated, a wide range of different oblique lateral projections of the jaws are possible. However, all the variations rely on the same basic principles regarding the position of:

- The cassette (image receptor)
- The patient's head
- The X-ray tubehead.

Cassette position

The cassette is held by the patient against the side of the face overlying the area of the jaws under investigation. The exact position of the cassette is determined by the area of interest.

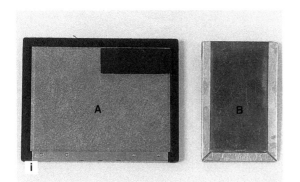
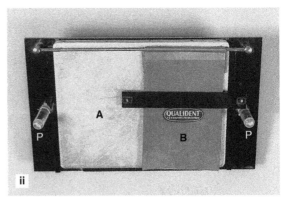

Fig. 10.3 Equipment used for oblique lateral radiography. (**i**) An 11 × 18 cm cassette **A** and lead shield **B**. (**ii**) An example of an angle board showing the cassette **A**, lead shield **B** and the plastic earpieces **P** for patient positioning.

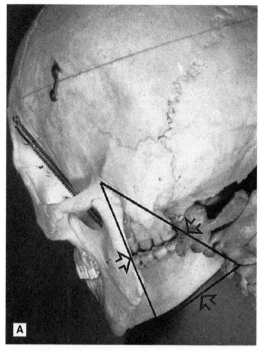 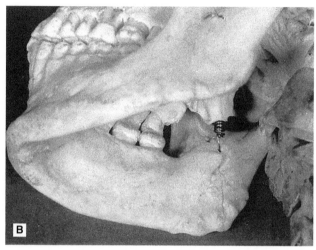

Fig. 10.4 A The view through the *radiographic keyhole* (arrowed) showing the right mandibular and maxillary posterior teeth. Note the anterior teeth are obscured by the left ramus of the mandible. **B** The view from underneath the left body of the mandible showing the right mandible and right posterior mandibular teeth. Note the right maxillary teeth are obscured by the left body of the mandible.

Patient's head position

The patient is normally seated upright in the dental chair and is then instructed to:

1. *Rotate the head to the side of interest.* This is done to bring the contralateral ramus forward, avoiding its superimposition and to increase the space available between the neck and shoulder in which to position the X-ray set.
2. *Raise the chin.* This is done to increase the triangular space between the back of the ramus and the cervical spine (the so-called *radiographic keyhole,* see Fig. 10.4) through which the X-ray beam will pass.

X-ray tubehead position

The X-ray tubehead is positioned on the opposite side of the patient's head to the cassette. There are two basic positions, depending on the area of the jaws under investigation:

- *Behind the ramus aiming through the radiographic keyhole.* The X-ray tubehead is positioned along the line of the occlusal plane, just below the ear, behind the ramus aiming through the *radiographic keyhole* at the particular maxillary **and** mandibular teeth under investigation. The view from this position is illustrated in Fig. 10.4A. As shown, the X-ray beam will not pass directly between the contact areas of the posterior teeth. This may result in some overlapping of the crowns.
- *Beneath the lower border of the mandible.* The X-ray tubehead is positioned beneath the lower border of the contralateral body of the mandible, directly opposite the particular mandibular teeth under investigation, aiming slightly upwards. The view from this position is illustrated in Fig. 10.4B. As shown, the X-ray beam will now pass between the contact areas of the teeth. However, there will still be some distortion of the image in the vertical plane owing to the upward angulation of the X-ray beam. In addition, the shadow of the body of the mandible will be superimposed over the maxillary teeth.

Once these principles are understood, the technique becomes straightforward and can be modified readily for different anatomical regions and clinical situations.

Positioning examples for various oblique lateral radiographs

Examples of the required positioning for different oblique laterals and the resultant radiographs are shown in Figs 10.5–10.8. Illustrations show the positioning for both adults and children.

Important points to note

- For stability, a small child is usually rotated through 90° in the chair, so the shoulder is supported and the cassette and head can be rested on the headrest.
- The area under investigation determines the position of the cassette and the X-ray tubehead.
- An X-ray request for an oblique lateral must specify the **exact** region of the jaws required.

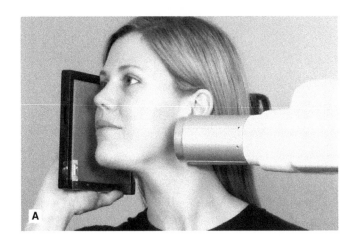

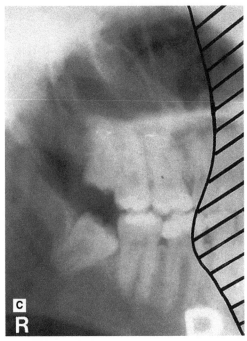

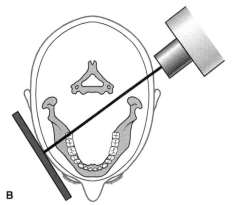

Fig. 10.5 A Cassette and X-ray tubehead positions for the RIGHT mandibular **and** maxillary molars on an adult. **B** Diagram of the positioning from above showing the cassette overlying the molar teeth and the X-ray beam passing between the cervical spine and mandibular ramus. **C** A typical resultant radiograph. The shadow of the superimposed left ramus, overlying the premolars, has been drawn in to emphasize its position. Compare with Fig. 10.4A. Note the radiograph is mounted and viewed as if the observer is looking at the right side of the patient's face.

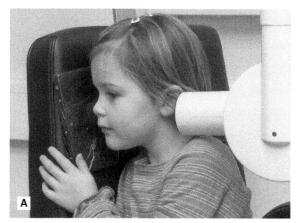

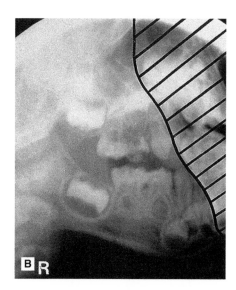

Fig. 10.6 A Positioning of a child, cassette and X-ray tubehead for the RIGHT deciduous maxillary and mandibular molars. **B** A typical resultant radiograph. The shadow of the superimposed left ramus has been drawn in.

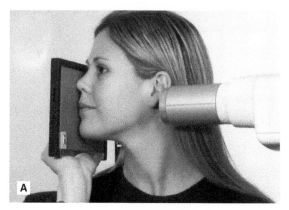

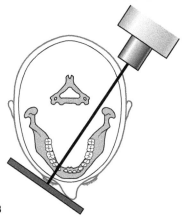

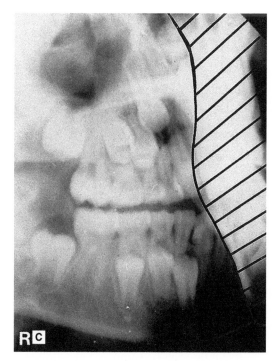

Fig. 10.7 A Cassette and X-ray tubehead positions for the RIGHT mandibular and maxillary canines. Note the displacement of the nose needed to achieve the desired position for the cassette. **B** Diagram of the positioning from above, showing the cassette overlying the canine teeth and the X-ray tubehead aimed through the *radiographic keyhole*. **C** A typical resultant radiograph of a patient in the mixed dentition. The shadow of the superimposed left ramus has been drawn in – it now overlies the lateral incisors. Again note the orientation of the radiograph and how it is mounted.

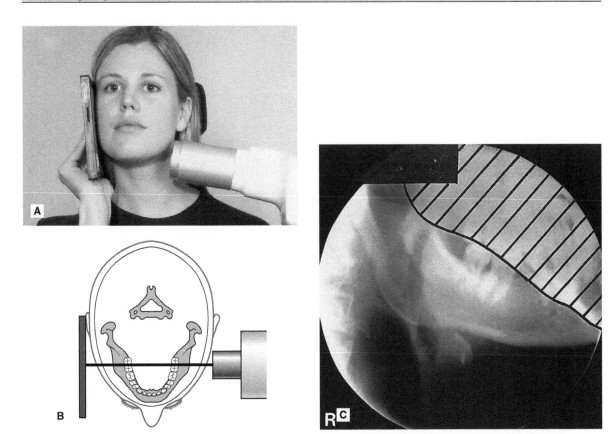

Fig. 10.8 A Cassette and X-ray tubehead position for the RIGHT mandibular molars. Note the upward angulation of the X-ray tubehead and its position beneath the left body of the mandible. **B** Diagram of the positioning from above. Note the position of the X-ray tubehead and compare with Fig. 10.5B. **C** A typical resultant radiograph showing the right mandibular molars. The superimposed shadow of the left mandibular body has been drawn in overlying the maxillary molars. Compare with Fig. 10.4B.

Bimolar technique

As mentioned earlier, *bimolar* is the term used for the radiographic projection showing oblique lateral views of the right and left sides of the jaws on the different halves of the **same** radiograph, as shown in Fig. 10.9.

The technique can be summarized as follows:

1. The patient is positioned with one side of the face in the middle of one half of the cassette, with the nose towards the midline. The precise positioning depends on which teeth or area of the jaws are being examined (like any other oblique lateral).
2. The other half of the cassette is covered by a lead shield to prevent exposure of this side of the film.

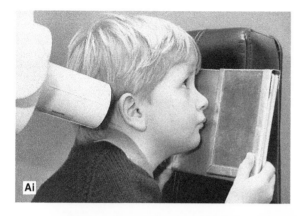

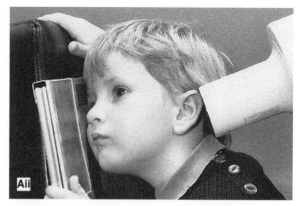

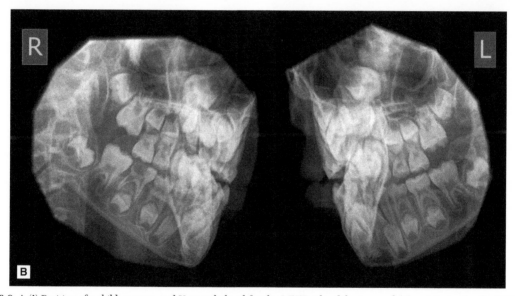

Fig. 10.9 A (**i**) Position of a child, cassette and X-ray tubehead for the LEFT side of the jaws and (**ii**) positioning for the RIGHT side. Note the lead shield covering the half of the cassette not being used. **B** An example of a child's bimolar.

3. The X-ray tubehead is positioned to show the desired area, and the exposure is made.
4. The lead shield is then placed over the other side of the cassette to protect the part of the film already exposed.
5. The patient is then positioned in a similar manner with the cassette held on the other side of the face.
6. The X-ray tubehead is repositioned and a second exposure made.

To access the self assessment questions for this chapter please go to www.whaitesessentialsdentalradiography.com

11 Cephalometric radiography

Cephalometric radiography is a standardized and reproducible form of skull radiography used extensively in orthodontics to assess the relationships of the teeth to the jaws and the jaws to the rest of the facial skeleton. Standardization was essential for the development of *cephalometry* – the measurement and comparison of specific points, distances and lines within the facial skeleton, which is now an integral part of orthodontic assessment. The greatest value is probably obtained from these radiographs if they are traced or digitized and this is essential when they are being used for the monitoring of treatment progress.

Main indications

The main clinical indications can be considered under two major headings – orthodontics and orthognathic surgery.

Orthodontics

- Initial diagnosis – confirmation of the underlying skeletal and/or soft tissue abnormalities
- Treatment planning
- Monitoring treatment progress, e.g. to assess anchorage requirements and incisor inclination
- Appraisal of treatment results, e.g. 1 or 2 months before the completion of active treatment to ensure that treatment targets have been met and to allow planning of retention.

When considering these indications, it should be remembered that all radiographs must be clinically justified – a legislative requirement in most countries. In the UK, indications and selection criteria for cephalometric radiographs are clearly identified in the British Orthodontic Society's 2008 booklet *Orthodontic Radiographs – Guidelines for the Use of Radiographs in Clinical Orthodontics* (3rd edn) and in the Faculty of General Dental Practice (UK)'s 2013 booklet *Selection Criteria for Dental Radiography* (3rd Edition). These guidelines are designed to assist in *the justification* process so as to avoid the use of unnecessary radiographs.

Orthognathic surgery

- Preoperative evaluation of skeletal and soft tissue patterns
- To assist in treatment planning
- Postoperative appraisal of the results of surgery and long-term follow-up studies.

Equipment

Several different types of equipment are available for cephalometric radiography, either as separate units, or as additional attachments to dental panoramic units. In some equipment, the patients are seated, while in others they remain standing.

Traditional equipment was designed to use indirect-action radiographic film in an extraoral cassette as the image receptor. The advent of digital imaging, using phosphor plates and solid-state sensors, has seen the development of new dedicated digital equipment. The basic components of these different types of equipment are described below.

Traditional film-based equipment

This consists of either an additional attachment to a panoramic unit as shown in Fig. 11.1, or as a completely separate dedicated unit as shown in Fig. 11.2. The basic components include:

- *X-ray generating apparatus* that should:
  - Be in a fixed position relative to the cephalostat and film so that successive radiographs are reproducible and comparable. To minimize the effect of magnification the focus-to-film distance should be greater than 1 m and ideally in the range 1.5–1.8 m (see Fig. 11.2).
  - Include a light beam diaphragm to facilitate the collimation. The beam should be collimated to an approximately triangular shape to restrict the area of the patient irradiated to the required cranial base and facial skeleton, so avoiding the skull vault and cervical spine and thyroid gland (see Fig. 11.2).
  - Be capable of producing an X-ray beam that is sufficiently penetrating to reach the film and parallel in nature.

- *Cephalostat (or craniostat)* (see Fig. 11.3) comprising:
  - Head positioning and stabilizing apparatus with ear rods to ensure a standardized patient position. Additional positioning guides can include forehead supports and infraorbital guide rods.
  - Cassette holder.
  - Optional fixed anti-scatter grid to stop photons scattered within the patient reaching the film and degrading the image. This is not usually included in combined panoramic/cephalostat units.
- Cassette (usually 18 × 24 cm) containing rare-earth intensifying screens and indirect action film.
- Aluminium wedge filter designed to attenuate the X-ray beam selectively in the region of the facial soft tissues to enable the soft tissue profile to be seen on the final radiograph. This is either attached to the tubehead, covering the anterior part of the beam (the preferred position) or it is included as part of the cephalostat and positioned between the patient and the anterior part of the cassette.

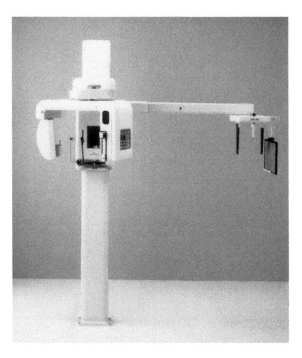

Fig. 11.1 An example of a traditional combined panoramic and cephalostat unit suitable for film-based or phosphor plate imaging.

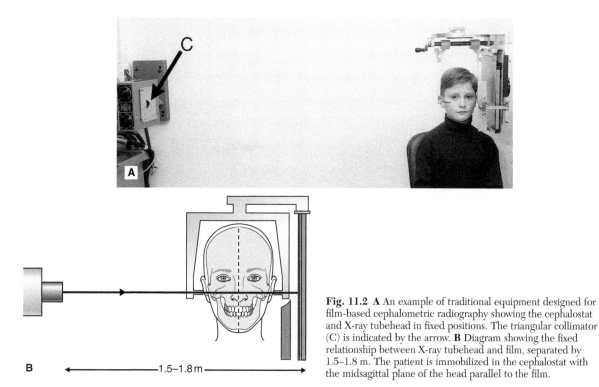

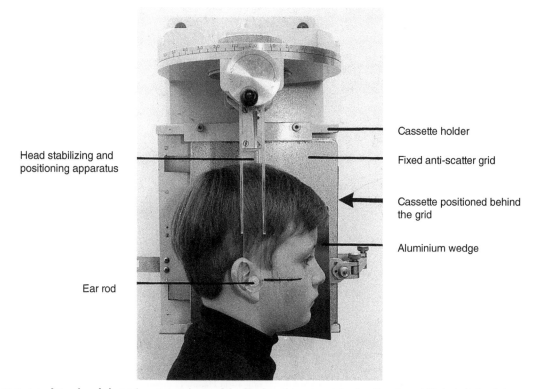

Fig. 11.2 **A** An example of traditional equipment designed for film-based cephalometric radiography showing the cephalostat and X-ray tubehead in fixed positions. The triangular collimator (C) is indicated by the arrow. **B** Diagram showing the fixed relationship between X-ray tubehead and film, separated by 1.5–1.8 m. The patient is immobilized in the cephalostat with the midsagittal plane of the head parallel to the film.

Fig. 11.3 A traditional cephalostat (craniostat) designed for film-based imaging. A fixed anti-scatter grid is included and the aluminium wedge filter positioned between the patient and the grid. The Frankfort plane is marked on the patient's face.

Digital equipment

Equipment variations exist depending on the type of digital image receptor chosen.

Using phosphor plates

Equipment such as combined panoramic/cephalostat units can be converted to digital by simply replacing the film and intensifying screens in the cassette with a suitably sized phosphor plate.

Using solid-state sensors

Several manufacturers have developed combined panoramic/cephalostat units utilizing specially designed solid-state sensors. An example is shown in Fig. 11.4. Sensor design was discussed in Chapter 3 and is illustrated in Fig. 3.19.

The sensor is obviously not the same size as an 18×24 cm cassette and the image cannot be captured in the same way. During the exposure, the X-ray beam and sensor **move** either *horizontally* or *vertically* to scan the patient, as shown in Fig. 11.5. The final image therefore takes a few seconds to build up. To ensure that the X-ray beam is the same shape as the CCD array in the sensor and that they are aligned exactly, the beam passes through a secondary collimator, which also moves throughout the exposure, as shown in Fig. 11.5.

Other features to note include:

- An aluminium wedge filter is not usually included. Soft tissue profile is enhanced by using computer software.
- Triangular beam collimation to avoid the skull vault and cervical spine and thyroid gland is not usually included.
- There is no anti-scatter grid.

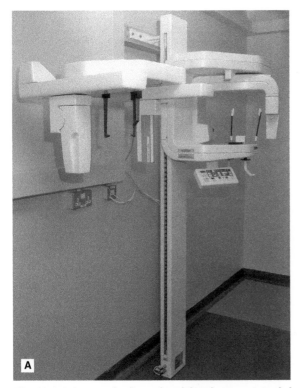

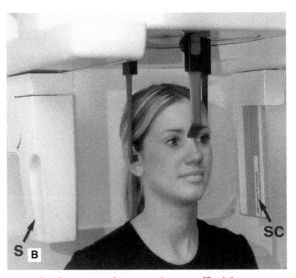

Fig. 11.4 A An example of a combined digital panoramic/cephalostat unit – the Planmeca Proline using the Dimax³® solid-state sensor. **B** Patient positioned and immobilized within the cephalostat unit. Note the solid-state sensor (S) and the secondary collimator (SC) (arrowed).

Main radiographic projections

These include:

- True cephalometric lateral skull
- Cephalometric posteroanterior of the jaws (PA jaws).

True cephalometric lateral skull

As stated in Chapter 10, the terminology used to describe lateral skull projections is somewhat confusing, the adjective *true*, as opposed to *oblique*, being used to describe lateral skull projections when:

- The image receptor is parallel to the sagittal plane of the patient's head
- The X-ray beam is perpendicular to the image receptor and sagittal plane.

In addition, the word *cephalometric* should be included when describing the *true lateral skull* radiograph taken in the cephalostat. This enables differentiation from the non-standardized *true lateral skull* projection taken in a skull unit. It is now an accepted convention to view orthodontic lateral skull radiographs with the patient facing to the right, as shown in Fig. 11.6.

Technique and positioning

This can be summarized as follows:

1. The patient is positioned within the cephalostat, with the sagittal plane of the head vertical and parallel to the image receptor and with the Frankfort plane horizontal. The teeth should generally be in maximum intercuspation.
2. The head is immobilized carefully within the apparatus with the plastic ear rods being inserted gradually into the external auditory meati.
3. The aluminium wedge, if used, is positioned to cover the anterior part of the image receptor.
4. The equipment is designed to ensure that, when the patient is positioned correctly, the X-ray beam is horizontal and centred on the ear rods (see Fig. 11.6).

Cephalometric tracing/digitizing

This produces a diagrammatic representation of certain anatomical points or landmarks evident on the lateral skull radiograph (see Fig. 11.7). These points are traced onto an overlying sheet of paper or acetate or digitally recorded. Either method allows precise measurements to be made.

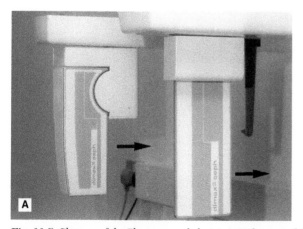 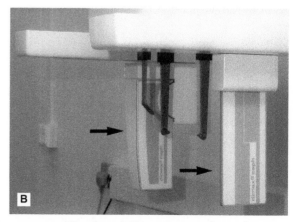

Fig. 11.5 Close up of the Planmeca cephalostat. **A** At the start of the exposure and **B** at the end. This equipment is designed to scan the patient *horizontally* with the X-ray beam, secondary collimator and sensor moving horizontally throughout the exposure (arrowed).

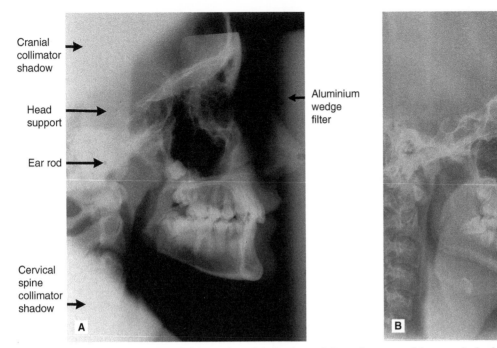

Cranial collimator shadow

Head support

Ear rod

Cervical spine collimator shadow

Aluminium wedge filter

A

B

Fig. 11.6 A An example of a true cephalometric lateral skull radiograph. Note the images of the ear rods should ideally appear superimposed on one another. The various shadows of the cephalostat equipment and the collimator are indicated. **B** A modern digitally captured example. Note there is no aluminium wedge shadow and no evidence of triangular collimation.

As a basic system these could include:

- The outline and inclination of the anterior teeth
- The positional relationship of the mandibular and maxillary dental bases to the cranial base
- The positional relationship of the dental bases to one another, i.e. the skeletal patterns
- The relationship between the bones of the skull and the soft tissues of the face.

Main cephalometric points

The definitions of the main cephalometric points (as indicated in a clockwise direction on the tracing shown in Fig. 11.7) include:

Sella (S). The centre of the sella turcica, (determined by inspection).

Orbitale (Or). The lowest point on the infraorbital margin.

Nasion (N). The most anterior point on the frontonasal suture.

Anterior nasal spine (ANS). The tip of the anterior nasal spine.

Subspinale or point A. The deepest midline point between the anterior nasal spine and prosthion.

Prosthion (Pr). The most anterior point of the alveolar crest in the premaxilla, usually between the upper central incisors.

Infradentale (Id). The most anterior point of the alveolar crest, situated between the lower central incisors.

Supramentale or point B. The deepest point in the bony outline between the infradentale and the pogonion.

Pogonion (Pog). The most anterior point of the bony chin.

Gnathion (Gn). The most anterior and inferior point on the bony outline of the chin, situated equidistant from pogonion and menton.

Menton (Me). The lowest point on the bony outline of the mandibular symphysis.

Gonion (Go). The most lateral external point at the junction of the horizontal and ascending rami of the mandible.

Note: The gonion is found by bisecting the angle formed by tangents to the posterior and inferior borders of the mandible.

Posterior nasal spine (PNS). The tip of the posterior spine of the palatine bone in the hard palate.

Articulare (Ar). The point of intersection of the dorsal contours of the posterior border of the mandible and temporal bone.

Porion (Po). The uppermost point of the bony external auditory meatus, usually regarded as coincidental with the uppermost point of the ear rods of the cephalostat.

Main cephalometric planes and angles

The definitions of the main cephalometric planes and angles shown in Fig. 11.8 include:

Frankfort plane. A transverse plane through the skull represented by the line joining porion and orbitale.

Mandibular plane. A transverse plane through the skull representing the lower border of the horizontal ramus of the mandible.

There are several definitions:

- A tangent to the lower border of the mandible
- A line joining gnathion and gonion
- A line joining menton and gonion.

Maxillary plane. A transverse plane through the skull represented by a joining of the anterior and posterior nasal spines.

SN plane. A transverse plane through the skull represented by the line joining sella and nasion.

SNA. Relates the anteroposterior position of the maxilla, as represented by the A point, to the cranial base.

SNB. Relates the anteroposterior position of the mandible, as represented by the B point, to the cranial base.

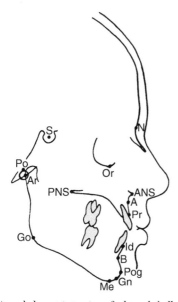

Fig. 11.7 A cephalometric tracing of a lateral skull radiograph showing the main cephalometric points.

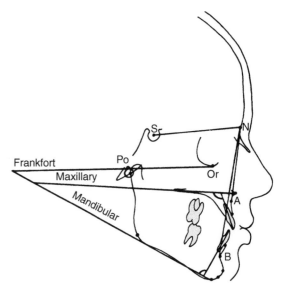

Fig. 11.8 A cephalometric tracing of a lateral skull radiograph showing the main cephalometric planes and angles.

ANB. Relates the anteroposterior position of the maxilla to the mandible, i.e. indicates the anteroposterior skeletal pattern – Class I, II or III.

Maxillary incisal inclination. The angle between the long axis of the maxillary incisors and the maxillary plane.

Mandibular incisal inclination. The angle between the long axis of the mandibular incisors and the mandibular plane.

All the definitions are those specified in the British Standards Glossary of Dental Terms (BS4492: 1983).

Cephalometric posteroanterior of the jaws (PA jaws)

This posteroanterior (PA) view of the jaws, like the lateral view, is standardized and reproducible. This makes it suitable for the assessment of facial asymmetries and for preoperative and postoperative comparisons in orthognathic surgery involving the mandible.

Technique and positioning

This can be summarized as follows:

1. The head-stabilizing apparatus of the cephalostat is rotated through 90°.
2. The patient is positioned in the apparatus with the head tipped forwards and with the radiographic baseline horizontal and perpendicular to the image receptor, i.e. in the *forehead–nose* position.
3. The head is immobilized within the apparatus by inserting the plastic ear rods into the external auditory meati.
4. The fixed X-ray beam is horizontal with the central ray centred through the cervical spine at the level of the rami of the mandible (see Figs 11.9 and 11.10).

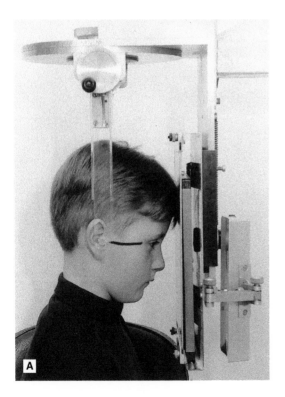

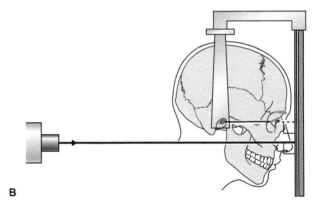

B

Fig. 11.9 A Positioning for the cephalometric PA jaws projection. The patient is in the *forehead–nose* position, with the radiographic baseline (marked on the face) horizontal and perpendicular to the film. **B** Diagram of the patient positioning and showing the X-ray beam horizontal and centred through the rami.

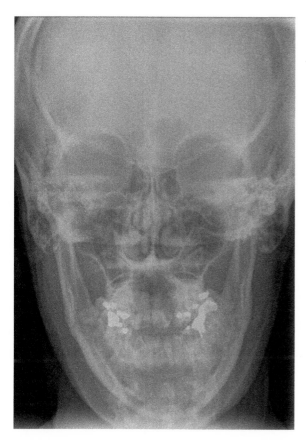

Fig. 11.10 An example of a cephalometric PA jaws radiograph.

To access the self assessment questions for this chapter please go to www.whaitesessentialsdentalradiography.com

12 Tomography and panoramic radiography

Introduction

Conventional *tomography* is a specialized radiographic technique developed originally for producing radiographs that showed only a *section* or *slice* of a patient. A useful analogy is to regard the technique as one that enables the patient to be imaged in slices – like a loaf of sliced bread (see Fig. 12.1). Each individual tomographic image (or slice) shows the tissues within that section sharply defined and in focus. The section is thus referred to as the *focal plane* or *focal trough*. Tissues and structures outside the tomographic section are not visible because they are very blurred and out of focus.

Production of each conventional tomographic slice required controlled, accurate movement of both the X-ray tubehead and the film during the exposure, thereby making it different from all the routine radiographic techniques described in previous chapters. As will be described later in this chapter, by varying the size of the X-ray beam and the type of equipment movement employed it proved possible to change the shape of the tomographic layer from a straight (linear) line (see Fig. 12.2) to a curve, and ultimately to the approximate horseshoe shape of the dental arch, providing an overall panoramic image of all the teeth and their supporting structures – the so-called dental panoramic tomograph (DPT) or panoramic radiograph (see Fig. 12.3).

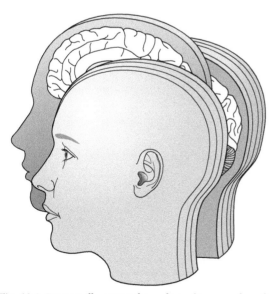

Fig. 12.1 Diagram illustrating the analogy of tomography – the patient is imaged and can be viewed in slices like a loaf of sliced bread.

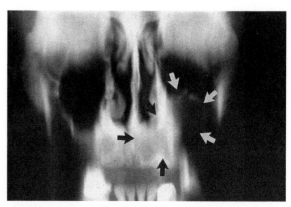

Fig. 12.2 A linear tomograph in the coronal plane. The slice passes through and contains part of the antra and facial skeleton and shows an antral tumour (arrowed).

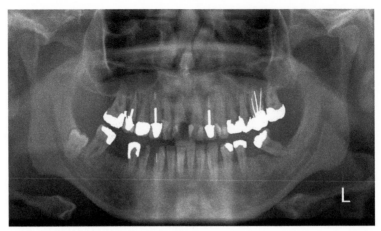

Fig. 12.3 A dental panoramic radiograph depicting a curved tomographic slice. The curved, horseshoe-shaped slice is approximately the shape of the dental arch and contains the teeth and their supporting structures. In both examples the tissues imaged in the tomographic slices are sharply defined and in focus, while the unwanted structures are blurred out.

While panoramic tomography remains very popular, conventional linear tomography has essentially been superseded in radiography by computed tomography, which enables computer-generated tomographic sectional images to be created. Cone beam computed tomography (CBCT) is described in Chapter 13.

Tomographic theory

The theory of panoramic tomography is complicated. Nevertheless, an understanding of how the resultant radiographic image is produced and which structures are in fact being imaged, is necessary for a critical evaluation and the interpretation of this type of radiograph.

As an explanatory introduction to how the approximately horseshoe-shaped, curved tomographic slice or focal trough in panoramic tomography is produced, the theory of tomographic movement and three methods for producing linear and curved tomographic slices are first described. These include:

- Linear tomography using a wide or broad X-ray beam
- Linear tomography using a narrow or slit X-ray beam
- Rotational curved tomography using a narrow slit X-ray beam.

Principle of tomographic movement

As stated, tomography requires controlled, accurate movement of both the X-ray tubehead and the film. They are therefore linked together. During the exposure, the X-ray tubehead moves in one direction while the film moves in the opposite direction, as shown in Fig. 12.4. The **point** at the centre of this rotating movement will appear in focus on the resultant radiograph, since its shadow will appear in the same place on the film throughout the exposure. All other points will appear blurred or out of focus.

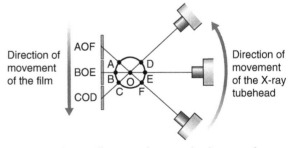

Fig. 12.4 Diagram illustrating the principle of tomographic movement. The X-ray tubehead moves in one direction while the film moves in the opposite direction. Points A, B, C, D, E and F will all appear on different parts of the film and thus will be blurred out, while point O, the centre of rotation, will appear in the same place on the film throughout the exposure and will therefore be sharply defined.

Broad-beam linear tomography

The principle of tomography illustrated in Fig. 12.4 shows a very thin X-ray beam producing one point (O) – the centre of rotation – in focus on the film. To produce a section or slice of the patient in focus, a broad X-ray beam is used. For each part of the beam, there is a separate centre of rotation, all of which lie in the same focal plane. The resultant tomography will therefore show all these points sharply defined. The principle of broad-beam tomography is illustrated in Fig. 12.5.

Slit or narrow-beam linear tomography

A similar straight linear tomograph can also be produced by modifying the equipment and using a narrow or slit X-ray beam. The equipment is designed so that the narrow beam traverses the film exposing different parts of the film during the tomographic movement. Only by the end of the tomographic movement has the entire film been exposed. The following equipment modifications are necessary:

- The X-ray beam has to be collimated from a broad beam to a narrow beam.
- The film cassette has to be placed behind a protective metal shield. A narrow opening in this shield is required to allow a small part of the film to be exposed to the X-ray beam at any one instant.
- A cassette carrier, incorporating the metal shield, has to be linked to the X-ray tubehead to ensure that they move in the **opposite** direction to one another during the exposure. This produces the synchronized tomographic movement in the *vertical* plane.
- Within this carrier, the film cassette itself has to be moved in the **same** direction as the tubehead. This ensures that a different part of the film is exposed to the X-ray beam throughout the exposure.

The principle of narrow-beam linear tomography using this equipment is illustrated in Fig. 12.6.

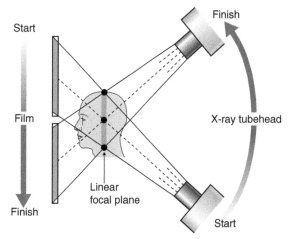

Fig. 12.5 Diagram showing the principle of broad-beam tomography. Using a broad beam there will be multiple centres of rotation (three are indicated: •) all of which will lie in the shaded zone. As all the centres of rotation will be *in focus*, this zone represents the *focal plane* or section of the patient that will appear sharply defined on the resultant tomograph.

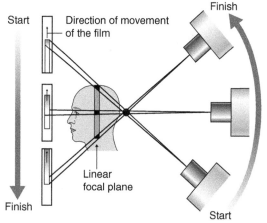

Fig. 12.6 Diagram showing the theory of narrow-beam linear tomography to produce a vertical coronal section. The tomographic movement is produced by the synchronized movement of the X-ray tubehead and the cassette carrier, in the vertical plane. The film, placed behind the metal protective front of the cassette carrier, also moves during the exposure, in the same direction as the X-ray tubehead. The narrow X-ray beam traverses the patient and film, exposing a different part of the film throughout the cycle.

Narrow-beam rotational tomography

In this type of tomography, narrow-beam equipment is again used, but the synchronized movement of the X-ray tubehead and the cassette carrier are designed to rotate in the *horizontal* plane, in a *circular* path around the head, with a *single* centre of rotation. The resultant focal trough is curved and forms the arc of a circle, as shown in Fig. 12.7.

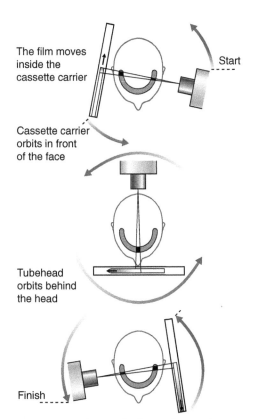

The film moves inside the cassette carrier

Start

Cassette carrier orbits in front of the face

Tubehead orbits behind the head

Finish

Fig. 12.7 Diagrams showing the theory of narrow beam rotational tomography. The tomographic movement is provided by the circular synchronized movement of the X-ray tubehead in one direction and the cassette carrier in the opposite direction, in the horizontal plane. The equipment has a single centre of rotation. The film also moves inside the cassette carrier so that a different part of the film is exposed to the narrow beam during the cycle, thus by the end the entire film has been exposed. The focal plane or trough (shaded) is curved and forms the arc of a circle.

Important points to note

- The X-ray tubehead orbits around the **back** of the head while the cassette carrier with the film orbits around the **front** of the face.
- The X-ray tubehead and the cassette carrier appear to move in **opposite** directions to one another.
- The film moves in the **same** direction as the X-ray tubehead, behind the protective metal shield of the cassette carrier.
- A different part of the film is exposed to the X-ray beam at any one instant, as the equipment orbits the head.
- The simple circular rotational movement with a single centre of rotation produces a curved **circular** focal trough.
- As in conventional tomography, shadows of structures not within the focal trough will be out of focus and blurred owing to the tomographic movement.

Panoramic tomography

The dental arch, though curved, is not the shape of an arc of a circle. To produce the required elliptical, horseshoe-shaped focal trough, panoramic tomographic equipment employs the principle of narrow-beam rotational tomography, but uses two or more centres of rotation.

There are several dental panoramic units available; they all work on the same principle but differ in how the rotational movement is modified to image the elliptical dental arch. Four main methods (see Fig. 12.8) have been used including:

- Two stationary centres of rotation, using two separate circular arcs
- Three stationary centres of rotation, using three separate circular arcs
- A continually moving centre of rotation using multiple circular arcs combined to form a final elliptical shape
- A combination of three stationary centres of rotation and a moving centre of rotation.

However, the focal troughs are produced, it should be remembered that they are three-dimensional. The focal trough is thus sometimes described as a *focal corridor*. All structures within

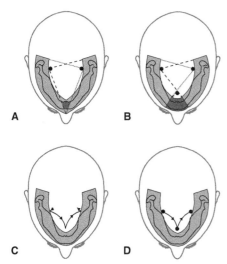

Fig. 12.8 Diagrams showing the main methods that have been used to produce a focal trough that approximates to the elliptical shape of the dental arch using different centres of rotation. **A** 2 stationary, **B** 3 stationary, **C** continually moving, **D** combination of 3 stationary and moving centre.

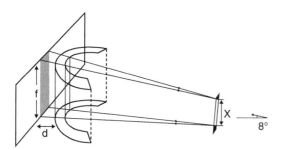

Fig. 12.9 Diagram showing how the height of the three-dimensional focal corridor is determined. The height (x) of the X-ray beam is collimated to just cover the height (f) of the film. The separation of the focal trough and the film (d), coupled with the 8° upward angulation of the X-ray beam results in the final image being slightly magnified.

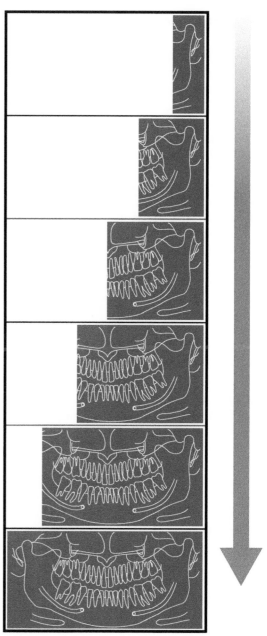

Fig. 12.10 Diagram showing the gradual build-up of a panoramic tomograph over an 18-second cycle, illustrating how a different part of the patient is imaged at different stages in the cycle.

the corridor, including the mandibular and maxillary teeth, will be in focus on the final radiograph. The vertical height of the corridor is determined by the shape and height of the X-ray beam and the size of the film, as shown in Fig. 12.9.

As in other forms of narrow-beam tomography, a different part of the focal trough is imaged throughout the exposure. The final radiograph is thus built up of sections (see Fig. 12.10), each created separately, as the equipment orbits around the patient's head.

Unfortunately, although the final radiograph shows all the teeth and their supporting structures, the tomographic image quality is generally inferior to that obtained using intraoral radiographic techniques and interpretation is more complicated.

Selection criteria

In the UK, the 2013 *Selection Criteria for Dental Radiography* booklet suggests panoramic radiography in general practice in the following circumstances:

- Where a bony lesion or unerupted tooth is of a size or position that precludes its complete demonstration on intraoral radiographs
- In the case of a grossly neglected mouth
- In assessment of periodontal bone support often supplemented with periapical radiographs
- For the assessment of wisdom teeth prior to planned surgical intervention. Routine radiography of unerupted third molars is not recommended
- As part of an orthodontic assessment where there is a clinical need to know the state of the dentition and the presence/absence of teeth. The use of clinical criteria to select patients rather than routine screening of patients is essential.

In addition, in dental hospitals panoramic radiographs are also used to assess:

- Fractures of all parts of the mandible except the anterior region
- Antral disease – particularly to the floor, posterior and medial walls of the antra
- Destructive diseases of the articular surfaces of the TMJ
- Vertical alveolar bone height as part of pre-implant planning.

The 2013 *Selection Criteria* specifically states that 'panoramic radiographs should only be taken in the presence of specific clinical signs and symptoms', and goes on to say that 'there is no justification for review panoramic radiography at arbitrary intervals'.

Equipment

Although varying in design and appearance, all panoramic units consist of four main components:

- An *X-ray tubehead*, producing a narrow fan-shaped X-ray beam, angled upwards at approximately 8° to the horizontal (see Fig. 12.9)
- *Control panel* (see Fig. 12.11)

- *Patient-positioning apparatus*, including chin and appropriate head immobilizing supports and light beam markers
- *An image receptor* (film or digital), with or without an associated carriage assembly.

Traditional panoramic equipment was designed to use indirect-action radiographic film in an extraoral cassette as the image receptor. With the advent of digital imaging several variations in image receptor now exist, including:

- Cassettes containing indirect-action film and rare-earth intensifying screens
- Cassettes containing a digital phosphor plate
- Flat cassette-sized solid-state sensors designed to fit into existing equipment
- Specially designed solid-state sensors – an integral part of new equipment (see Ch. 3).

Two examples are shown in Fig. 12.12. Ideally:

- Equipment should have a range of tube potential settings, preferably 60–90 kV.
- The beam height at the receiving slit of the cassette holder should not be greater than the film in use (normally 125 mm or 150 mm). The width of the beam should not be greater than 5 mm.
- Equipment should be provided with adequate patient-positioning aids incorporating light beam markers.
- Equipment should provide facilities for field-limitation techniques.

Control panel

The control panel design also varies but a typical panel is shown in Fig. 12.11. The main features usually allow the operator to:

- Select the field size
- Select a limited range of arch shapes and sizes
- Select the mA and kV exposure factors
- Adjust the AP position of the bite-peg
- Select the size of the patient to be X-rayed
- Adjust the height of the equipment
- Select a range of field limitation options.

Equipment movement

Figure 12.13 shows diagrammatically how a typical panoramic machine, using film or digital phosphor plate as the image receptor, functions.

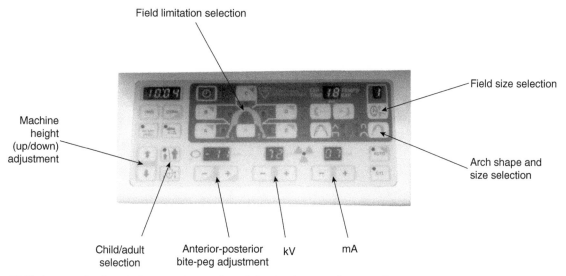

Field limitation selection

Field size selection

Machine
height
(up/down)
adjustment

Arch shape and
size selection

Child/adult
selection

Anterior-posterior
bite-peg adjustment

kV

mA

Fig. 12.11 An example of a typical panoramic control panel showing the main adjustment features.

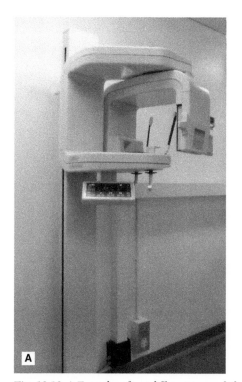

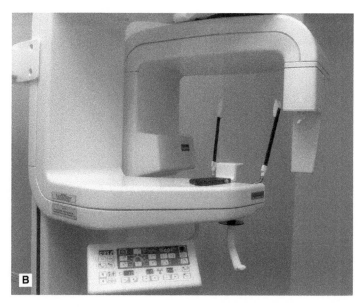

Fig. 12.12 A Examples of two different types of Planmeca panoramic radiography machines. **A** Traditional unit incorporating a cassette suitable for film-based or digital phosphor plate imaging. **B** Dedicated digital unit with specifically designed built-in solid-state digital sensor. The basic components including the X-ray tubehead, the control panel and the patient positioning apparatus are common to both units.

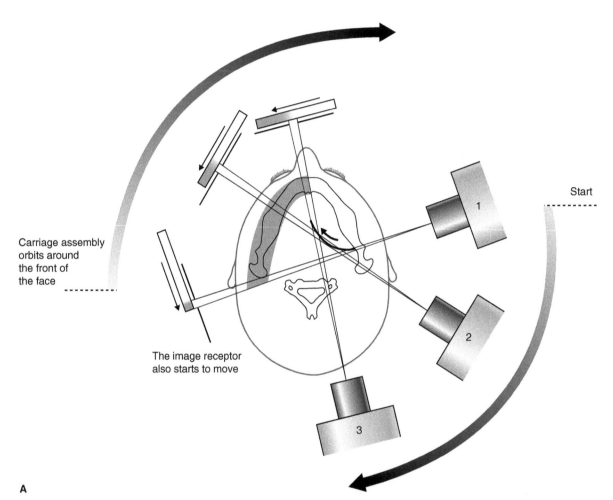

A

Fig. 12.13A Diagram from above, showing the relative movements of the X-ray tubehead, carriage assembly and image receptor (film or phosphor plate) during the first half of the panoramic cycle when the left side of the jaw is imaged. As the X-ray tubehead moves behind the patient's head to image the anterior teeth, the carriage assembly moves in front of the patient's face and the centre of rotation moves forward along the dark arc (arrowed) towards the midline. Note that the X-ray beam has to pass through the cervical spine.

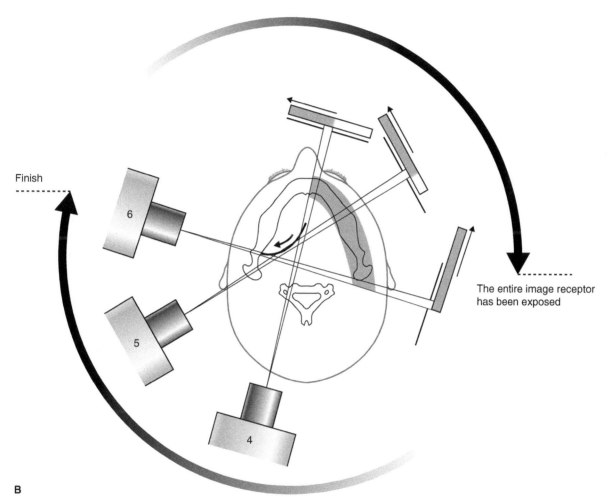

Finish

The entire image receptor has been exposed

B

Fig. 12.13B Diagram from above, showing the relative movements during the second half of the panoramic cycle when the right side of the jaw is imaged. The X-ray tubehead and carriage assembly continue to move around the patient's head to image the opposite side, and the centre of rotation moves backwards along the dark arc (arrowed) a way from the midline. Throughout the cycle the film or phosphor plate is also continuously moving as illustrated, so that a different part of the image receptor is exposed at any one time.

Technique and positioning

The exact positioning techniques vary from one machine to another. However, there are some general requirements that are common to all machines and these can be summarized as follows:

Patient preparation

- Patients should be asked to remove any earrings, jewellery, hair pins, spectacles, dentures or orthodontic appliances.
- The procedure and equipment movements should be explained, to reassure patients and if necessary use a test exposure to show them the machine's movements.

Equipment preparation

- The cassette containing the film or phosphor plate should be inserted into carriage assembly (if appropriate).
- The operator should put on suitable protective gloves (e.g. latex or nitrile) (see Ch. 6).
- The collimation should be set to the size of field required.
- The appropriate exposure factors should be selected according to the size of the patient – typically in range 70–90 kV and 4–12 mA.

Patient positioning

- The patient should be positioned in the unit so that their spine is straight and instructed to hold any stabilizing supports or handles provided (see Fig. 12.14).
- The patient should be instructed to bite their upper and lower incisors edge-to-edge on the bite-peg with their chin in good contact with the chin support.
- The head should be immobilized using the temple supports.
- The light beam markers should be used so that the mid-sagittal plane is vertical, the Frankfort plane is horizontal and the canine light lies between the upper lateral incisor and canine.
- The patient should be instructed to close their lips and press their tongue on the roof of their mouth so that it is in contact with their hard palate and not to move throughout the exposure cycle (approximately 15–18 seconds).

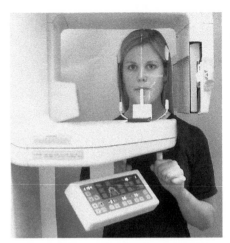

Fig. 12.14 Patient positioned in the Planmeca PM2002. Note the bite-peg, chin and temple supports and the three light-beam markers to facilitate accurate positioning.

Important points to note

- Panoramic radiography is generally considered to be unsuitable for children under six years old, because of the length of the exposure and the need for the patient to keep still.
- A protective lead apron should not be used. In the UK the 2001 *Guidance Notes* confirm that there is no justification for using a protective lead apron. If used, it can interfere with the final image (see Fig. 12.27H).

After exposure

- The temple supports should release automatically to enable the patient to leave the machine.
- The equipment should be wiped down with a surface disinfectant and the bite-peg sterilized (see Ch. 6).
- Gloves should be discarded as clinical waste.
- The film or phosphor plate should be processed.

The importance of accurate patient positioning

The positioning of the patient's head within this type of equipment is critical – it must be positioned accurately so that the teeth lie within the *focal trough*. The effects of placing the head too far forward, too far back or asymmetrically in relation to the focal trough are shown in Fig. 12.15. The parts of the jaws outside the focal trough will be out of focus. The fan-shaped X-ray beam causes patient malposition to be represented mainly as distortion in the horizontal plane, i.e. teeth appear too wide or too narrow rather than foreshortened or elongated. Thus, if the patient is rotated to the left (as shown in Fig. 12.15C), the left teeth are nearer the film and will be narrower, while the teeth on the right will be further away from the film and wider. These and other positioning errors are shown later (see Fig. 12.28).

However accurately the patient's head is positioned, the inclination of the incisor teeth, or the underlying skeletal base pattern, may make it impossible to position both the mandibular **and** maxillary teeth ideally within the focal corridor (see Fig. 12.16).

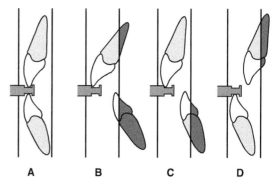

Fig. 12.16 Diagrams showing the vertical walls of the focal trough in the incisor region and the relative positions of the teeth with different underlying dental or skeletal abnormalities. **A** Class I. **B** Gross class II division 1 malocclusion with large overjet. **C** Angle's class II skeletal base. **D** Angle's class III skeletal base. The shaded areas outside the focal trough will be blurred and out of focus.

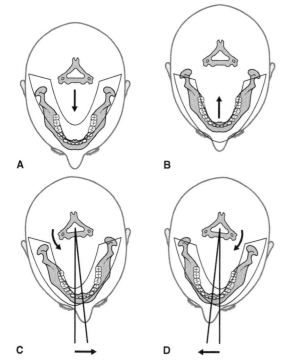

Fig. 12.15 Diagrams showing the position of the mandible in relation to the focal trough when the patient is not positioned correctly. **A** The patient is too close to the film and in front of the focal trough. **B** The patient is too far away from the film and behind the focal trough. **C** and **D** The patient is placed asymmetrically within the machine.

Technique variations

There are a number of technique variations possible with modern equipment, including:

- *Edentulous patient positioning* – the chin support is used instead of the bite-peg and the canine positioning light beam is centred on the corner of the mouth
- *TMJ programmes*
- *Cross-sectional imaging* for implant assessment
- *Collimation* – restricting the size of the beam so restricting the field of view, e.g. the height of the beam is automatically reduced when selecting the settings for children
- *Field limitation* techniques – only preselected parts of the patient are exposed and imaged on the final film as illustrated in Fig. 12.17.

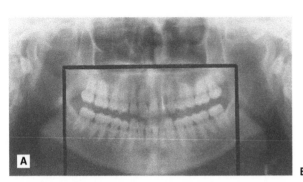
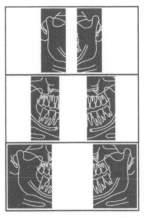
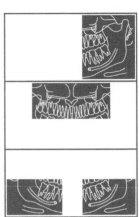

Fig. 12.17 **A** The effect of selecting collimation to reduce the height of the beam and field limitation techniques to exclude the rami and parotid producing the so-called *dentition only* image. This has been reported to reduce the effective dose by approximately 50%. **B** Diagram showing a selection of images that can be obtained by using collimation and field limitation techniques.

Normal anatomy

The normal anatomical shadows that are evident on panoramic radiographs vary from one machine to another, but in general they can be subdivided into:

- *Real* or *actual shadows* of structures in, or close to, the focal trough

- *Ghost* or *artefactual shadows* created by the tomographic movement and cast by structures on the opposite side or a long way from the focal trough. The 8° upward angulation of the X-ray beam means that these ghost shadows appear at a higher level than the structures that have caused them.

These two types of shadows are clearly demonstrated in Figs 12.18 and 12.19.

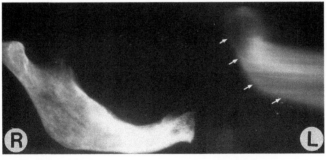

Fig. 12.18 A panoramic radiograph taken of the *right* half of a hemisectioned mandible. The **real shadows** are clearly shown on the *right*. The ghost shadow of the mandible is shown on the *left* (arrowed). Note these **ghost** shadows are at a higher level on the film than the real shadows because of the 8° rising X-ray beam that is used.

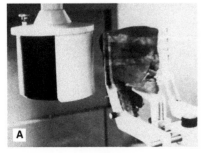
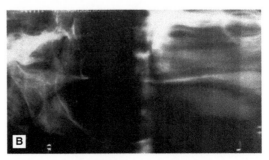

Fig. 12.19 **A** Hemisected cadaver head positioned in a dental panoramic machine. **B** Resultant radiograph showing the **real hard and soft tissue** shadows on the right and the **ghost** shadows on the left. (Reproduced from *Oral Radiology* (2nd edn, 1987), by kind permission of Paul W. Goaz and Stuart C. White and The C.V. Mosby Company.)

Real or actual shadows

Important hard tissue shadows include: (see Figs 12.20 and 12.21)

- Teeth
- Mandible
- Maxilla, including the floor, medial and posterior walls of the antra
- Hard palate
- Zygomatic arches
- Styloid processes
- Hyoid bone
- Nasal septum and conchae
- Orbital rim
- Base of skull.

Important air shadows include:

- Mouth/oral opening
- Oropharynx.

Important soft tissue shadows include:

- Ear lobes
- Nasal cartilages
- Soft palate
- Dorsum of tongue
- Lips and cheeks
- Nasolabial folds.

Ghost or artefactual shadows

(see Fig. 12.22)

The more important ghost shadows include:

- Cervical vertebrae
- Body, angle and ramus of the contralateral side of the mandible
- Palate.

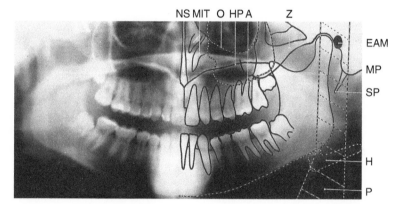

Fig. 12.20 A panoramic radiograph showing the main real hard tissue shadows, including the plastic head support, drawn in on one side of the radiograph, **NS** – nasal septum, **MIT** –middle and inferior turbinates, **O** – orbital margin, **HP** – hard palate, **A** – floor of antrum, **Z** – zygomatic arch, **EAM** – external auditory meatus, **MP** – mastoid process, **SP** –styloid process, **H** – hyoid, **P** – plastic head support.

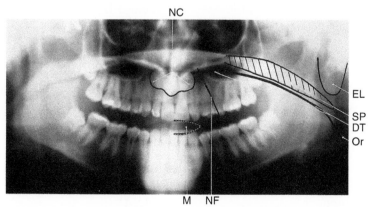

Fig. 12.21 A panoramic radiograph showing the main **real soft tissue** and **air** shadows drawn in on one side of the radiograph, **NC** – nasal cartilages, **EL** – ear lobe, **SP** – soft palate, **DT** – dorsum of tongue, **Or** – oropharynx, **NF** – naso-labial fold, **M** – mouth.

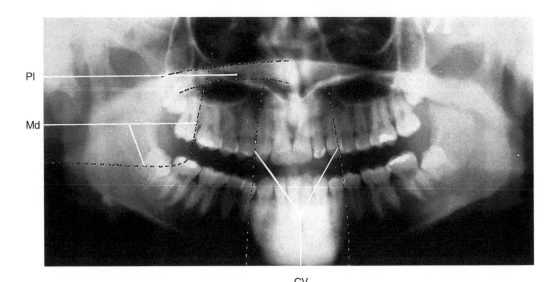

Fig. 12.22 A panoramic radiograph showing the main anatomical **ghost** or **artefactual shadows** drawn in on one side of the radiograph, **Pl** – palate, **Md** – mandible, **CV** – cervical vertebrae.

Advantages and disadvantages

Advantages

- A large area is imaged and all the tissues within the focal trough are displayed, including the anterior teeth, even when the patient is unable to open the mouth.
- The image is easy for patients to understand, and is therefore a useful teaching aid.
- Patient movement in the vertical plane distorts only that part of the image being produced at that instant.
- Positioning is relatively simple and minimal expertise is required.
- The overall view of the jaws allows rapid assessment of any underlying, possibly unsuspected, disease.
- The view of both sides of the mandible on one film is useful when assessing fractures and is comfortable for the injured patient.
- The overall view is useful for evaluation of periodontal status and in orthodontic assessments.
- The antral floor, medial and posterior walls are well shown.
- Both condylar heads are shown on one film, allowing easy comparison.
- The radiation dose (*effective dose*) may be lower than a full-mouth survey of intraoral images in some cases (see Ch. 4).

- Development of field limitation techniques which result in further dose reduction.

Disadvantages

- The tomographic image represents only a section of the patient. Structures or abnormalities not in the focal trough may not be evident (Fig. 12.23).
- Soft tissue and air shadows can overlie the required hard tissue structures (Fig. 12.24).
- Ghost or artefactual shadows can overlie the structures in the focal trough (Fig. 12.25).
- The tomographic movement together with the distance between the focal trough and image receptor produce distortion and magnification of the final image (approx. × 1.3).
- The use of indirect-action film and intensifying screens results in some loss of image quality but image resolution can be improved by using digital image receptors.
- The technique is not suitable for children under six years or on some disabled patients because of the length of the exposure cycle.
- Some patients do not conform to the shape of the focal trough and some structures will be out of focus.
- Movement of the patient during the exposure can create difficulties in image interpretation (Fig. 12.26).

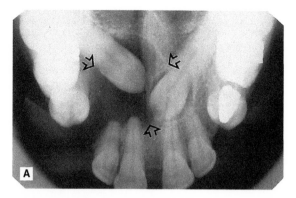

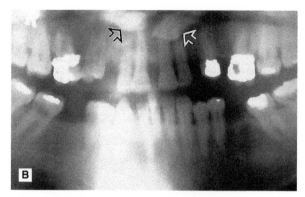

Fig. 12.23 A Upper standard occlusal showing unerupted 3|3 and a large dentigerous cyst -(arrowed) associated with 3| .
B Panoramic radiograph showing the two unerupted canines out of focus (arrowed) and only a suggestion of the dentigerous cyst, because they are all outside the focal trough.

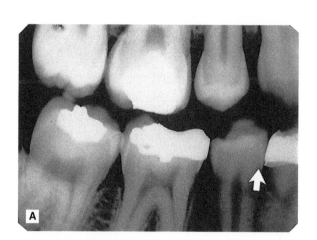

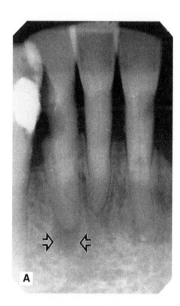

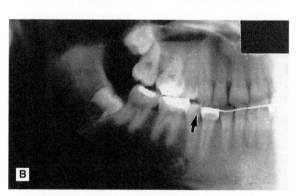

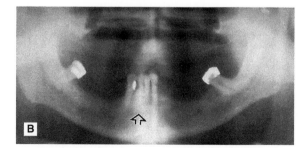

Fig. 12.24 A Right bitewing showing no evidence of mesial caries in 5| (arrowed). **B** Panoramic radiograph showing an apparent lesion in this tooth (arrowed). This appearance is created by the overlying air shadow of the corner of the mouth.

Fig. 12.25 A Periapical of 21|12 region showing an area of radiolucency at the apex of 1| (arrowed). **B** Panoramic radiograph showing no evidence of the lesion (arrowed) owing to superimposition of the shadow of the cervical vertebrae.

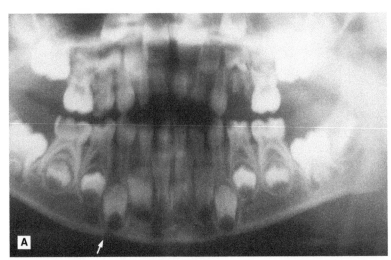
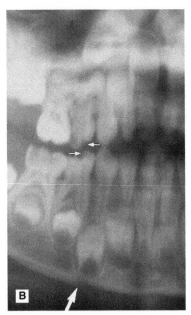

Fig. 12.26 A Panoramic radiograph of a young child, who had fallen over, showing a step deformity (arrowed) in the lower border suggesting a fracture. **B** Same radiograph enlarged showing the step deformity (large arrow), but also notice the step deformities in the crowns of the upper and lower first deciduous molars (small arrows). Sudden slight vertical movement of the patient makes interpretation difficult.

Assessment of image quality

As mentioned in previous chapters, in relation to all other radiographs, image quality assessment essentially involves three separate stages, namely:

- Comparison of the image against ideal quality criteria
- Subjective rating of image quality using published standards
- Detailed assessment of rejected films to determine the source of error.

Ideal quality criteria

Irrespective of the type of image receptor being used, typical quality criteria for a full field of view panoramic radiograph include:

- All the upper and lower teeth and their supporting alveolar bone should be clearly demonstrated
- The whole of the mandible should be included

- Magnification in the vertical and horizontal planes should be equal
- The right and left molar teeth should be equal in their mesiodistal dimension
- The density across the image should be uniform with no air shadow above the tongue creating a radiolucent (black) band over the roots of the upper teeth
- The image of the hard palate should appear above the apices of the upper teeth
- Only the slightest ghost shadows of the contralateral angle of the mandible and the cervical spine should be evident
- There should be no evidence of artefactual shadows due to dentures, earrings and other jewellery
- The patient identification label should not obscure any of the above features
- The image should be clearly labelled with the patient's name and date of the examination
- The image should be clearly marked with a **R**ight and/or **L**eft letter.

Subjective rating of image quality

The simple three-point subjective rating scale published in the UK's 2001 *Guidance Notes* was introduced in Chapter 7 and is discussed in detail, together with the errors associated with exposure factors and chemical processing, in Chapter 14. The summary is shown again in Table 12.1. Panoramic patient preparation and positioning errors are described below.

Assessment of rejected films and determination of errors

Patient preparation errors (Fig. 12.27)

These can include:

- Failure to remove jewellery
  - Earrings
  - Necklaces
  - Piercings
- Failure to remove dentures
- Failure to remove orthodontic appliances
- Failure to remove spectacles
- Inappropriate use of the lead apron.

Patient positioning errors
(Figs 12.28 and 12.29)
These can include:

- Failure to ensure that the spine is straight (ghosting shadow error)
- Failure to ensure the incisors are biting edge-to-edge on the bite-peg (anteroposterior error)
- Failure to use the light beam marker to ensure midsagittal plane is vertical and the head is not rotated (horizontal error)
- Failure to use the light beam marker to ensure the Frankfort plane is horizontal (vertical error)
- Failure to instruct the patient to press the tongue against the roof of the mouth (air shadow error)
- Failure to instruct the patient to remain still throughout the exposure (movement error).

Equipment positioning errors (Fig. 12.30)
These can include:

- Failure to set height adjustment correctly
- Failure to select correct exposure settings
- Failure to use the cassette correctly.

Table 12.1 Subjective quality rating criteria for film-captured images published in the 2001 *Guidance Notes for Dental Practitioners on the Safe Use of X-ray Equipment*

Rating	Quality	Basis
1	Excellent	No errors of patient preparation, exposure, positioning, processing or film handling
2	Diagnostically acceptable	Some errors of patient preparation, exposure, positioning, processing or film handling, but which do not detract from the diagnostic utility of the radiograph
3	Unacceptable	Errors of patient preparation, exposure, positioning, processing or film handling, which render the radiograph diagnostically unacceptable

Footnote

Panoramic radiographs should not be considered an alternative to high-resolution intraoral radiographs. However, they are commonly considered as an alternative to right and left *oblique lateral* radiographs or the bimolar projection (see Ch. 10) mainly because it is assumed that less operator expertise is required to produce panoramic images of adequate diagnostic quality. Unfortunately, the multiple and varied causes of error in panoramic radiography make the technique very operator-dependent, no matter how sophisticated the equipment and the image receptors become. The use of digital sensors (solid-state or phosphor plate) improves the resolution of panoramic images when compared to those captured using indirect-action film and intensifying screen combinations. In addition, digital images can be enhanced and manipulated using computer software (see Ch. 3).

The diagnostic value of all panoramic images is increased considerably if clinicians understand that the image created is a tomograph (whatever the image receptor) and are aware of the limitations that this imposes. A suggested systematic approach to interpretation of panoramic images is outlined in Chapter 16.

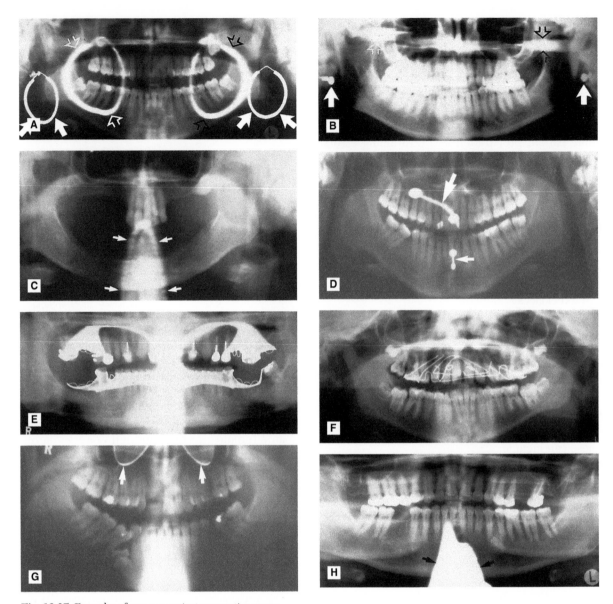

Fig. 12.27 Examples of common patient preparation errors.

A Failure to remove large ring-shaped earrings – note each earring casts two shadows, one real (in focus, solid arrows) and one ghost (blurred, open arrows). The ghost shadow of the LEFT earring is marked with white open arrows, that of the RIGHT earring with black open arrows.

B Failure to remove stud earring, real shadows (solid arrows) with ghost shadows (open arrows).

C Failure to remove a necklace – blurred ghost shadow (arrowed).

D Failure to remove piercing in the tongue (large arrow) and lower lip (small arrow).

E Failure to remove upper and lower metallic partial dentures.

F Failure to remove an upper orthodontic appliance.

G Failure to remove spectacles (arrowed).

H Inappropriate use of a protective lead apron – too high on the neck casting a dense radiopaque shadow (arrowed) over the anterior part of the mandible.

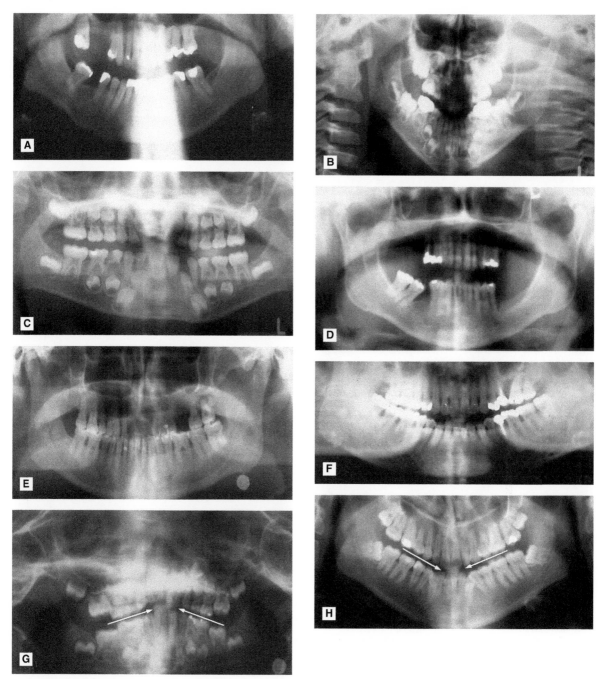

Fig. 12.28 Examples of common patient positioning errors. **A** Failure to position the neck correctly – extension of the neck causing excessive spinal ghosting shadows over the anterior teeth. **B** Anteroposterior error – patient positioned too far forwards (too close to the image receptor) and vertical error – Frankfort plane not horizontal (chin tipped down) creating narrow, out of focus anterior teeth, distorted occlusal plane (so-called *smiley face*) and excessive peripheral spinal shadowing. **C** Anteroposterior error – patient positioned too far back (too far away from the image receptor) creating widened, magnified and out of focus anterior teeth. **D** Anteroposterior error – patient positioned too far forwards (too close to the image receptor) creating narrowed incisors **and** failure to instruct patient to keep their tongue in contact with the palate creating the radiolucent band across the film. **E** Horizontal error – patient asymmetrical, rotated to the RIGHT. The RIGHT molars are closer to the image receptor and smaller, the LEFT molars are further away from the image receptor and larger. **F** Vertical error – Frankfort plane not horizontal (chin tipped down) creating out of focus lower incisors and excessive ghosting shadows of the contralateral angles of the mandible. **G** Vertical error – Frankfort plane not horizontal (chin tipped up) creating out-of-focus upper incisors and distorted occlusal plane (arrowed) (so-called *grumpy face*). **H** Vertical error – Frankfort plane not horizontal (chin tipped down) creating out of focus lower incisors and distorted occlusal plane (arrowed) (so-called *smiley face*).

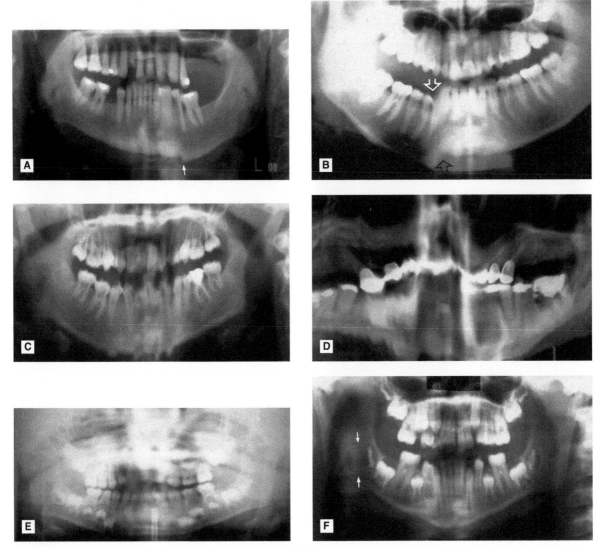

Fig. 12.29 Examples of failure to instruct the patient to keep still during the full panoramic cycle.
A Sudden movement in the vertical plane – distortion of the image 45 region creating a step-deformity in the lower border (see also Fig. 12.23).
B Movement in the vertical plane caused by the patient opening their mouth causing distortion in the $\overline{43|}$ region (arrowed).
C Multiple vertical movements while the anterior teeth were being imaged.
D Continuous shaking movements throughout the cycle.
E Sudden side-to-side horizontal movement while the anterior teeth were being imaged causing them to be blurred.
F Horizontal movement towards the end of the cycle causing horizontal elongation and stretching of the shadow of the developing lower right third molar (arrowed).

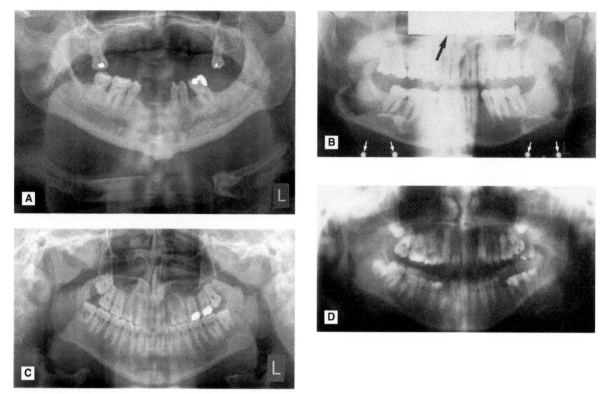

Fig. 12.30 Examples of equipment positioning errors. **A** The X-ray tubehead and image receptor carriage assembly positioned too low relative to the patient – the antra and condyles are not imaged. **B** Cassette positioned back-to-front in the carriage assembly. Name plate and hinge screws are evident (arrowed). **C** Modern cassette positioned back-to-front. **D** Cassette inadvertently used twice and double-exposed.

To access the self assessment questions for this chapter please go to www.whaitesessentialsdentalradiography.com

13 Cone beam computed tomography (CBCT)

Cone beam computed tomography (CBCT) has been developed in recent years specifically for use in the dental and maxillofacial regions and is gradually establishing itself as the imaging modality of choice in certain clinical situations. It is also referred to as *digital volume tomography* or *cone beam volumetric imaging*. As described later, the size of the *volume* or *field of view* (FOV) of the maxillofacial skeleton imaged varies; as a result CBCT scans are often described by their *field of view*:

- *Small, limited or dento-alveolar* (approx. 4 cm^3)
- *Medium or maxillofacial* (approx. 8 cm^3)
- *Large* or *craniofacial* including the cranial base ± the skull vault.

As this type of equipment is gradually being installed in dental practice, as well as in dental hospitals, it is likely that dental care professionals will increasingly encounter it in the future. This chapter is therefore included to provide an introduction and overview to this new technology.

Main indications

Considerable controversy exists as to the main indications for CBCT and robust clinical research justifying its use is limited. Some authorities argue that CBCT should be regarded as almost routine for all dental and maxillofacial applications, while others argue that CBCT should not be used unless the results of the examination are going to alter patient management as the technique delivers a higher dose than conventional two-dimensional imaging. In 2011 the European-wide *Safety and Efficacy of a New and Emerging Dental X-ray Modality* SEDENTEXCT project published guidelines based on what evidence was available at that time. These guidelines, and a more cautious approach to the justified use of CBCT, are endorsed by the authors. Hence the indications summarised below are based broadly on the SEDENTEXCT recommendations.

The developing dentition

CBCT may be indicated for:

- Localization of an unerupted tooth (small FOV)
- Assessment of external resorption in relation to unerupted teeth (small FOV)
- Localized assessment of an impacted tooth (small FOV)
- Assessment of cleft palate (small or medium FOV)
- Planning complex orthodontic/surgical management of maxillofacial skeletal abnormalities (medium or large FOV).

CBCT is generally not indicated for:

- Planning the placement of temporary anchorage in orthodontics
- Routine orthodontic diagnosis.

Restoring the dentition

If conventional imaging proves inadequate CBCT may be indicated for:

- Assessment of periodontal infra-bony defects and furcation lesions (small FOV)
- Periapical assessment (small FOV)
- Assessment of root canal anatomy in multi-rooted teeth (small FOV)
- Planning surgical endodontic procedures (small FOV)
- Endodontic treatment complicated by resorption lesions, combined perio-endo lesions, perforations and atypical pulp anatomy (small FOV)
- Assessment of dental trauma (suspected root fracture) (small FOV).

CBCT is generally not indicated for:

- Diagnosis of dental caries
- Routine imaging of periodontal support
- Routine diagnosis of periapical disease
- Routine assessment of root canal anatomy.

Surgical applications

CBCT may be indicated for:

- Assessment of lower third molars where an intimate relationship with the inferior dental canal is suspected (small FOV)
- Assessment of unerupted teeth (small FOV)
- Cross-sectional imaging prior to implant placement (small or medium FOV)
- Assessment of pathological lesions affecting the jaws (small or medium FOV) including cysts, tumours, giant cell lesions and osseous dysplasias
- Assessment of facial fractures where soft tissue detail is not required (medium or large FOV)
- Planning orthognathic surgery to obtain three-dimensional datasets of the craniofacial skeleton (medium or large FOV)
- Assessment of the bony elements of the TMJ (small or medium FOV)
- Assessment of the bony walls of the maxillary antra.

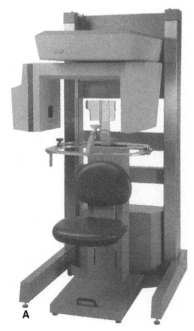
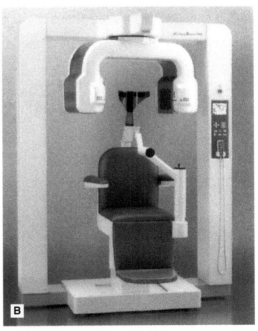

Fig. 13.1 Examples of two CBCT machines specially designed for imaging the maxillofacial skeleton. **A** The i-CAT (imaging Sciences International, Inc., USA) and **B** the 3-D Accuitomo (J. Morita, Japan).

Equipment and theory

Multiple CBCT machines are currently available with new, upgraded models launched regularly by most manufacturers of X-ray equipment. Almost all modern machines resemble panoramic units, as shown in Fig. 13.1.

All equipment employs a cone-shaped X-ray beam and a special detector (e.g. an image intensifier linked to a charge-coupled device (CCD) or, more commonly, an amorphous silicon flat panel). The scanning/image creation process divides into three stages:

- Data acquisition
- Primary reconstruction
- Secondary or multiplanar reconstruction

Stage 1 – Data acquisition

The patient is positioned with the unit (as described later). The equipment orbits around the patient in a 180°, 270° or 360° rotation, taking approximately 5–40 seconds, and in one cycle or scan, images a cylindrical or spherical *volume* referred to as the *field of view* (FOV). As all the information/data is obtained in the single scan, the patient must remain stationary throughout the exposure. As described earlier, the FOV can vary in size enabling small, medium or large volumes of a patient to be imaged. Using a large field of view (e.g. 15 cm^3) most of the maxillofacial skeleton fits within the cylindrical or spherical shape and is imaged in the one scan as shown in Fig. 13.2.

Stage 2 – Primary reconstruction

Having obtained data from the one scan, the computer then divides the volume into tiny cubes or *voxels* (ranging in size between 0.076 mm^3 and 0.4 mm^3) and calculates the X-ray absorption in each voxel. As with *pixels* in two-dimensional digital imaging, described in Chapter 3, each voxel is allocated a number and then allocated a colour from the grey scale from black through to white. Typically one scan contains over 100 million voxels. The overall image resolution clinically of hard tissues (teeth and bones) is generally very good in CBCT imaging, although measured spatial resolution (3–4 line pairs/mm) is not yet as good as two-dimensional film-based or digital imaging (10–25 lp/mm) (see Chapter 3). Using a smaller voxel size potentially increases the spatial resolution but increases the radiation dose. Even so CBCT cannot be used to examine the soft tissues in detail because of the size of the kV and types of detectors used and the amount of scatter. Essentially all that can be seen is the outline of the soft tissues where it interfaces with air.

Stage 3 – Secondary or multiplanar reconstruction

Following the primary reconstruction, the computer software then allows the operator to select voxels in the three anatomical orthogonal planes to create sagittal, coronal or axial images – as shown in Fig. 13.2. A set of sagittal, coronal and axial images appear simultaneously on the computer monitor. The software then enables these image data sets to be scrolled through in real time. For example, by selecting and moving the horizontal cursor up and down on the coronal image, all the axial images can be scrolled through from top to bottom.

Using a small field of view (e.g. 4 cm^3) just two or three teeth and their supporting structures fit within the cylindrical or spherical shape. The same three stages of data acquisition, primary reconstruction and secondary or multiplanar reconstruction are employed to create images in the sagittal, coronal and axial planes, as shown in Fig. 13.3.

Multiplanar reconstruction also allows voxels in other planes to be selected. For example, it is possible to plot the curvature and shape of the dental arch to enable the computer to construct a panoramic image made up of the voxels that coincide with the plotted arch shape – either mandibular or maxillary (see Fig. 13.4).

In addition, it is also possible to reconstruct cross-sectional (also referred to as *transaxial*) images of any part of the jaw, and with appropriate software to produce so-called *volume rendered* or *surface rendered* images, as shown in Fig. 13.5.

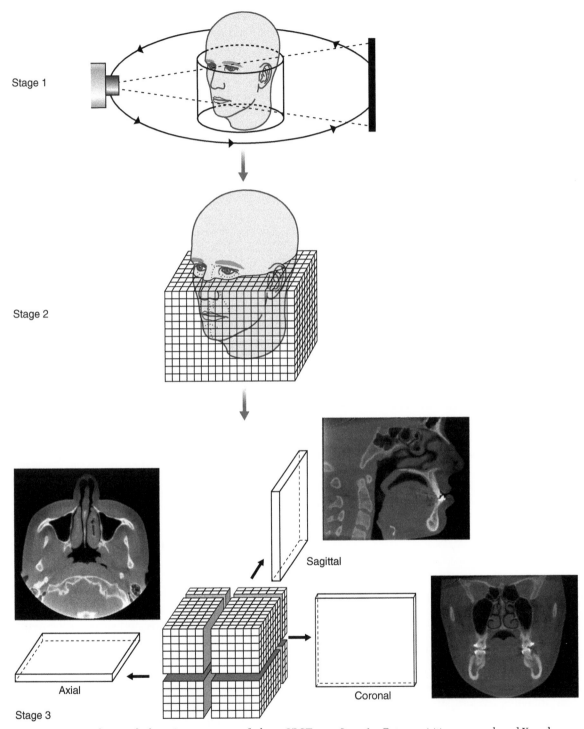

Stage 1

Stage 2

Axial

Sagittal

Coronal

Stage 3

Fig. 13.2 Diagram showing the basic 3-stage concept of a large CBCT scan. Stage 1 – *Data acquisition*: a cone-shaped X-ray beam is used which orbits around the patient obtaining information/data in a cylindrical volume. The patient's maxillofacial skeleton is positioned within the cylinder. Stage 2 – *Primary reconstruction*: the computer divides the cylinder into tiny cubes or voxels. Stage 3 – *Secondary or multiplanar reconstruction*: the computer creates separate images in the sagittal, coronal and axial anatomical planes.

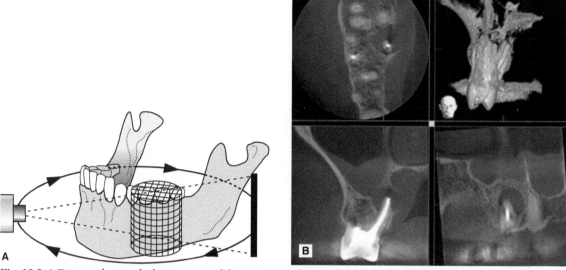

Fig. 13.3 A Diagram showing the basic concept of *data acquisition* for a small field of view CBCT. A cone-shaped X-ray beam orbits once round the patient acquiring data within a small cylinder containing two or three teeth. **B** An example of a small volume CBCT scan showing axial, coronal and sagittal images and a 3-D reconstructed image following *secondary* or *multiplanar reconstruction*.

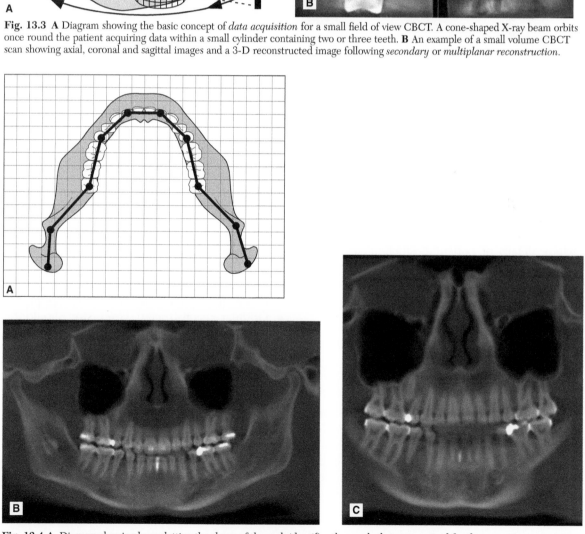

Fig. 13.4 A Diagram showing how plotting the shape of the arch identifies the voxels that are required for the computer to generate a panoramic image. Panoramic image based on **B** the curved shape of the mandibular arch and **C** the maxillary arch.

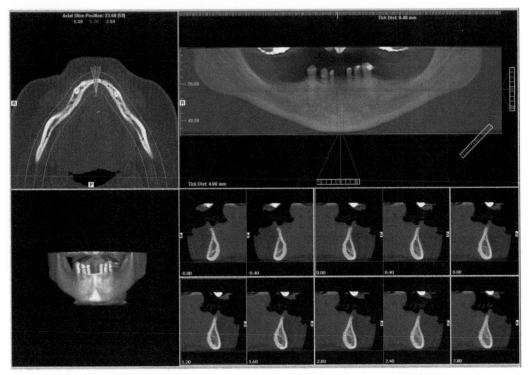

Fig. 13.5 An example of the i-CAT *implant planning screen*, showing an axial slice allowing the arch shape to be defined resulting in the panoramic image, together with 10 transaxial/cross-sectional images through the midline of the mandible and a 3-D image.

Technique and positioning

As in panoramic radiography, described in Chapter 12, the exact patient positioning techniques vary from one machine to another, but whatever the machine, written protocols for each CBCT examination should be provided which include details of patient positioning, exposure parameters and volume size. There are, however, some general requirements that are common to all machines and these include:

- Patient preparation.
- Equipment preparation.
- Patient positioning.

Patient preparation

- Patients should be asked to remove any earrings, jewellery, hair pins, spectacles, dentures or orthodontic appliances.
- The procedure and equipment movements should be explained to reassure patients and the importance of remaining stationary throughout the scan should be stressed.

Equipment preparation

- The smallest volume size needed to answer the clinical question should be used to reduce the radiation dose to the patient. Using a smaller volume reduces scatter and potentially improves image quality.
- Optimal exposure factors should be selected to satisfy the diagnostic requirements of the examination. Higher exposure factors may be chosen if a higher spatial resolution is required.
- Optimal reconstructed voxel size should be selected. If choosing a larger voxel size results in a reduced patient dose (due to lower exposure factors being used) then this should be considered as long as the lower resolution is compatible with the aims of the radiographic examination.
- Some machines offer a 'quick scan' where the rotation arc is reduced. This feature reduces the number of projections taken and therefore reduces the dose. If the required diagnostic information can be obtained using this scan protocol then it should be selected.

Patient positioning

- The patient should be positioned using the manufacturer's guidelines to ensure that the correct region of interest is captured. A *scout* view may be useful to ensure the right part of the jaw is imaged, as shown in Fig. 13.6.
- Once positioned correctly, using the light beam markers, immobilization chin cups and head straps must be used to prevent any patient movement as shown in Fig. 13.7.

- There is no need for the routine use of a protective lead apron.
- There is no need for the routine use of a protective thyroid collar as the thyroid gland does not normally lie in the primary beam, however its use should be considered on a case by case basis, particularly in children. If used, it must be positioned so that it does not interfere with the primary beam since this could lead to significant artefacts.

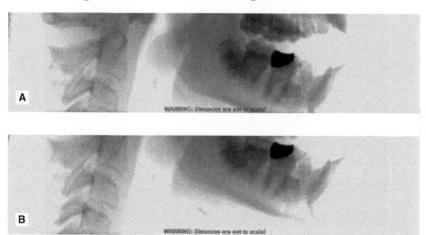

Fig. 13.6 Examples of *scout* views taken on the i-CAT Classic. **A** The first scout view of the mandible shows that the lower part of the mandible has been missed. The set-up was altered and the scout view repeated. **B** The second scout view following alteration of the set-up. The whole body of the mandible is now included, and the full scan can now be carried out in the knowledge the complete region of interest will be imaged.

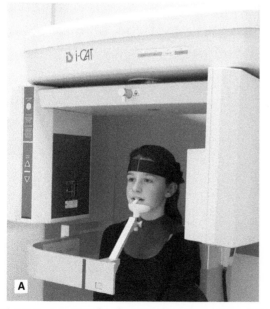
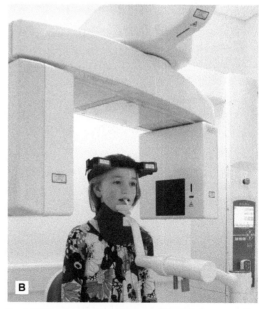

Fig. 13.7 A Patient positioned in the i-CAT Next Generation and **B** in the 3-D Accuitomo. Note the use of the light beam markers and immobilizing chin cup and head strap to prevent movement. Both children have protective thyroid collars in place.

Normal anatomy (Figs 13.8–13.12)

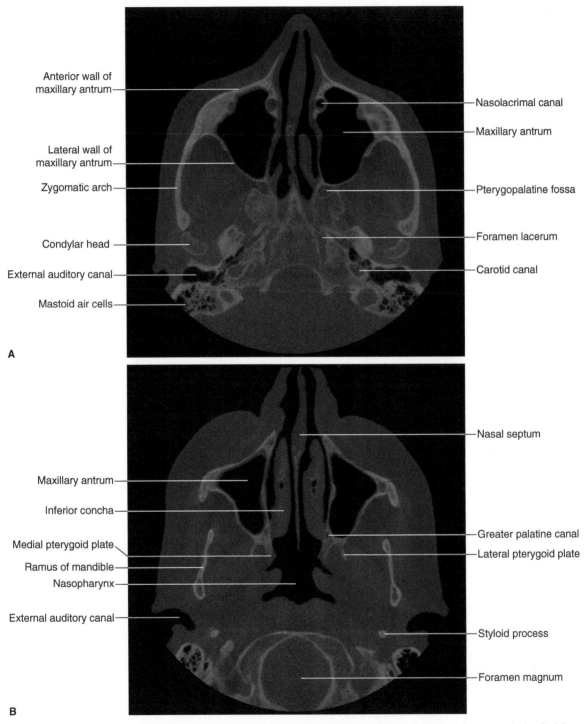

Anterior wall of maxillary antrum

Lateral wall of maxillary antrum

Zygomatic arch

Condylar head

External auditory canal

Mastoid air cells

Nasolacrimal canal

Maxillary antrum

Pterygopalatine fossa

Foramen lacerum

Carotid canal

A

Maxillary antrum

Inferior concha

Medial pterygoid plate

Ramus of mandible

Nasopharynx

External auditory canal

Nasal septum

Greater palatine canal

Lateral pterygoid plate

Styloid process

Foramen magnum

B

Fig. 13.8 Examples of large volume CBCT images with the main anatomical features indicated. **A** An axial image at the level of the condyle. **B** An axial image at the level of the ramus of the mandible.

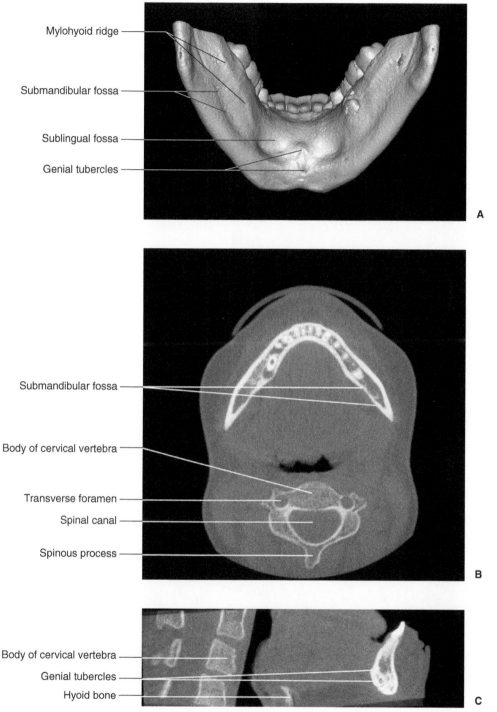

Fig. 13.9 Examples of CBCT images of the mandible showing the main anatomical features. **A** A 3-D surface rendered reconstruction of the mandible viewed from the lingual side (© Materialise Dental NV – SimPlant®). **B** An axial image through roots of the mandibular teeth. **C** A sagittal image through the midline of the mandible.

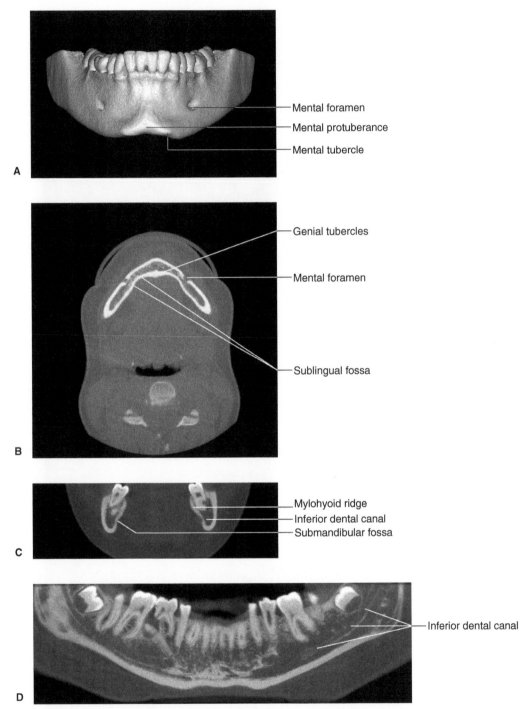

Fig. 13.10 Further examples of CBCT images of the mandible showing the main anatomical features. **A** A 3-D surface rendered reconstruction of the mandible viewed from the front (© Materialise Dental NV – SimPlant®). **B** An axial image at the level of the mental foramina. **C** A coronal image through the molar teeth. **D** A panoramic type reconstruction along the course of the inferior dental canal.

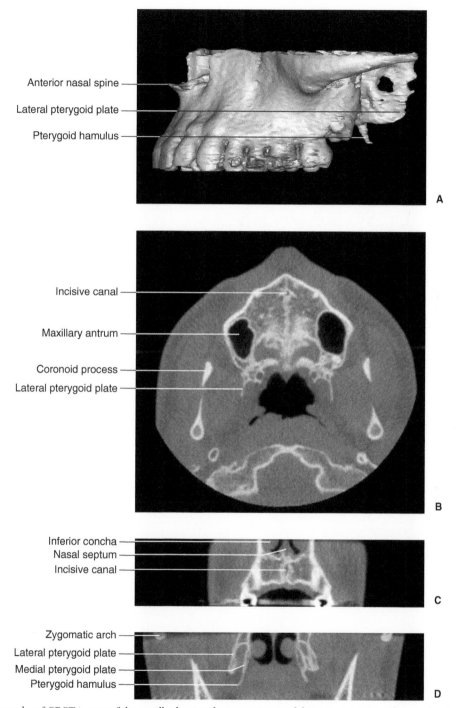

Anterior nasal spine

Lateral pterygoid plate

Pterygoid hamulus

A

Incisive canal

Maxillary antrum

Coronoid process

Lateral pterygoid plate

B

Inferior concha
Nasal septum
Incisive canal

C

Zygomatic arch
Lateral pterygoid plate
Medial pterygoid plate
Pterygoid hamulus

D

Fig. 13.11 Examples of CBCT images of the maxilla showing the main anatomical features. **A** A 3-D surface rendered reconstruction of the left side of the maxilla (© Materialise Dental NV – SimPlant®). **B** An axial image through the base of the maxillary antra. **C** A coronal image through the incisive canal. **D** A coronal image through the pterygoid plates.

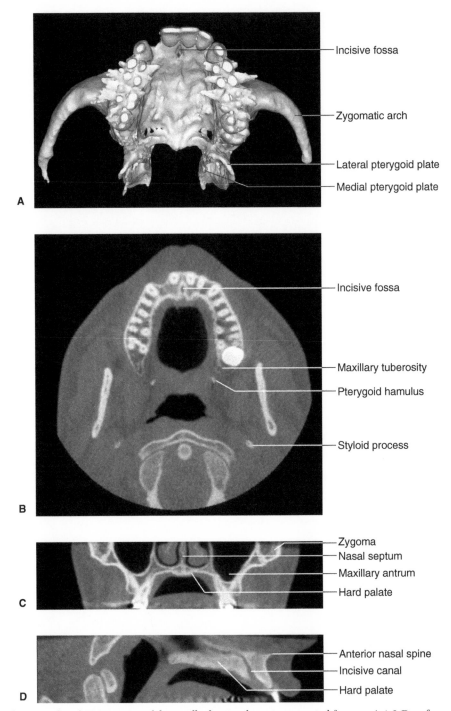

Fig. 13.12 Further examples of CBCT images of the maxilla showing the main anatomical features. **A** A 3-D surface rendered reconstruction of the maxilla viewed from below (© Materialise Dental NV – SimPlant®). **B** An axial image through the roots of the maxillary teeth. **C** A coronal image through the maxillary antra. **D** A sagittal image through the midline of the maxilla.

Radiation dose

The exposure factors on some CBCT machines are fixed by the manufacturer. However, on other units operators are able to adjust the exposure factors – typically in the range 60–120 kV and in the range 1–20 mA – allowing optimization of the dose. As mentioned the scan time varies between 5 and 40 seconds, but the equipment may use a *pulsed* beam rather than a *continuous* beam. As a result, during a scan lasting 20 seconds the patient may be exposed to ionizing radiation for about 3.5 seconds only.

The effective dose from different CBCT machines varies considerably. It depends on a number of factors including:

- The exposure factors (kV, mA and time of exposure)
- The volume size – *field of view*
- The type of equipment used
- The part of the jaw/maxillofacial skeleton being imaged.

Typically doses are lower than medical CT but higher than conventional dental radiography.

However, some new CBCT units are producing very small *field of view*, high resolution images with doses equivalent to that of a few periapical radiographs. The effective doses from CBCT imaging and other investigations, initially shown in Chapter 4, are shown again in Table 13.1.

Advantages and disadvantages

Advantages

- Multi-planar reformatting and data manipulation allowing anatomy/pathological conditions to be viewed in different planes
- Lower radiation dose than medical CT
- Geometrically accurate images
- Very good spatial resolution
- Fast scanning time
- Compatible with implant and cephalometric planning software.

Disadvantages

- The patient has to remain absolutely stationary throughout the scan to avoid movement artefacts (see Fig. 13.13)
- Soft tissues not imaged in detail
- Computer constructed panoramic type images are not directly comparable with conventional panoramic radiographs – particular care is needed in their interpretation
- Radiodense objects such as restorations and root filling materials can produce so-called beam hardening artefacts as well as the streak or star artefacts shown in Fig. 13.14.

Table 13.1 Table showing the effective dose from a range of different radiographic examinations including CBCT

X-ray examination	Effective dose (E) mSv
Bitewing/periapical radiograph	0.0003–0.022
Panoramic radiograph	0.0027–0.038
Upper standard occlusal	0.008
Lateral cephalometric radiograph	0.0022–0.0056
Skull radiograph (PA)	0.02
Skull radiograph (lateral)	0.016
Chest (PA)	0.014
Chest (lateral)	0.038
CT head	1.4
CT chest	6.6
CT abdomen	5.6
CT mandible and maxilla	0.25–1.4
Barium swallow	1.5
Barium enema	2.2
Dento-alveolar CBCT	0.01–0.67
Craniofacial CBCT	0.03–1.1

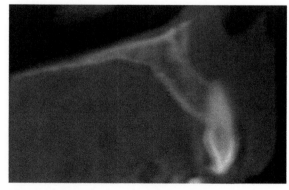

Fig. 13.13 Sagittal section through the upper incisor region resulting from severe patient movement. The scan is non-diagnostic and needs to be retaken.

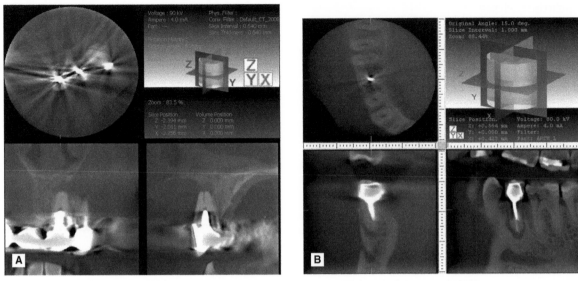

Fig. 13.14 Examples showing beam hardening and streak or star artefacts caused by radiodense (metallic) objects.

Assessment of image quality

In the UK the 2010 Health Protection Agency's guidelines included slightly modified image quality criteria and ratings from those recommended for conventional two-dimensional dental radiographs and shown in several earlier chapters. The recommended subjective image quality ratings and minimum targets for CBCT are shown in Table 13.2.

Table 13.2 Subjective image quality ratings and targets for CBCT recommended by the Health Protection Agency in the UK in 2010

Quality rating	Basis	Target
Grade 1 – Diagnostically acceptable	No errors or minimal errors in either patient preparation, exposure, positioning or image reconstruction and of sufficient image quality to answer the clinical question	Not less than 95%
Grade 2 – Diagnostically unacceptable	Errors in either patient preparation, exposure, positioning or image reconstruction which render the image diagnostically unacceptable	Not greater than 5%

To access the self assessment questions for this chapter please go to www.whaitesessentialsdentalradiography.com

The quality of radiographic images and quality assurance

Introduction

The factors that can affect the quality of radiographic images depends on:

- How the image was taken (radiographic technique)
- What image receptor was used (film or digital)
- How the visual image was created
  - Chemical processing (film)
  - Computer processing (digital).

The effects of poor radiographic technique are the same whatever type of image receptor is used. These technique errors have already been covered in detail in relation to the three main projections used in dentistry, namely: periapicals (Ch. 7), bitewings (Ch. 8) and panoramic radiographs (Ch. 12).

The creation of the visual *digital* image was described in Chapter 3, together with how computer software can be used to alter and manipulate the image with regards to contrast, brightness (degree of blackening), magnification, inversion, enhancement and pseudocolourization.

Creation of the black/white/grey image on *film* using chemical processing was also described in Chapter 3. These various images can, however, be affected by many other factors. This chapter therefore is designed for revision, bringing together and summarizing from earlier chapters all these various factors. It also includes a quick reference section as an aid to fault-finding of film-captured images. Various image faults are illustrated together with their possible causes. This is followed by a section on

quality assurance and suggested quality control measures.

Film-based image quality

As mentioned in Chapter 1, image quality and the amount of detail shown on a radiograph depend on several factors including:

- Contrast
- Image geometry
- Characteristics of the X-ray beam
- Image sharpness and resolution.

Contrast

Radiographic contrast, i.e. the final visual difference between the various black, white and grey shadows, depends on:

- Subject contrast
- Film contrast
- Fog and scatter.

Subject contrast

This is the difference caused by different degrees of attenuation as the X-ray beam is transmitted through different parts of the patient's tissues. It depends upon:

- Differences in tissue thickness
- Differences in tissue density
- Differences in tissue atomic number (photoelectric absorption $\propto Z^3$ (see Ch. 2))
- Quality (voltage (kV)) or penetrating power of the radiation beam.

Film contrast

This is an inherent property of the film itself (see Ch. 3). It determines how the film will respond to the different exposures it receives after the X-ray beam has passed through the patient. Film contrast depends upon four factors:

- The characteristic curve of the film
- Optical density or degree of blackening of the film
- Type of film – direct or indirect action
- Processing.

Fog and scatter

Stray radiation reaching the film either as a result of background fog, or owing to scatter from within the patient, produces unwanted film density (blackening), and thus reduces radiographic contrast.

Image geometry

As mentioned and illustrated in Chapter 1, the geometric accuracy of an image depends upon the position of the X-ray beam, object and image receptor (film or digital) satisfying certain basic geometrical requirements:

- The object and the image receptor should be in contact or as close together as possible
- The object and the image receptor should be parallel to one another
- The X-ray tubehead should be positioned so that the beam meets the object and the image receptor at right angles.

Characteristics of the X-ray beam

The ideal X-ray beam used for imaging should be:

- Sufficiently penetrating to pass through the patient, to a varying degree, and react with the film emulsion to produce good *contrast* between the various black, white and grey shadows (see earlier)
- Parallel, i.e. non-diverging, to prevent magnification of the image (see Ch. 3)

- Produced from a point source to reduce blurring of the image margins and the *penumbra effect* (see Ch. 3).

Image sharpness and resolution

Sharpness is defined as the ability of the X-ray film to define an edge. The main causes of loss of edge definition include:

- Geometric unsharpness including the *penumbra effect* (see above)
- Motion unsharpness, caused by the patient moving during the exposure
- Absorption unsharpness – caused by variation in object shape, e.g. cervical *burn-out* at the neck of a tooth (see Chs 8 and 17)
- Screen unsharpness, caused by the diffusion and spread of the light emitted from intensifying screens (see Ch. 3)
- Poor resolution. Resolution, or resolving power of the film, is a measure of the film's ability to differentiate between different structures and record separate images of small objects placed very close together, and is determined mainly by characteristics of the film including:
  - type – direct or indirect action
  - speed
  - silver halide emulsion crystal size. Resolution is measured in line pairs per mm.

Practical factors influencing film-based image quality

In practical terms, the various factors that can influence overall film-captured image quality can be divided into factors related to:

- The X-ray equipment
- The image receptor – film or film/screen combination
- Processing
- The patient
- The operator and radiographic technique.

As a result of all these variables, film faults and alterations in image quality are inevitable. However, since the diagnostic yield from radiography is related directly to the quality of the image, regular checks and monitoring of these variables are essential to achieve and maintain good quality radiographs. It is these checks which form the basis of *quality assurance (QA) programmes* (see later).

Dental care professionals need to be able to recognize the cause of the various film faults so that appropriate corrective action can be taken.

Typical film faults

Examples of typical film faults are shown below and summarized later in Table 14.1.

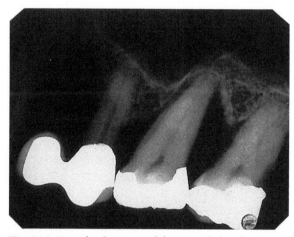

Fig. 14.1 Example of a periapical that is too dark with poor contrast.

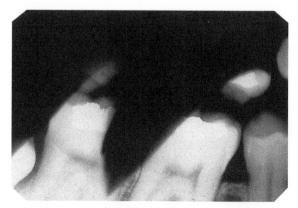

Fig. 14.2 Example of a fogged (blackened) film. Bitewing fogged in the darkroom by inadvertently exposing the upper part of the film to light. The lower part was protected by the operator's fingers.

Film too dark (Figs 14.1 and 14.2)

Possible causes

- Overexposure owing to:
  - Faulty X-ray equipment, e.g. timer
  - Incorrect exposure time setting by the operator
- Overdevelopment owing to:
  - Excessive time in the developer solution
  - Developer solution too hot
  - Developer solution too concentrated
- Fogging owing to:
  - Poor storage conditions:
    - Allowing exposure to stray radiation
    - Too warm
  - Old film stock i.e. films used after expiry date
  - Faulty cassettes allowing ingress of stray light
  - Faulty darkroom/processing unit:
    - Allowing leakage of stray light
    - Faulty safe-light
- Thin patient tissues.

Film too pale (Fig. 14.3)

Possible causes

- Underexposure owing to:
  - Faulty X-ray equipment, e.g. timer
  - Incorrect exposure time setting by the operator
  - Failure to keep timer switch depressed throughout the exposure

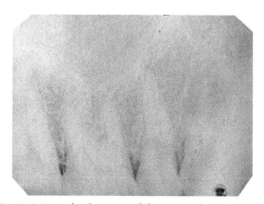

Fig. 14.3 Example of a periapical that is too pale with poor contrast.

- Underdevelopment owing to:
  - Inadequate time in the developer solution
  - Developer solution too cold
  - Developer solution too dilute
  - Developer solution exhausted
  - Developer contaminated by fixer
- Excessive thickness of patient's tissues
- Film packet back to front (film also marked).

Film with inadequate or low contrast
(Figs 14.1, 14.2, 14.3)

Possible causes

- Processing error owing to:
  - Underdevelopment (film also pale)
  - Overdevelopment (film also dark)
  - Developer contaminated by fixer
  - Inadequate fixation time
  - Fixer solution exhausted
- Fogging owing to:
  - Poor storage conditions:
    - Allowing exposure to stray radiation
    - Too warm
  - Poor stock control and film used after expiry date
  - Faulty cassettes allowing the ingress of stray light
  - Faulty darkroom/processing unit.

Image unsharp and blurred (Fig. 14.4)

Possible causes

- Movement of the patient during the exposure (see also Chs 7, 8 and 12)
- Excessive bending of the film packet during the exposure (see also Ch. 7)
- Poor film/screen contact within a cassette
- Film type – image definition is poorer with indirect-action film than with direct-action film
- Speed of intensifying screens – fast screens result in loss of detail
- Overexposure – causing *burn-out* of the edges of a thin object
- Poor positioning in panoramic radiography (see Ch. 12).

Film marked (Fig. 14.5)

Possible causes

- Film packet bent by the operator
- Careless handling of the film in the darkroom resulting in marks caused by:
  - Finger prints
  - Finger nails
  - Bending
  - Static discharge

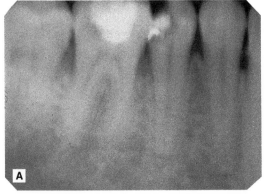 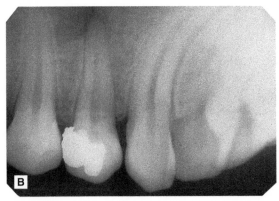

Fig. 14.4 Examples of unsharp and blurred films. **A** As a result of patient movement. **B** As a result of excessive bending of the film packet during the exposure.

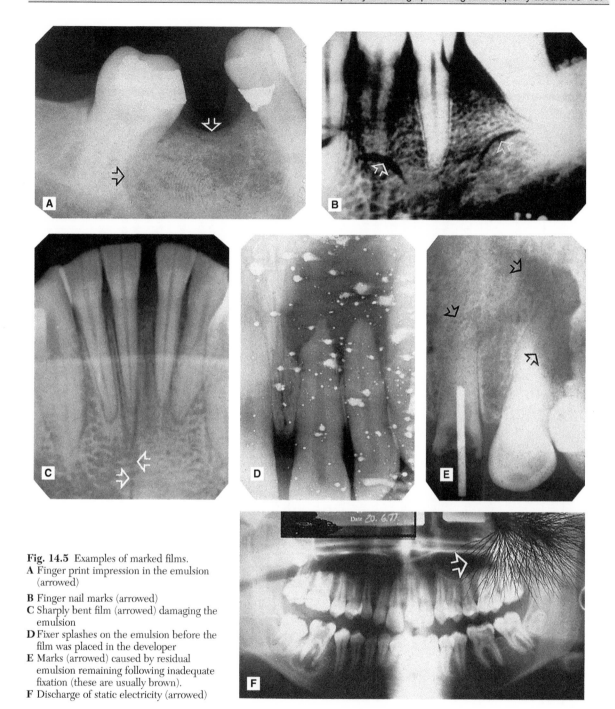

Fig. 14.5 Examples of marked films.

A Finger print impression in the emulsion (arrowed)

B Finger nail marks (arrowed)

C Sharply bent film (arrowed) damaging the emulsion

D Fixer splashes on the emulsion before the film was placed in the developer

E Marks (arrowed) caused by residual emulsion remaining following inadequate fixation (these are usually brown).

F Discharge of static electricity (arrowed)

- Processing errors owing to:
  - Chemical spots
  - Underfixation – residual silver halide emulsion remaining
  - Roller marks
  - Protective black paper becoming stuck to the film
  - Insufficient chemicals to immerse films fully
- Patient biting too hard on the film packet
- Dirty intensifying screens in cassettes.

Table 14.1 Summary of common film quality problems and their possible causes

Reason for rejection	Possible causes		Remedy to each particular fault
	General	**Particular**	
Film too dark	Processing fault (overdevelopment)	Developer concentration too high	Dilute or change chemicals
		Development time too long	Adjust as necessary
		Developer temperature too high	Adjust as necessary
	Excessive X-ray exposure	Incorrect exposure setting	Adjust and repeat examination
		Faulty timer on X-ray set	Arrange service and repair of X-ray set
		Thin patient tissues	Decrease exposure and repeat
	Fogged film	Light leak in darkroom	Check and correct
		Faulty safelighting	Inspect safelights visually, coin test, and correct any fault detected
		Old film stock	Discard film
		Poor film storage	Discard film and re-assess storage facilities
		Light leak in cassette	Check hinges and catches and repair or replace if required
Film too pale	Processing fault (underdevelopment)	Overdiluted developer	Change chemicals
		Inadequate development time	Adjust as necessary
		Developer temperature too low	Adjust as necessary
		Exhausted developer	Change chemicals
		Developer contaminated by fixer	Change chemicals
	Inadequate X-ray exposure	Incorrect exposure setting	Adjust and repeat
		Faulty timer on X-ray set	Arrange service and repair of X-ray set
		Excessive thickness of patient's tissues	Increase exposure and repeat
	Technique error	Film back to front	Adjust and repeat
Inadequate or low contrast	Processing fault	Overdevelopment (plus dark films)	Check development and time/temperature relationship
		Underdevelopment (plus pale films)	As above
		Developer contaminated by fixer	Change chemicals
		Inadequate fixation time (films opaque; milky sheen)	Adjust as necessary
		Fixer exhausted (films opaque; milky sheen)	Change fixer solution
	Fogged film	See above	See above

Unsharp image	Technique error	Patient movement Excessive bending of the film packet during exposure Poor patient positioning (in panoramic radiography)	Assess and instruct patient carefully Adjust and repeat Greater care in positioning and full use of positioning aids
	Cassette error	Poor film/screen contact Incorrect intensifying screen speed	Check cassette and repair or replace if necessary Change screens
	Excessive X-ray exposure	Incorrect exposure setting for thin object causing *burn-out*	Decrease exposure setting and repeat
Film marked	Handling fault	Film packet bent Careless handling in darkroom	Careful handling As above
	Processing fault	Chemical spots Insufficient chemicals to allow full immersion of film Automatic roller marks Patient biting too hard on the film Dirt on intensifying screens	Careful chemical handling Check chemical tanks and adjust Clean processor Instruct patient correctly and repeat Clean screens regularly
Poor positioning	Film packet incorrectly positioned	Film back to front (plus pale film) Not covering area of interest Film used twice (plus dark film)	Use film holders for intraoral radiography when possible As above Greater care in film handling
	X-ray tubehead incorrectly positioned	Too steep an angle producing foreshortening Too shallow an angle producing elongation	Use beam-aiming devices when possible As above
	Patient incorrectly positioned	Patient incorrectly placed (in panoramic unit)	Greater care in positioning and full use of positioning aids

Reproduced, with modifications, from *Dental Update* with kind permission of Professor K. Horner and George Warman Publications.

Patient preparation and positioning (radiographic technique) errors (Fig. 14.6)

These errors can happen whatever image receptor is being used and were described in detail and illustrated in Chapters 7, 8 and 12. They are summarized below and can be divided into intraoral and panoramic technique errors.

Intraoral technique errors

These can include:

- Failure to position the image receptor correctly to capture the area of interest
- Failure to position the image receptor correctly causing it to bend (if flexible) creating geometrical distortion
- Failure to orientate the image receptor correctly and using it back to front
- Failure to align the X-ray tubehead correctly in the horizontal plane causing:
  - coning off or cone cutting
  - overlapping and geometrical distortion
  - superimposition
- Failure to align the X-ray tubehead correctly in the vertical plane causing:
  - coning off or cone cutting
  - foreshortening and geometrical distortion
  - elongation and geometrical distortion
- Failure to instruct the patient to remain still during the exposure with subsequent movement resulting in blurring

- Failure to set correct exposure settings (image too dark or too pale – see earlier)
- Careless inadvertent use of the image receptor twice.

Panoramic technique errors

These can include:

- Failure to remove jewellery
- Failure to remove dentures
- Failure to remove orthodontic appliances
- Failure to remove spectacles
- Inappropriate use of a protective lead apron
- Failure to ensure the spine is straight
- Failure to ensure the incisors are biting on the bite-peg (anteroposterior error)
- Failure to use the light beam markers to ensure midsagittal plane is vertical and Frankfort plane is horizontal (horizontal and vertical errors)
- Failure to instruct the patient to press the tongue against the roof of the mouth
- Failure to instruct the patient to remain still throughout the exposure cycle
- Failure to set machine height adjustment correctly
- Failure to set correct exposure settings (image too dark or too pale – see earlier)
- Failure to use the cassette/image receptor correctly.

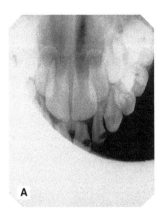 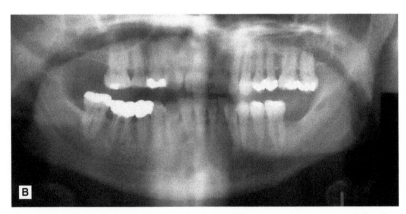

Fig. 14.6 Two examples of positioning (radiographic technique) errors. **A** Intraoral – *coning off* or *cone cutting* – X-ray tubehead incorrectly positioned, anterior part of image receptor not exposed. **B** Panoramic – patient too far away from the image receptor – incisor teeth magnified (anteroposterior error) and patient rotated to the LEFT, left molars narrowed, right molars widened (horizontal error).

Quality assurance in dental radiology

The World Health Organization has defined radiographic quality assurance (QA) programmes as '... an organised effort by the staff operating a facility to ensure that the diagnostic images produced by the facility are of sufficiently high quality so that they consistently provide adequate diagnostic information at the lowest possible cost and with the least possible exposure of the patient to radiation'.

Quality control measures are therefore as essential in a general dental practice *facility,* as they are in a specialized radiography department. This importance of **quality** is acknowledged in the UK in the Ionising Radiations Regulations 1999, which make quality assurance in dental radiography a mandatory requirement. This chapter is based broadly on the recommendations *Guidance Notes for Dental Practitioners on the Safe Use of X-ray Equipment.*

Terminology

The main terms in quality procedures include:

- *Quality control* – the specific measures for ensuring and verifying the quality of the radiographs produced
- *Quality assurance* – the arrangements to ensure that the quality control procedures are effective and that they lead to relevant change and improvement
- *Quality audit* – the process of external reassurance and assessment that quality control and quality assurance mechanisms are satisfactory and that they work effectively.

Quality assurance programme

A basic principle of quality assurance is that, within the overall QA programme, all necessary procedures should be laid down in writing and in particular:

- Implementation should be the responsibility of a named person.
- Frequency of operations should be defined.
- The content of the essential supporting records should be defined and the frequency for the formal checking of such records.

As stated in the 2001 *Guidance Notes* and implied by the WHO definition, a well-designed QA programme should be comprehensive but inexpensive to operate and maintain. The standards should be well researched but once laid down would be expected to require only infrequent verification or modification. The procedures should amount to little more than 'written down common sense'. The aims of these programmes can be summarized as follows:

- To produce diagnostic radiographs of consistently high standard
- To reduce the number of repeat radiographs
- To determine all sources of error to allow their correction
- To increase efficiency
- To reduce costs
- To ensure that radiation doses to patients and staff are kept as low as reasonably practicable (ALARP).

Quality control procedures for film-based radiography

The essential quality control procedures relate to:

- Image quality and film reject analysis
- Patient dose and X-ray equipment
- Darkroom, image receptors and processing
- Working procedures
- Staff training and updating
- Audits.

Image quality and film reject analysis

Image quality assessment is an important test of the entire QA programme. Hence the need for clinicians to be aware of all the various factors, outlined earlier, that affect image quality and to monitor it on a regular basis. This assessment should include:

- A day-to-day comparison of the quality of every radiograph to a high standard reference film positioned permanently on the viewing screen and an investigation of any significant deterioration in quality.
- A formal analysis of film quality, either retrospective or prospective, approximately every 6 months. The 2001 *Guidance Notes* recommended the simple three-point subjective rating scale shown in Table 14.2, and shown previously in Chapters 7, 8 and 12, be used for film-based intraoral and extraoral dental radiography.
- Based on these quality ratings, performance targets can be set. Suitable targets recommended in the *Guidance Notes* are shown in Table 14.3 with the advice that practices should aim to achieve these targets within 3 years of implementing the QA programme. The 'interim targets' should be regarded as the minimum achievable standard in the shorter term.
- Analysis of all unacceptable films given a rating of 3, sometimes referred to as *film reject analysis* (see below).

Film reject analysis

This is a simple method of identifying all film faults and sources of error and amounts to a *register of reject radiographs*. To do this, it is necessary to collect all rejected (grade 3) radiographs and record:

- Date
- Nature of the film fault/error, as shown earlier, e.g.:
  - Film too dark
  - Film too pale
  - Low or poor contrast
  - Unsharp image
  - Poor positioning
- Known or suspected cause of the error or fault and corrective action taken (see Table 14.1)
- Number of repeat radiographs (if taken)
- Total number of radiographs taken during the same time period. This allows the percentage of faulty films to be calculated.

Regular review of film reject analysis records is an invaluable aid for identifying a range of problems, including a need for equipment maintenance,

additional staff training as well as processing faults that could otherwise cause unnecessary radiation exposure of patients and staff.

Patient dose and X-ray equipment

One of the aims of quality assurance stated earlier is to ensure that radiation doses are kept as low as reasonably practicable. X-ray equipment must comply with national current recommendations. Dental care professionals should familiarize themselves with the equipment and the supporting documentation. Typical equipment QA measures include:

- An initial *critical examination and report* – carried out by the installer
- An *acceptance test* – carried out by the radiation protection adviser/medical physicist before equipment is brought into clinical use, which should include measurement of patient dose

Table 14.2 Subjective quality rating criteria for film-captured images published in 2001 *Guidance Notes for Dental Practitioners on the Safe Use of X-ray Equipment*

Rating	Quality	Basis
1	Excellent	No errors of patient preparation, exposure, positioning, processing or film handling
2	Diagnostically acceptable	Some errors of patient preparation, exposure, positioning, processing or film handling, but which do not detract from the diagnostic utility of the radiograph
3	Unacceptable	Errors of patient preparation, exposure, positioning, processing or film handling, which render the radiograph diagnostically unacceptable

Table 14.3 Minimum and interim targets for radiographic quality from the 2001 *Guidance Notes**

Rating	Target	Interim target
1	Not less than 70%	Not less than 50%
2	Not greater than 20%	Not greater than 40%
3	Not greater than 10%	Not greater than 10%

*Percentage of radiographs taken.

- A *re-examination report* following any relocation, repair or modification of equipment that may have radiation protection implications
- Regular checks of important features that could affect radiation protection, including:
  - correct functioning of warning lights and audible alarms
  - correct operation of safety devices
  - satisfactory performance of the counterbalance for maintaining the correct position of the tubehead
  - correct alignment of the beam collimation
  - X-ray equipment output. This can be performed in dental practice using one of the recently developed devices shown in Fig. 14.7.
- Written records and an equipment log should be maintained and include:
  - all installer's formal written reports describing the checks made, the results obtained and action taken
  - results of all equipment checks in chronological order
  - details of all routine or special maintenance
- An up-to-date inventory of each item of X-ray equipment should be maintained, and available, at each practice and contains:
  - name of the manufacturer
  - model number

- serial number or other unique identifier
- year of manufacture
- year of installation
- Compliance with any national medical physics recommendations, for example in the UK the *Recommended Standards for the Routine Performance Testing of Diagnostic X-ray Imaging Systems*, Report 91 of the Institute of Physics and Engineering in Medicine (IPEM) published in 2005.

Darkroom, image receptors and processing
Darkroom

The QA programme should include instructions on all the regular checks that should be made, and how frequently, with all results recorded in a log. Important areas include:

- General cleanliness (daily), but particularly of work surfaces and film hangers (if used)
- Light-tightness (yearly), by standing in the darkroom in total darkness with the door closed and safelights switched off and visually inspecting for light leakage
- Safelights (yearly), to ensure that these do not cause fogging of films. Checks are required on:
  - Type of filter – this should be compatible with the colour sensitivity of film used, i.e. blue, green or ultraviolet (see Ch. 3)

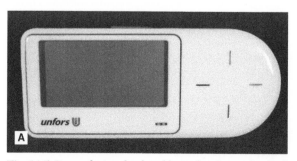

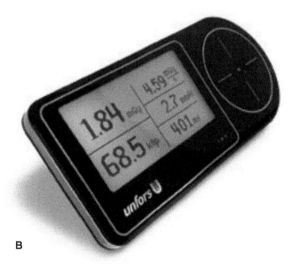

Fig. 14.7 Recent devices developed by Unfors for regular checks on X-ray equipment output. **A** The Raysafe to simply check satisfactory output and **B** the more complex Thin-X that produces actual measurements of output. (Kindly provided by Mr Mark Chapman).

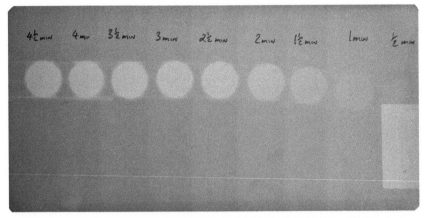

Fig. 14.8 An example of the coin test. The film, with nine coins on it, has been gradually uncovered every 30 seconds. The coin-covered part of the film remains white while the surrounding film is blackened or fogged. The longer the film is exposed to the safelight the darker it becomes.

- Condition of filters – scratched filters should be replaced
- Wattage of the bulb – ideally it should be no more than 25 W
- Their distance from the work surface – ideally they should be at least 1.2 m (4 ft) away
- Overall safety (i.e. their fogging effect on film) – the simple quality control measure for doing this is known as the *coin test*:
  1. Expose a piece of screen film in a cassette to a very small even exposure of X-rays (so-called *flash* exposure) to make the emulsion ultrasensitive to subsequent light exposure.
  2. In the darkroom, remove the film from the cassette and place on the worksurface underneath the turned-off safelight.
  3. Place a series of coins (e.g. seven) in a row on the film and cover them all with a piece of card.
  4. Turn on the safelight and then slide the card to reveal the first coin and leave for approximately 30 seconds.
  5. Slide the card along to reveal the second coin and leave again for approximately 30 seconds.
  6. Repeat until all the coins have been revealed.
  7. Process the film in the normal way.

A typical result is shown in Fig. 14.8. Fogging (blackening) of the film owing to the safelight will then be obvious when compared to the clear area protected by the coin. The part of the film adjacent to the first coin will have been exposed to the safelight for the longest time and will be the darkest. In practice, the normal film-handling time under the safelight can be measured and the effect of safelight fogging established.

Note: The *coin test* can also be used to assess the amount of light transmission through the safety glass of automatic processors by performing the test within the processor under the safety glass under normal daylight loading conditions.

Image receptors
The QA programme requires written information, usually obtained from the suppliers, on film speed, expiry date and storage conditions as well as details regarding the maintenance and cleaning instructions of cassettes and intensifying screens. Typical requirements could include:

X-ray film requires:
- Ideal storage conditions – cool, dry and away from all sources of ionizing radiation – as recommended by the manufacturers
- Strict stock control with records to ensure usage before the expiry date
- Careful handling.

Cassettes require:
- Regular cleaning of intensifying screens with a proprietary cleaner

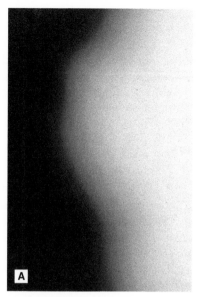

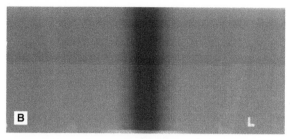

Fig. 14.9B An example of a panoramic image following the graph paper test for film/screen contact. Good film screen contact enables the detailed pattern of the graph paper to be seen.

Fig. 14.9A Radiograph from a faulty cassette being checked for light-tightness. The light that has got into the cassette has blackened one side of the film.

Chemical solutions. These should be:

- Always made up to the manufacturers' instructions taking special precautions to avoid even trace amounts of contamination of the developer by the fixer, e.g. always fill the fixer tank first so that any splashes into the developer tank can be washed away **before** pouring in the developer
- Always at the correct temperature
- Changed or replenished regularly – ideally every 2 weeks – and records should be kept to control and validate these changes
- Monitored for deterioration. This can be done easily using radiographs of a *step-wedge phantom:*
    1. Make a simple step-wedge phantom using the lead foil from inside intraoral film packets, as shown in Fig. 14.10.

- Regular checks for light-tightness, as follows:
    1. Load a cassette with an unexposed film and place the cassette on a window sill in the daylight for a few minutes.
    2. Process the film – any ingress of light will have fogged (darkened) the film (see Fig. 14.9A).
- Regular checks for film/screen contact, as follows:
    1. Load a cassette with an unexposed film and a similar sized piece of graph paper.
    2. Expose the cassette to X-rays using a very short exposure time.
    3. Process the film – any areas of poor film/screen contact will be demonstrated by loss of definition of the image of the graph paper (see Fig. 14.9B).
- A simple method of identification of films taken in similar-looking cassettes, e.g. a Letraset letter on one screen.

Processing

The QA programme should contain written instructions about each of the following:

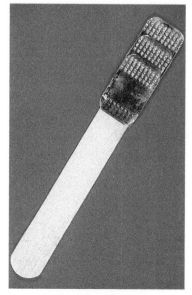

Fig. 14.10 A simple step-wedge phantom constructed using pieces of lead foil taped to a tongue spatula.

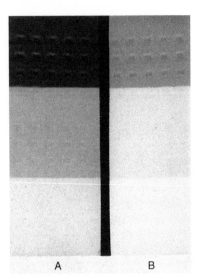

Fig. 14.11 A The *standard reference* film of the step-wedge phantom on DAY ONE processed using newly made-up chemical solutions. **B** Test film processed in chemical solutions 1 week old – note the reduced amount of blackening of the second film owing to the weakened action of the developer.

2. Radiograph the step-wedge using known exposure factors.
3. Process the film in **fresh** solutions to produce a *standard reference film*.
4. Repeat, using the same exposure factors, every day as the solutions become exhausted.
5. Compare each day's film with the standard reference film to determine objectively any decrease in blackening of the processed film which would indicate deterioration of the developer (see Fig. 14.11).
6. Record the results.

Processing equipment

- Manual processing requires the use of accurate timers, thermometers and immersion heaters. Instructions on their proper use should be provided.
- Automatic processors require regular replenishment of chemical solutions and regular cleaning, especially of the rollers. All cleaning procedures should be written down including how often they should be carried out.
- Record log confirming that all cleaning procedures have been carried out should be kept.

Working procedures

These include:

- *Local rules* – required in the UK under the Ionising Radiations Regulations 1999 (see Ch. 6). These rules should contain the procedural and operational elements that are essential to the safe use of X-ray equipment, including guidance on exposure times, and as such should contain much of what is relevant to the maintenance of good standards in QA.
- Employers' *written procedures* – required in the UK under the Ionising Radiation (Medical Exposure) Regulations 2000.
- *Operational procedures or systems of work* – these include written procedures that provide for all actions that indirectly affect radiation safety and diagnostic quality, e.g. instructions for the correct preparation and subsequent use of processing chemicals (as explained earlier).
- *Procedures log* – the QA programme should include the maintenance of a procedures log to record the existence of appropriate *Local Rules* and *Employers' Written Procedures*, together with a record of each occasion on which they are reviewed or modified (ideally every 12 months).

Staff training and updating

It is a legal requirement in the UK and many other countries that all practitioners and operators (dental care professionals) are adequately trained and that continuing professional development (CPD) is undertaken. The QA programme should incorporate a register of all staff involved with any aspect of radiography and should include the following information:

- Name
- Responsibility
- Date, nature and details of training received
- Recommended date for a review of training needs.

Audits

Each procedure within the QA programme will include a requirement for written records to be made by the responsible person at varying intervals. In addition, the person with overall responsibility for the QA programme should check the full programme at intervals not exceeding 12 months. This is an essential feature of demonstrating effective implementation of the programme. Clinical audits may include:

- The QA programme and associated records
- The justification and authorization of radiographs
- The appropriateness of requests/investigations
- The clinical evaluation of radiographs.

Digital image quality

As with film-based image quality described earlier, digital image quality and the amount of detail shown on a digital radiographic image depends on several factors, including:

- Subject contrast – the black/white and grey difference in the visual caused by different degrees of attenuation as the X-ray beam is transmitted through different parts of the patient's tissues and dependent upon:
  - Differences in tissue thickness
  - Differences in tissue density
  - Difference in tissue atomic number
  - Quality of the X-ray beam
- Image geometry – the geometric accuracy of any image depends upon the position of the X-ray beam, object and image receptor satisfying certain basic geometrical requirements:
  - The object and the digital image receptor should be in contact or as close together as possible
  - The object and the digital image receptor should be parallel to one another
  - The X-ray tubehead should be positioned so that the X-ray beam meets both the object and the digital image receptor at right angles
- Characteristics of the X-ray beam – the beam should be:
  - Sufficiently penetrating to pass through the patient, to a varying degree, to interact differentially with the digital image receptor

(solid-state or phosphor plate) to produce a good contrasted black/white/grey image
  - Parallel, i.e. non-diverging, to prevent magnification of the image (see Ch. 3)
  - Produced from a point source to reduce blurring of the image margins and the penumbra effect (see Ch. 3)
- Type of digital image receptor – solid-state or phosphor plate and their resolution and ability to define image sharpness (see Ch. 3)
- Quality of viewing monitor (see Ch. 16)
- Image enhancement software (see Ch. 3).

Practical factors influencing digital image quality

In practical terms, the various factors that can influence overall digital image quality can be divided into factors related to:

- The X-ray equipment
- The image receptor – solid-state or phosphor plate
- Image processing and manipulation using computer software (see Ch. 3)
- The patient
- The operator and the radiographic technique
- The quality of the viewing monitor (see Ch. 16).

As a result of all these variables, digital image faults and alterations in digital image quality are inevitable and not all these faults can be corrected by manipulating the image using image enhancement software, as described in Chapter 3. Quality assurance (QA) programmes are still required.

Dentists and dental care professionals using digital imaging need to be able to recognize the cause of the various image faults so that appropriate corrective action can be taken.

Typical digital image faults

Examples of some typical digital image faults, other than those as a result of poor radiographic technique described in Chapters 7, 8 and 12, are shown below.

Solid-state detectors

Faults include:

- *Blooming* – caused by overexposure and overloading/flooding the CCDs
- Cracked sensor
- Sensor used back to front
- Loss of uniformity.

(See Figs 14.12–14.14.)

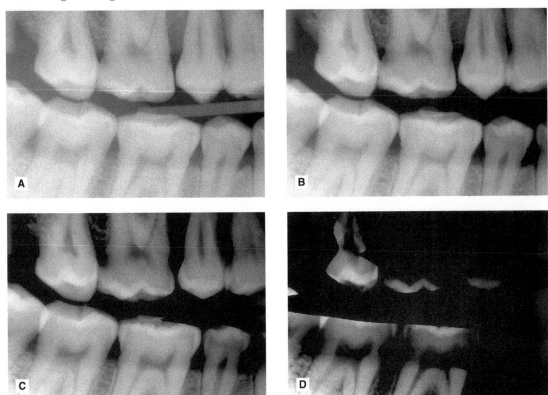

Fig. 14.12 The effect of *blooming*. Four bitewing images taken using a CCD solid-state sensor. **A** Underexposed. **B** Ideally exposed. **C** Overexposed. **D** Considerably overexposed. In images C and D some of the CCDs have become over-loaded or flooded and parts of the image have become completely black. Blooming cannot be reversed by using image manipulation software. (Kindly provided by Mr Jonathan Davies.)

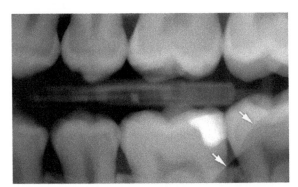

Fig. 14.13 Example of a bitewing radiograph taken using a solid-state detector that has been dropped and cracked (arrowed). (Kindly provided by Mr Jonathan Davies.)

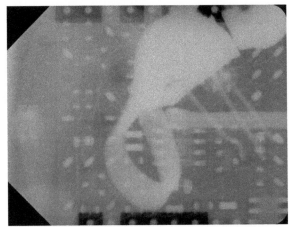

Fig. 14.14 Example of the resultant image when a solid-state sensor is used back to front rendering the internal electronics visible.

Photostimulable phosphor plates

Faults include:

- Phosphor plate used back-to-front
- Light leakage/fogging
- Debris on the plate
- Scratched plate
- Loss of uniformity.

(See Figs 14.15–14.18.)

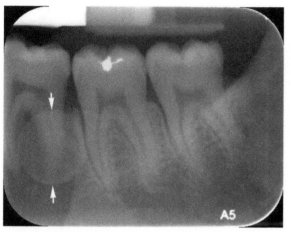

Fig. 14.15 Example of the resultant image when a Digora phosphor plate is used back to front. The circular shadow cast by the magnet is visible (arrowed). (Kindly provided by Mr Jonathan Davies.)

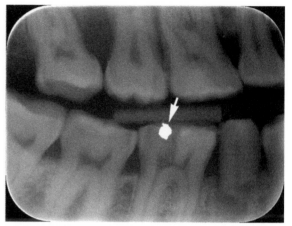

Fig. 14.17 Example of a bitewing radiograph taken with a dirty phosphor plate (see also Fig. 14.20C). The debris on the plate results in an opaque artefact (arrowed).

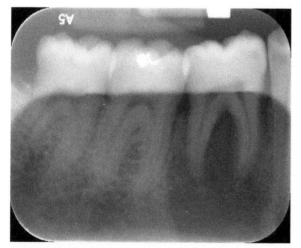

Fig. 14.16 Example of a light-fogged phosphor plate image. The top part of the image was exposed to light which has partially cleared the image before the plate was placed in the reader. (Kindly provided by Mr Jonathan Davies.)

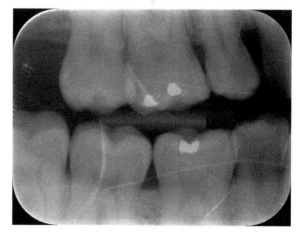

Fig. 14.18 Example of a bitewing taken with a scratched phosphor plate (see also Fig. 14.20B and D).

Computer software malfunction

As with any computer software, occasional glitches and malfunctions happen. When they do, the digital image can be completely distorted, as shown in Fig. 14.19.

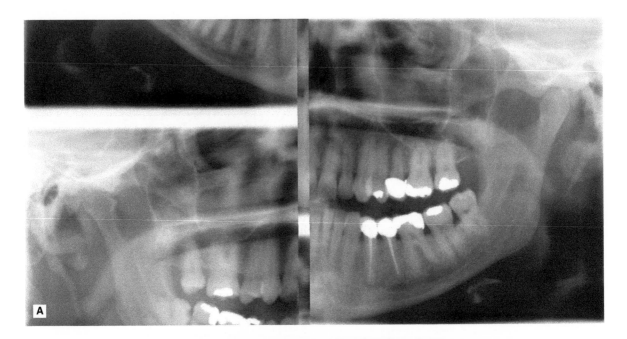

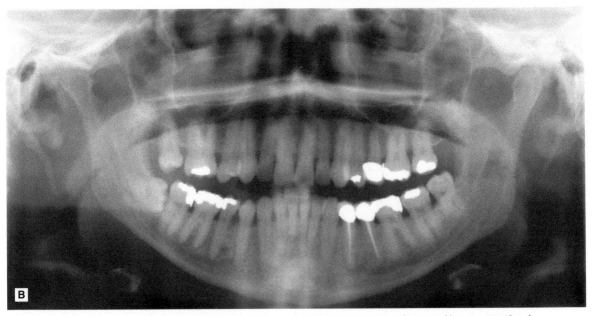

Fig. 14.19 A Example of a grossly distorted panoramic image resulting from a computer software malfunction. **B** What the panoramic should have looked like! (Kindly provided by Mr John Llewellyn.)

Quality control procedures for digital radiography

The overall quality control procedures for digital radiography are similar, and in some instances identical, to those required for film-based radiography. They relate to:

- Image quality assessment
- Patient dose and X-ray equipment
- Image processing and manipulation
- Working procedures
- Staff training and updating
- Audits.

Those QA procedures specifically relevant to digital imaging, including digital image quality assessment and digital equipment, are described below.

Table 14.4 Suggested subjective quality rating criteria for digitally captured images

Rating	Quality	Basis
1	Excellent	No errors of patient preparation, positioning or digital receptor handling
2	Diagnostically acceptable	Some errors in patient preparation, positioning or digital receptor handling but which do not detract from the diagnostic utility of the image
3	Unacceptable	Errors of patient preparation, positioning, digital receptor handling or exposure (which cannot be corrected by computer software) which render the image diagnostically unacceptable

Digital image quality assessment and image reject analysis

This assessment should include:

- Investigation of any significant deterioration in quality and instigation of appropriate corrective action
- Recording all investigations together with the identified cause of deterioration and the action taken
- Regular annotation (approx. every 3 months) of the image quality record to indicate that the day-to-day checks have been carried out and, where appropriate, that no significant deterioration in image quality has been observed
- Subjective assessment of the quality of each radiograph. The NRPB/DoH's 2001 guidelines recommended a simple three-point scale for film that can be used, but the basis of the decision needs to be amended (Table 14.4).

All images should be assessed in this way and the results recorded so that the overall quality of radiography can be evaluated and measured against the NRPB/DoH targets (see earlier in Table 14.3).

Image reject analysis

Assess all rejected (category 3) images and record:

- Date
- Nature of the digital image fault/error, as shown earlier, e.g.:
  - Image too dark, e.g. 'blooming'
  - Image too pale – sensor underexposed
  - Image marked – sensor damaged
  - Unsharp or blurred image – patient movement
  - Poor positioning
- Known or suspected cause of the error or fault and corrective action taken
- Number of repeat images (if taken).

Digital equipment

Solid-state sensors

These require:

- Regular checks to ensure no evidence of cracks or damage to the cable and sensor casing (see Fig. 14.20A)
- Regular assessment for non-uniformity of receptor.

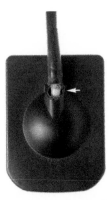

Fig. 14.20 A solid-state detector showing damage to the cable (arrowed) (kindly provided by Peter Ash).

Phosphor plates

These require:

- Regular checks for visible scratches and dirt (see Figs 14.21)
- Being passed daily through the reader to detect scratches (see Fig. 14.21)
- Regular cleaning following the manufacturer's instructions
- Regular assessment for non-uniformity of receptor (see Fig. 14.21).

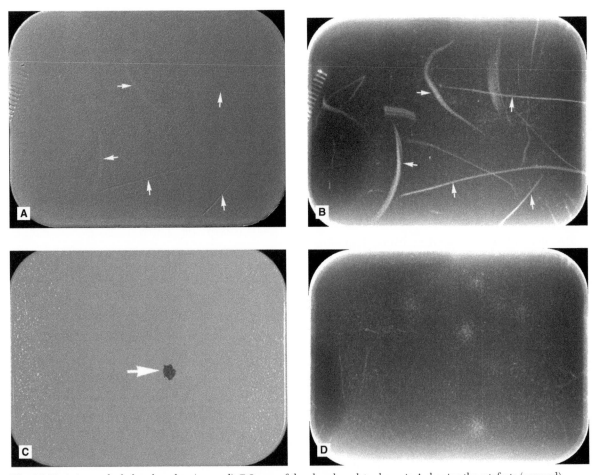

Fig. 14.21 A A scratched phosphor plate (arrowed). **B** Image of the phosphor plate shown in **A** showing the artefacts (arrowed) created by the scratches. **C** Debris on a phosphor plate (arrowed) (see also Fig. 17.16). **D** Image showing the result of a uniformity test on a photostimulable phosphor plate. There are several regions of non-uniformity as well as several scratches. This image receptor has failed the test and should not be put back into clinical use.

Monitors

These require

- Regular cleaning
- Regular QA calibration/checks for distortion, grey scale reproduction, limiting resolution (at both high and low contrast) and uniformity. This can be done using specific test patterns designed for this purpose such as the Technical Group 18 QC (TG18-QC) test pattern produced by the American Association of Physicists in Medicine, as shown in Fig. 14.22A or the SMPTE test pattern designed by the Society of Motion Pictures and Television Engineers, as shown in Fig. 14.22B. Alternatively, specifically designed QA calibration tools and software can be used, as shown in Fig. 14.22C.

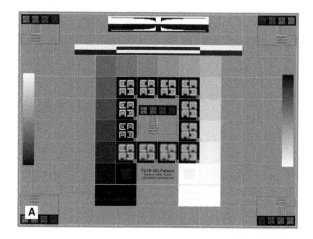

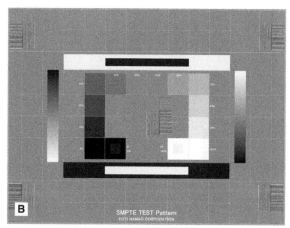

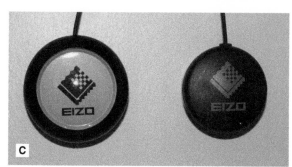

Fig. 14.22 A The TG18-QC monitor test pattern (kindly provided by the American Association of Physicists in Medicine) and **B** the SMPTE monitor test pattern (kindly provided by SMPTE www.smpte.org). **C** The specially designed EIZO QA calibration tools – RadiCS™ RX1 and RadiCS™ UX1 – for use with appropriate software.

Footnote

The requirement for quality assurance and quality control measures, for both film-based and digital imaging, in general dental practice applies equally to specialized hospital radiography departments. However, in view of the cost implications, the expensive, sophisticated equipment, available for precise quality assurance measurements and monitoring used in hospital X-ray departments, is often inappropriate to general dental practice. The practical suggestions in this chapter are designed to satisfy the WHO definition of QA by bringing an element of objectivity to quality assurance in practice, but at the same time being simple, easily done and inexpensive.

To access the self assessment questions for this chapter please go to www.whaitesessentialsdentalradiography.com

Radiographic assessment and localization of unerupted maxillary canines

Assessment of unerupted maxillary canines

The upper canines are often misplaced and fail to erupt as a result of their long path of eruption, the timing of their eruption and the frequency of upper arch overcrowding. Many of the factors that influence the treatment of this anomaly can be obtained from the radiographic assessment, the purpose of which is two-fold:

- To determine the size and shape of the canine and any related disease
- To determine the position of the canine.

Assessment of the canine size and shape and the surrounding tissues

Radiographic views used (see Fig. 15.1)

The usual radiographs used include:

- Periapicals
- Upper standard occlusal
- Panoramic radiograph.

Radiographic interpretation

The specific features that need to be examined relate to:

- The crown
- The root
- Surrounding structures.

Note: These views, on their own, do not provide information as to the position of the canines.

The crown
Note in particular:

- Crown size (in relation to the space available in the arch)
- Crown shape
- The presence and severity of resorption
- The presence of any related disease, such as a dentigerous cyst
- The effect on adjacent teeth, such as resorption.

The root
Note in particular:

- Root size
- Root shape
- Stage of development.

Surrounding structures
Note in particular:

- The deciduous canine
  - root length
  - degree of resorption
- The presence of an odontome or supernumerary
- The condition of the surrounding bone.

Assessment of the position of the canine – localization

There are several methods available for localization. They can be used for canines and other unerupted teeth as well as odontomes and

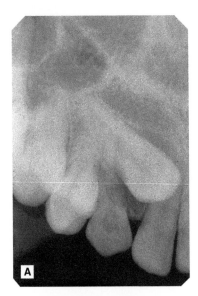

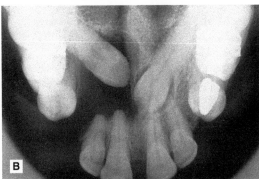

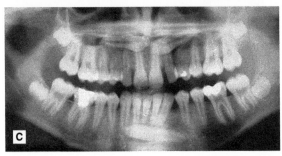

Fig. 15.1 Examples of the radiographs used typically to assess unerupted canines and the surrounding structures. **A** Periapical showing unerupted 3| with retained. **B** Upper standard occlusal showing both upper canines unerupted, a dentigerous cyst associated with 3|, extensive destruction of the alveolar bone and resorption of |3. **C** Panoramic radiograph showing unerupted 3|3 and |3.

supernumeraries. Although emphasis in this section is on canines, examples of localization of other unerupted developmental anomalies are also shown.

Main localization methods

- Parallax in the horizontal plane
- Parallax in the vertical plane
- Cross-sectional tomography
- Cone beam CT (see Ch. 13).

The principle of parallax

Parallax is defined as *the apparent displacement of an object because of different positions of the observer.* In other words, if two objects, in two separate planes, are viewed from two different positions, the objects will appear to move in different directions in relation to one another, from one view to the next, as shown in Fig. 15.2.

Using the principle of parallax, if two views of an unerupted canine are taken with the X-ray tubehead in two different positions, the resultant radiographs will show a difference in the position of the unerupted canine relative to the incisors, as follows:

- If the canine is **palatally** positioned, it will appear to have moved in the *same* direction as the X-ray tubehead.
- If the canine is **buccally** positioned, it will appear to have moved in the **opposite** direction to the X-ray tubehead.
- If the unerupted canine is in the **same plane** as the incisors, i.e. in the line of the arch, it will appear **not to have moved** at all.

A useful acronym to remember the movements of parallax is SLOB, standing for:

Same
Lingual
Opposite
Buccal.

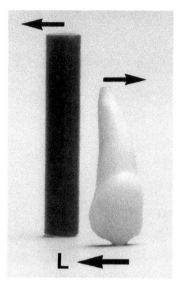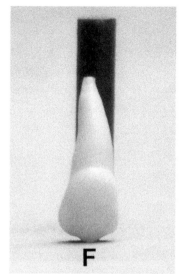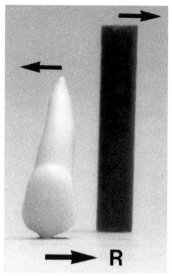

Fig. 15.2 The principle of parallax. Photographs of a small black cylinder positioned behind a tooth. From directly in front (F), the tooth and cylinder are superimposed. With the camera moved to the left (L), the tooth and cylinder are both visible and appear to have moved in different directions. The cylinder, being further away from the camera, appears to have moved in the same direction as the camera, i.e. to the left, while the tooth appears to have moved in the opposite direction. With the camera moved to the right (R) a similar apparent movement of the tooth and cylinder relative to the camera takes place, with the cylinder appearing to have moved to the right and the tooth to the left.

Parallax in the horizontal plane

The movement of the X-ray tubehead is in the horizontal plane, for example:

- 2 periapicals – one centred on the upper central incisor and the other centred on the canine region, as shown in Fig. 15.3
- An upper standard occlusal, centred in the midline plus a periapical or an upper oblique occlusal, centred on the canine region.

Examples are shown in Figs 15.4–15.6.

Note: The advantage of the upper standard occlusal for the initial view is that it shows both sides of the arch and unerupted canines are often bilateral.

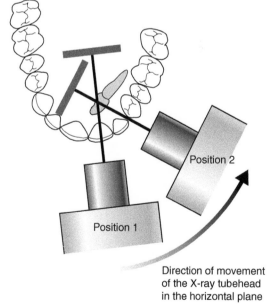

Direction of movement
of the X-ray tubehead
in the horizontal plane

Fig. 15.3 Diagram showing the two different tubehead positions required for parallax in the horizontal plane: Position (1) centres on the upper central incisor. Position (2) centres on the canine region.

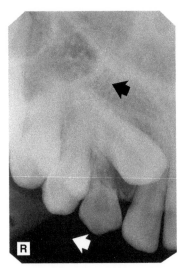
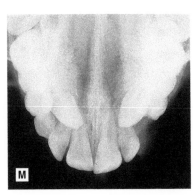
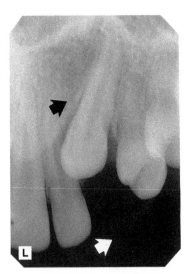

Fig. 15.4 An upper standard occlusal (the midline view) and two periapicals centred on the unerupted canines on either side. The teeth can be localized as follows:

1. Examine the midline view radiograph (M), centred on the upper central incisors. The tip of the RIGHT canine appears opposite the root canal of 1|; the tip of the LEFT canine appears opposite the mesial aspect |2.
2. Examine radiograph (R), the periapical centred on the RIGHT canine region (i.e. the X-ray tubehead has been moved distally in the direction of the white arrow). The tip of the canine appears opposite the mesial aspect of |2|. Therefore, it appears to have moved distally in the direction of the black arrow, i.e. in the *same* direction as the X-ray tubehead was moved.
3. Examine radiograph (L), the periapical centred on the LEFT canine region. The tip of the canine appears opposite the root canal of |2. Again both the X-ray tubehead (white arrow) and the canine (black arrow) appear to have moved in the *same* direction.
Thus the crowns of both the right and left canines are *palatally* positioned in relation to the incisors.

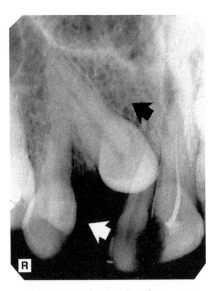
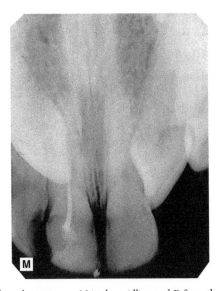

Fig. 15.5 Two periapicals showing the relative positions of the unerupted 3| to the incisors – M in the midline and R from the right. The X-ray tubehead (white arrow) and the canine (black arrow) appear to have moved in the *same* direction. The canine is thus palatally positioned.

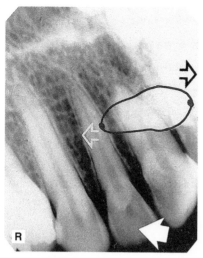 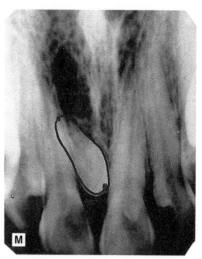

Fig. 15.6 Two periapicals showing an unerupted mesiodens. It can be localized as follows:

1. Examine the midline radiograph (M). The tip of the mesiodens' crown appears opposite the mesial aspect of $\underline{1}$, while its apex appears opposite the root canal of $\underline{1}$.
2. Examine the periapical centred on the RIGHT canine region (R). The tip of the mesiodens crown appears opposite the root canal of $\underline{1}$, while its apex appears opposite the mesial aspect of $\underline{2}$.
3. The X-ray tubehead was moved distally in the direction of the large white solid arrow.
4. The crown of the mesiodens appears to have moved mesially (black open arrow), i.e. in the *opposite* direction to the tubehead. It is thus buccally placed.
5. The apex appears to have moved in the *same* direction (white open arrow) as the tubehead and is thus palatally placed. The mesiodens thus lies across the arch, between the central incisors, with its crown buccally positioned and its apex palatally positioned.

Parallax in the vertical plane

The movement of the X-ray tubehead is in the vertical plane, for example:

- A panoramic radiograph – the X-ray beam is aimed upwards at 8° to the horizontal
- An upper standard occlusal – the X-ray beam is aimed downwards at 65°–70°

to the horizontal, as shown in Figs 15.7 and 15.8.

Note: This combination of views is used frequently in orthodontics, when patients with unerupted canines are usually assessed. Use of these films to their full potential may obviate the need for further films merely to localize the unerupted canines.

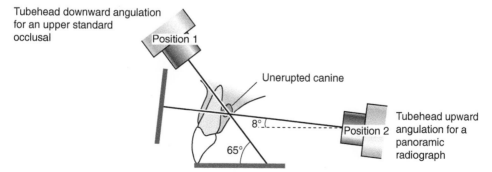

Fig. 15.7 Diagram showing the two different tubehead positions when taking a panoramic radiograph and an upper standard occlusal, allowing parallax in the vertical plane.

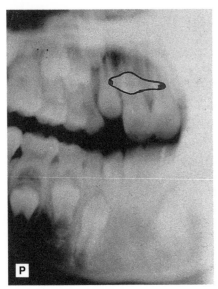
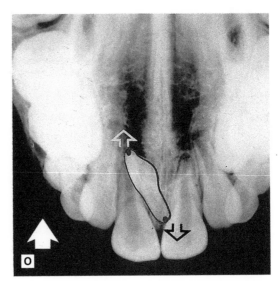

Fig. 15.8 Part of a panoramic radiograph and an upper standard occlusal showing an unerupted mesiodens. It can be localized as follows:

1. Examine the panoramic radiograph (P) taken with the tubehead aimed upwards at 8° to the horizontal. The tip of mesiodens' crown appears opposite the neck of the lateral incisor, while its apex appears opposite the root of 1̲ .
2. Examine the occlusal radiograph (O) taken with the tubehead aimed downwards at 65° to the horizontal. The tip of the mesiodens' crown now appears beyond the apex of 2̲ , while its apex now appears opposite the crown of 1̲ .
3. The X-ray tubehead has moved vertically upwards from view (P) to view (O) in the direction of the solid white arrow.
4. The crown of the mesiodens appears to have moved in the *same* direction (white open arrow) and is thus palatally placed.
5. The apex of the mesiodens appears to have moved in the *opposite* direction (black open arrow), and is thus buccally placed. The mesiodens thus lies across the arch between the central incisors, with its crown palatally positioned and its apex buccally positioned.

Localization using cross-sectional tomography and cone beam CT (see Ch. 13)

Localization of unerupted developmental anomalies using these more modern advanced imaging modalities is straightforward, if the facilities are available. They allow visualization of the unerupted abnormality in different planes. There is no need to use the principles of parallax. Two examples are shown in Figs 15.9 and 15.10.

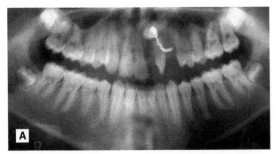
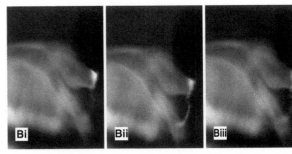

Fig. 15.9 A Panoramic radiograph and **B** three 2 mm cross-sectional tomographs showing the relative positions of bucally placed unerupted left canine (with orthodontic chain attached) and the left lateral incisor. The two teeth are clearly separated and there is no evidence of root resorption of the lateral incisor.

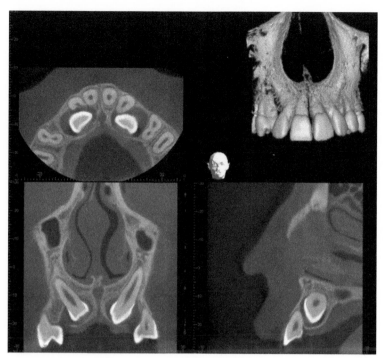

Fig. 15.10 Small volume CBCT showing palatally positioned maxillary canines.

To access the self assessment questions for this chapter please go to www.whaitesessentialsdentalradiography.com

Radiology

Part 4

16 Introduction to radiological interpretation

Interpretation of radiographs can be regarded as an unravelling process – uncovering all the information contained within the black, white and grey radiographic images. The main objectives are:

- To identify the presence or absence of disease
- To provide information on the nature and extent of the disease
- To enable the formation of a differential diagnosis.

To achieve these objectives and maximize the diagnostic yield, interpretation should be carried out under specified conditions, following ordered, systematic guidelines.

Unfortunately, interpretation is often limited to a cursory glance under totally inappropriate conditions. It is easy to fall victim to the problems and pitfalls produced by *spot diagnosis* and *tunnel vision*. This is in spite of knowing that in most cases radiographs are the main diagnostic aid.

This chapter provides an introductory approach to show dental care professionals how radiographs should be interpreted, specifying the viewing conditions required and suggesting systematic guidelines.

Essential requirements for interpretation

The essential requirements for interpreting dental radiographs can be summarized as follows:

- Optimum viewing conditions
- Understanding the nature and limitations of the black, white and grey radiographic image
- Knowledge of what the radiographs used in dentistry should look like, enabling a critical assessment of individual image quality

- Detailed knowledge of the range of radiographic appearances of normal anatomical structures
- Detailed knowledge of the radiographic appearances of the pathological conditions affecting the head and neck
- A systematic approach to viewing the entire radiograph and to viewing and describing specific lesions
- Access to previous images for comparison.

Optimum viewing conditions

For film-captured images these include:

- An even, uniform, bright light viewing screen (preferably of variable intensity to allow viewing of films of different densities) (see Fig. 16.1)
- A quiet, darkened viewing room
- The area around the radiograph should be masked by a dark surround so that light passes only through the film
- Use of a magnifying glass to allow fine detail to be seen more clearly on intraoral films
- The radiographs should be dry.

These ideal viewing conditions give the observer the best chance of perceiving all the detail contained within the radiographic image. With many simultaneous external stimuli, such as extraneous light and inadequate viewing conditions, the amount of information obtained from the radiograph is reduced. Radiographs should be viewed once they have dried as films still wet from processing may show some distortion of the image.

Digital images should be viewed on bright, high-resolution monitors in subdued lighting (see Fig. 16.2).

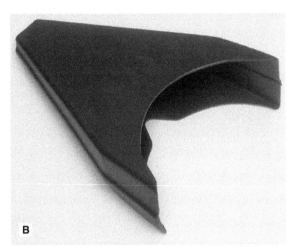

Fig. 16.1 A Wardray viewing box incorporating an additional central bright-light source for viewing overexposed dark films. **B** The SDI X-ray reader – an extraneous light excluding intraoral film viewer with built-in magnification.

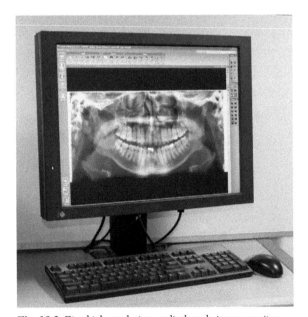

Fig. 16.2 Eizo high-resolution medical grade image monitor.

The nature and limitations of the radiographic images

The importance of understanding the nature of different types of radiographic images – film-captured or digital (depending on the type of image receptor used) – and their specific limitations was explained in Chapter 1. How the visual images are created by processing – chemical or computer – was explained in Chapter 3. Revision of both these chapters is recommended. To reiterate, the final image, whether captured on film or digitally, is 'a two-dimensional picture of three-dimensional structures superimposed on one another and represented as a variety of black, white and grey shadows' – a *shadowgraph*.

Critical assessment of radiographic quality

To be able to assess and interpret any radiograph correctly, dental care professionals have to know what that radiograph should look like and which structures should be shown. It is for this reason that the chapters on radiography included:

1. WHY each projection was taken.
2. HOW the projections were taken.
3. WHAT the resultant radiographs should look like and which anatomical features they showed.

With this practical knowledge of radiography, dental care professionals are in a position to make an overall critical assessment of individual film-captured and digital images.

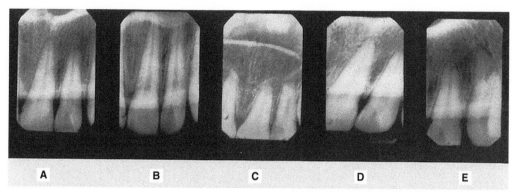

Fig. 16.3 Examples of how variations in radiographic technique can alter the images – film or digital – produced of the same object. **A** Correct projection. **B** Incorrect vertical angulation producing an elongated image. **C** Incorrect vertical angulation producing a foreshortened image. **D** and **E** Incorrect horizontal angulations producing distorted images.

Film-captured images

The practical factors that can influence *image quality* were discussed in Chapter 14, and included:

- The X-ray equipment
- The image receptor–film or film/screen combination
- Processing
- The patient
- The operator and radiographic technique.

A critical assessment of radiographs can be made by combining these factors and by asking a series of questions about the final image. These questions relate to:

- Radiographic technique
- Exposure factors and film density
- Processing.

Here are some typical examples.

Radiographic technique (see Fig. 16.3)

- Which technique has been used?
- How were the patient, film and X-ray tubehead positioned?
- Is this a good example of this particular radiographic projection?
- How much distortion is present?
- Is the image foreshortened or elongated?
- Is there any rotation or asymmetry?
- How good are the image resolution and sharpness?
- Has the film been fogged?
- Which artefactual shadows are present?
- How do these technique variables alter the final radiographic image?

Exposure factors and film density
(see Fig. 16.4)

- Is the radiograph correctly exposed for the specific reason it was requested?
- Is it too dark and so possibly overexposed?
- Is it too light/pale and so possibly underexposed?
- How good is the contrast?
- What effect will exposure factor variation have on the zone under investigation?

Processing

- Is the radiograph correctly processed?
- Is it too dark and so possibly overdeveloped?
- Is it too pale and so possibly underdeveloped?
- Is it dirty with emulsion still present and so underfixed?
- Is the film wet or dry?

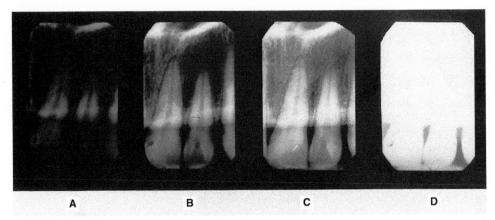

Fig. 16.4 The effect on the degree of blackening by altering exposure (mAs – current or exposure time) for film-captured images, OR by altering the *brightness* control for digital images.

Digitally captured images

The practical factors that can affect digitally captured images, how the images are created and how they can be altered using computer software were discussed in Chapter 3 and included:

- The image receptor – solid-state or photostimulable phosphor plate
- Computer image processing and enhancement
- The patient
- The operator and radiographic technique.

As with film-captured images a critical assessment of digital images can be made by combining these factors and by asking a series of questions about the final image. These questions relate to:

- Radiographic technique
- Image processing.

Radiographic technique

- Which technique has been used?
- How were the patient, digital receptor and X-ray tubehead positioned?
- Is this a good example of this particular radiographic projection?
- How much distortion is present?
- Has the whole area of interest been included?
- Is the image foreshortened or elongated?
- Is there any rotation or asymmetry?
- How good are the image resolution and sharpness?
- Which artefactual shadows are present?
- How do these technique variables alter the final radiographic image?

Note: These technique questions are almost identical to those relating to film-captured images. Image quality is totally dependent on high-quality practical radiography whatever image receptor is chosen.

Image processing

- Is the contrast optimal?
- Is the brightness optimal?
- Is the image enhancement optimal?
- Is the magnification optimal?

With experience, this critical assessment of image quality is not a lengthy procedure but it is never one that should be overlooked. A poor radiographic image is a poor diagnostic aid and sometimes may be of no diagnostic value at all. Dental care professionals used to using film-captured images who work with dentists who decide to 'go digital' should take time to understand the nature of the digital image, the effect on the image of using powerful computer software manipulation and the importance of viewing digital images on high resolution, calibrated monitors.

Detailed knowledge of normal anatomy

A detailed knowledge of the radiographic appearances of **normal** anatomical structures is necessary if dental care professionals are to be able to recognize the **abnormal** appearances of the many diseases that affect the jaws.

Not only is a comprehensive knowledge of hard and soft tissue anatomy required but also a knowledge of:

- The type of radiograph being interpreted (e.g. conventional radiograph or tomograph)
- The position of the patient, image receptor and X-ray tubehead.

Only with **all** this information can observers appreciate how the various normal anatomical structures, through which the X-ray beam has passed, will appear on any particular radiograph.

Detailed knowledge of pathological conditions

Radiological interpretation depends on recognition of the typical patterns and appearances of different diseases. The more important appearances that dental care professionals are likely to come across and should be able to recognize are described in Chapters 17–21.

Systematic approach

A systematic approach to viewing radiographs is necessary to ensure that no relevant information is missed. This systematic approach should apply to:

- The entire radiograph
- Specific lesions.

The entire radiograph

Any systematic approach will suffice as long as it is logical, ordered and thorough. Several suggested sequences are described in later chapters. By way of an example, a suggested systematic approach to the overall interpretation of panoramic radiographs (see Ch. 12) is shown in Fig. 16.5.

This type of ordered sequential viewing of radiographs requires discipline on the part of the observer. It is easy to be sidetracked by noticing something unusual or abnormal, thus forgetting the remainder of the radiograph.

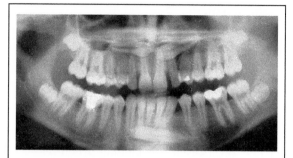

General overview of the entire image
1 Note the chronological and development age of the patient.
2 Trace the outline of all normal anatomical shadows and compare their shape and radiodensity.

The teeth
3 Note particularly:
  a. The number of teeth present
  b. Stage of development
  c. Position
  d. Condition of the crowns
    (i) Caries
    (ii) Restorations
  e. Condition of the roots
    (i) Length
    (ii) Fillings
    (iii) Resorption
    (iv) Crown/root ratio.

The apical tissues
4 Note particularly:
  a. The integrity of lamina dura
  b. Any radiolucencies or opacities associated with the apices.

The peridontal tissues
5 Note particularly:
  a. The width of the periodontal ligament
  b. The level and quality of crestal bone
  c. Any vertical or horizontal bone loss
  d. Any furcation involvements
  e. Any calculus deposits.

The body and ramus of the mandible
6 Note:
  a. Shape
  b. Outline
  c. Thickness of the lower border
  d. Trabeculae pattern
  e. Any radiolucent or radiopaque areas
  f. Shape of the condylar heads.

Other structures
7 These include:
  a. The antra, note:
    (i) The outline of the floor, medial and posterior walls
    (ii) Radiodensity
  b. Nasal cavity
  c. Styloid processes

Fig. 16.5 An example of a panoramic radiograph and a suggested systematic sequence for viewing this type of image.

Specific lesions

A systematic description of a lesion should include its:

- Site or anatomical position
- Size
- Shape
- Outline/edge or periphery
- Relative radiodensity and internal structure
- Effect on adjacent surrounding structures
- Time present, if known.

Making a radiological differential diagnosis depends on this systematic approach.

Comparison with previous images

The availability of previous images for comparative purposes is an invaluable aid to radiographic interpretation. The presence, extent and features of lesions can be compared to ascertain the speed of development and growth, or the degree of healing.

Note: Care must be taken that views used for comparison have been taken with a comparable technique **and** are of comparable density.

Conclusion

Successful interpretation of radiographs, no matter what the quality, relies ultimately on observers understanding the radiographic image, being able to recognize the range of normal appearances as well as knowing the salient features of relevant pathological conditions.

The following chapters are designed to emphasize these requirements and to reinforce the basic approach to interpretation outlined earlier.

To access the self assessment questions for this chapter please go to www.whaitesessentialsdentalradiography.com

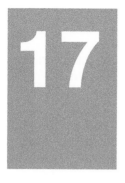

Dental caries and the assessment of restorations

Introduction

The word *caries* is used to describe both the invisible *caries process* and the potentially visible caries lesion. Understanding this difference is important if the role and value of radiography is to be understood.

The *caries process* is the interaction of the biofilm of plaque with the dental hard tissues. The *biofilm* consists of a community of metabolically active micro-organisms capable of fermenting sugars (e.g. sucrose or glucose) to produce acid, which can lower the pH to 5 in 1–3 minutes and produce *demineralization* of the dental hard tissues. The acid can be neutralized by saliva and mineral regained resulting in *remineralization*. Together these processes produce the *caries lesion*, which may or may not be visible clinically and/or radiographically. Being able to see the lesion depends on the extent and balance between demineralization and remineralization.

The first half of this chapter concentrates on the detection of caries in posterior teeth from bitewing radiographs. The second half summarizes the important features to observe when assessing restorations and outlines a systematic approach to interpreting bitewing radiographs.

Classification of caries

Lesions of caries are usually classified and/or described by the anatomical site of the tooth affected. Terminology used includes:

- Pit or fissure caries
- Smooth surface caries
- Enamel caries
- Root caries
- Primary caries – caries developing on unrestored surfaces
- Secondary or recurrent caries – caries developing adjacent to restorations
- Residual caries – demineralized tissue left behind before filling the tooth.

Lesions of caries are also classified and/or described by the activity of the *caries process*. Terminology used includes:

- Active caries
  - Rampant caries – multiple active lesions in the same patient, often on surfaces that are usually caries-free. In very small children this is sometimes referred to as *bottle caries* or *nursing caries*
  - Early childhood caries
- Arrested or inactive caries.

Levels of disease

Caries is also described by the extent or size of the lesion. Typically four levels of disease are used:

- D1 – Clinically detectable enamel lesions with intact surfaces
- D2 – Clinically detectable cavities limited to enamel
- D3 – Clinically detectable lesions in dentine
- D4 – Lesions into the pulp.

These distinctions are important with regard to management. Lesions at levels D1 and D2 are generally managed using preventative measures, whereas lesions at the D3 or D4 level are likely to require restorative treatment. Detection of lesions of caries and being able to assess the level of disease are therefore crucial in determining clinical treatment.

Diagnosis and detection of caries

Diagnosis has been defined as identifying a disease from its signs and symptoms. In caries diagnosis that would involve both detecting the lesion and determining the activity of the process. Dental radiography is one method used to detect the lesion but it gives no information on the activity of the process. Various detection methods are available for different sites.

Occlusal caries

- Clinical examination using direct vision of clean, dry teeth
- Bitewing radiography
- Laser fluorescence (DIAGNOdent (KaVo, Germany)
- Electrical conductance measurements (ECM).

Approximal caries

- Clinical examination using direct vision of clean, dry teeth
- Gentle probing
- Bitewing radiography in adults and children (posterior teeth)
- Paralleling technique periapical radiography (anterior teeth)
- Fibreoptic transillumination (FOTI)
- Light fluorescence (QLF)
- Elective temporary tooth separation
- Ultrasound.

Secondary or recurrent caries (caries developing adjacent to a restoration)

- Clinical examination using direct vision of clean, dry teeth
- Gently probing
- Bitewing radiography.

Radiographic detection of lesions of caries

Bitewing radiographic techniques, using both film packets and digital sensors (solid-state and phosphor plates) as the image receptor, were described in Chapter 8. For caries detection, film packets and phosphor plates are preferred as the imaging area of the equivalent sized solid-state sensors is smaller. It has been reported that on average three fewer interproximal tooth surfaces are shown per image.

Approximal lesions of caries are detectable radiographically only when there has been 30–40% demineralization, so allowing the lesion to be differentiated from normal enamel and dentine. The importance of optimum viewing conditions for both film and digital images, as described in Chapter 16, cannot be overemphasized when looking for these early subtle changes. Magnification is of particular importance, as shown in Fig. 17.1.

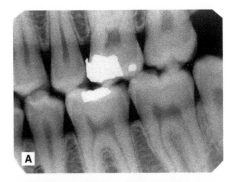

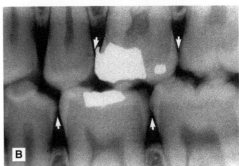

Fig. 17.1 The effect of magnification. **A** Bitewing radiograph showing almost invisible very early approximal lesions in the molar and premolar teeth. **B** Magnified central portion of the same bitewing showing the approximal lesions (arrowed) more clearly.

Radiographic assessment of caries activity

A single bitewing radiograph may illustrate one or more caries lesions but it gives no information on caries activity. As caries is a slowly progressing disease, this progression and therefore caries activity, can be assessed over time by periodic radiographic investigations.

In the UK, the 2013 Faculty of General Dental Practice (UK)'s booklet *Selection Criteria for Dental Radiography* recommends that the frequency of these follow-up radiographs be linked to the *caries risk* of the patient. There are three risk categories – high, moderate or low risk – for both children and adults. The *Selection Criteria* booklet contains a number of evidence-based recommendations, the main ones of which are summarised in Table 17.1. As can be seen for *high risk* children and adults 6-monthly time intervals are recommended, for *moderate risk* patients 12-monthly intervals and for *low risk* children 12–18 month intervals and for *low risk* adults 2-yearly intervals

Radiographs used to monitor the progression of caries lesions need to be geometrically identical – hence the need for image receptor holders and beam-aiming devices (see Ch. 8). They should also be similarly exposed to give comparable contrast and density.

Geometrically reproducible digital images can be superimposed and the information in one image subtracted from the other to create the subtraction image, which shows the changes that have taken place between the two investigations.

Radiographic appearance of caries lesions

As lesions of caries progress and enlarge, they appear as differently shaped areas of radiolucency in the crowns or necks of the teeth. These shapes are fairly characteristic and vary according to the site and size of the lesion. They are illustrated diagrammatically in Fig. 17.2 and examples are shown in Fig. 17.3.

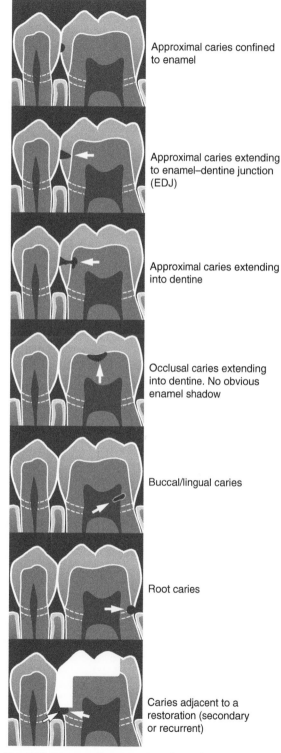

Approximal caries confined to enamel

Approximal caries extending to enamel–dentine junction (EDJ)

Approximal caries extending into dentine

Occlusal caries extending into dentine. No obvious enamel shadow

Buccal/lingual caries

Root caries

Caries adjacent to a restoration (secondary or recurrent)

Fig. 17.2 Diagrams illustrating the radiographic appearances and shapes of various lesions of caries.

Table 17.1 Summary of the main recommendations for using radiographs for the diagnosis of dental caries (linked to caries risk), based on the Faculty of General Practice (UK)'s 2013 *Selection Criteria for Dental Radiography* (3rd Ed)

Recommendation	Evidence-based grading*
All *children* designated as *high caries risk* should have six-monthly posterior bitewings taken until no new or active lesions are apparent and the individual has entered another risk category (*Bitewings should not be taken more frequently and it is imperative to reassess caries risk in order to justify using this interval again.*)	B
All *children* designated as *moderate caries risk* should have annual posterior bitewings taken until no new active lesions are apparent and the individual has entered another risk category	B
All *children* designated as *low caries risk* should have posterior bitewings taken at approximately 12–18 month intervals in primary dentition and at approximately two-yearly intervals in the permanent dentition. More extended radiographic recall intervals may be employed if there is explicit evidence of continuing low caries risk	B
All *adults* designated as *high caries risk* should have six-monthly posterior bitewings taken until no new or active lesions are apparent and the individual has entered another risk category (*Bitewings should not be taken more frequently and it is imperative to reassess caries risk in order to justify using this interval again. It is also important to remember that rates of caries progress in enamel and dentine will differ and that rates in adults may well be slower than in children*)	C
All *adults* designated as *moderate caries risk* should have annual posterior bitewings taken until no new or active lesions are apparent and the individual has entered another risk category	C
All *adults* designated as *low caries risk* should have posterior bitewings taken at approximately two-yearly intervals. More extended radiographic recall intervals may be employed if there is explicit evidence of continuing low caries risk.	C
The taking of 'routine' radiographs based solely on time elapsed since the last examinations is not supportable.	C
Intervals between subsequent radiographic examinations must be reassessed for each new period as patients can move in and out of caries risk categories over time.	C
CBCT should not be used as a routine method of caries diagnosis	B

*Evidence-based grading **B** = based on evidence from well conducted clinical studies but with no specific *in vitro* validation studies; **C** = based on evidence from expert committee reports or opinions and/or clinical experience of respected authorities and indicates an absence of directly applicable studies of good quality.

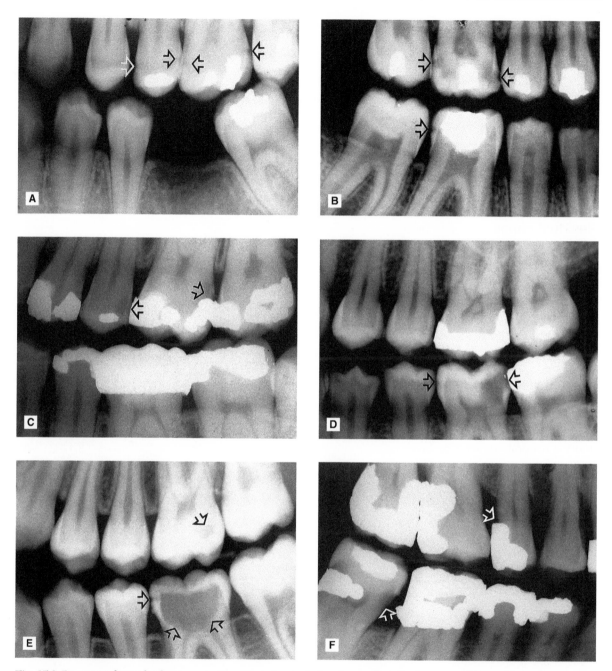

Fig. 17.3 Bitewing radiographs showing examples of typical caries lesions (arrowed). **A** Small approximal lesions |56. Large approximal lesions with extensive dentine involvement 6| and a small lesion 6|. **C** Approximal lesion extending into dentine |5 and recurrent caries |6. **D** Small and extensive approximal lesions 6|. **E** Small occlusal lesion |6 and extensive occlusal lesion 6|, apart from the small approximal enamel lesion, the enamel cap appears intact. **F** Root caries 7| and recurrent caries 5|.

Other important radiographic appearances

Radiographic detection of caries lesions is not always straightforward. It can be complicated by:

- Residual caries
- Radiodensity of adhesive restorations
- Cervical *burn-out* or cervical *translucency*
- Dentinal changes beneath amalgam restorations.

Residual caries

The rationale for removal of caries has changed in recent years. The primary aim nowadays when excavating dentine caries is to remove only the highly infected, irreversibly demineralized dentine in order to allow effective restoration of the cavity and surface anatomy of the tooth and to prevent disease progression. In other words, demineralized tissue (*residual caries*) is left behind in the base of the cavity and the tooth restored. Radiographically, this *inactive caries* may show a zone of radiolucency beneath the restoration. This appearance is identical to that of an *active caries lesion* under a restoration (see Fig. 17.4).

Radiodensity of adhesive restorations

The development of successful adhesive restorative materials in recent years, including dentine bonding agents and glass ionomer cements, has resulted in many teeth being restored with non-metallic fillings. These various adhesive materials vary considerably in their radiodensity and do not appear as white on radiographic images as traditional amalgam, as shown in Fig. 17.5. Identifying subtle radiolucent lesions of caries adjacent to these materials can be very difficult, if not impossible.

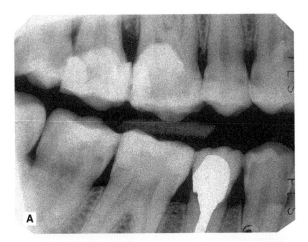

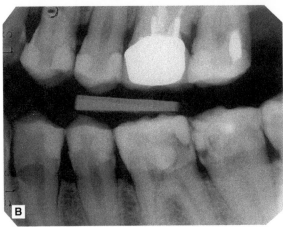

Fig. 17.5 A RIGHT and **B** LEFT bitewings showing numerous posterior teeth that have been restored with adhesive restorations. **Note:** the restorations look less radiopaque than amalgam, and as a result the reduced contrast difference between dentine and restoration makes identification of adjacent radiolucent caries difficult. (Kindly provided by Prof A. Banerjee.)

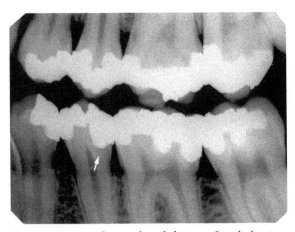

Fig. 17.4 Bitewing showing the radiolucency of residual caries beneath the restoration in $\overline{5}$ (arrowed). It is impossible to assess whether the lesion is *active* or *inactive*.

Cervical burn-out or cervical translucency

This radiolucent shadow is often evident at the neck of the teeth, as illustrated in Fig. 17.6. It is an artefactual phenomenon created by the anatomy of the teeth and the variable penetration of the X-ray beam.

Cervical *burn-out* can be explained by considering **all** the different parts of the tooth and supporting bone tissues that the same X-ray beam has to penetrate:

- In the crown – the dense enamel cap and dentine
- In the neck – only dentine
- In the root – dentine and the buccal and lingual plates of alveolar bone (see Fig. 17.7).

Thus, at the edges of the teeth in the cervical region, there is **less** tissue for the X-ray beam to pass through. Less attenuation therefore takes place and virtually no opaque shadow is cast of this area on the radiograph. It therefore appears radiolucent, as if some cervical tooth tissue does not exist or that it has been apparently *burnt out.*

Cervical *burn-out* is of diagnostic importance because of its similarity to the radiolucent shadows of cervical and recurrent caries. However, *burn-out* can usually be distinguished by the following characteristic features:

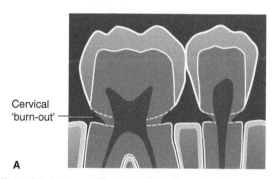

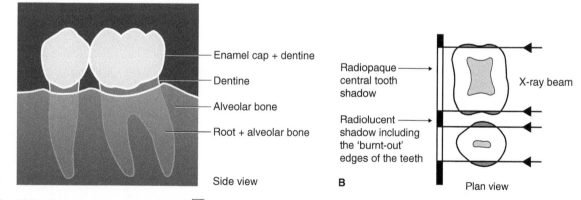

Fig. 17.6 A Diagram illustrating the radiographic appearance of cervical *burn-out.* **B** Bitewing radiograph showing extensive cervical *burn-out* of the premolars (arrowed). Compare this with the appearance of cervical caries on distal aspect 6|.

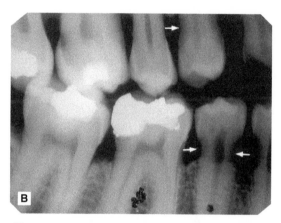

Fig. 17.7 A Diagrammatic representation of |56 from the side showing the three-dimensional structures involved in the formation of the radiographic image. Note that in the cervical region there is less tissue present. **B** Plan view at the level of the necks of the teeth. Through the centre of the teeth there is a large mass of dentine to absorb the X-ray beam, while at the edges there is only a small amount. The edges of the necks of the teeth are therefore not dense enough to stop the X-ray beam, so their normally opaque shadows do not appear on the final radiograph.

- It is located at the neck of the teeth, demarcated above by the enamel cap or restoration and below by the alveolar bone level.
- It is triangular in shape, gradually becoming less apparent towards the centre of the tooth.
- Usually all the teeth on the radiograph are affected, especially the smaller premolars.

In contrast, *root* and *recurrent caries lesions*, although they also often affect the cervical region, have no apparent upper and lower demarcating borders. These lesions are saucer-shaped and tend to be localized, as shown in Fig. 17.2. If in doubt, the diagnosis should be confirmed clinically by direct vision and gentle probing, having cleaned and dried the area.

Important points to note

- *Burn-out* is more obvious when the exposure factors are increased, as required ideally for detecting approximal caries.
- It is also more apparent by the perceptual problem of *contrast* if the tooth contains a metallic restoration, which may make the zone above the cervical shadow completely radiopaque (see Fig. 17.8 and Ch. 1, Fig. 1.16). As this area is also the main site for recurrent caries, diagnosis is further complicated.

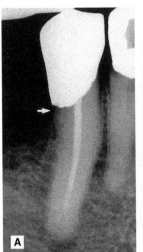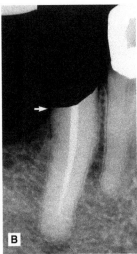

Fig. 17.8 The visual perceptual problem of contrast. **A** The zone at the distal cervical margin (arrowed), directly beneath the white metallic restoration shadow, appears radiolucent in the 5⌋. **B** The same image but with the white restoration blacked out. The zone beneath the restoration (arrowed) now appears less radiolucent.

Dentinal changes beneath amalgam restorations

Following attack by caries, posterior teeth are still commonly restored using dental amalgam. An *amalgam* is defined as an alloy of mercury with another metal or metals. In dental amalgam, mercury is mixed with an alloy powder. The alloy powders available principally contain silver, tin and copper with small amounts of zinc. It has been shown that, with time, tin and zinc ions are released into the underlying demineralized (but not necessarily infected) dentine producing a radio-opaque zone within the dentine which follows the S-shaped curve of the underlying tubules (see Fig. 17.9). The radiopacity of this zone may make the normal dentine on either side appear more radiolucent by contrast which may simulate the radiolucent shadows of caries and lead to difficulties in diagnosis.

In addition, the pulp may also respond to both the carious attack and subsequent restorative treatment by laying down *reparative secondary dentine* which reduces the size of the pulp chamber.

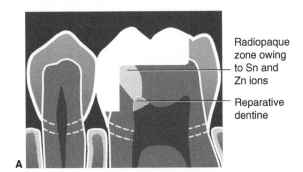

Radiopaque zone owing to Sn and Zn ions

Reparative dentine

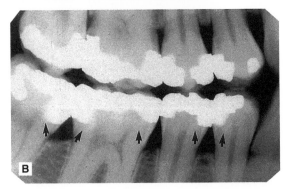

Fig. 17.9 A Diagram illustrating the S-shaped radiopaque zone caused by tin and zinc ions released into the underlying demineralized dentine beneath an amalgam restoration and the appearance of reparative dentine. **B** Bitewing radiograph showing the S-shaped radiopaque shadows (arrowed) in the heavily restored lower teeth.

Limitations of radiographic diagnosis of caries

In addition to the problems of diagnosis caused by the radiolucent and radiopaque shadows mentioned earlier, further limitations are imposed by the radiographic image. The main problems include:

- Caries lesions are usually larger clinically than they appear radiographically and very early lesions are not evident at all.
- Technique variations in image receptor and X-ray beam positions can considerably affect the image of the caries lesion – varying the horizontal tubehead angulation can make a lesion confined to enamel appear to have progressed into dentine (see Fig. 17.10) – hence the need for accurate, reproducible techniques as described in Chapter 8.
- Exposure factors can have a marked effect on the overall radiographic contrast (see Fig. 17.11) on film-captured images and thus affect the appearance or size of caries lesions on the radiograph.
- Superimposition and a two-dimensional image (film or digital) mean that the following features cannot always be determined:
  - The exact site of a caries lesion, e.g. buccal or lingual
  - The buccolingual extent of a lesion
  - The distance between the caries lesion and the pulp horns. These two shadows can appear to be close together or even in contact but they may not be in the same plane
  - The presence of an enamel lesion – the density of the overlying enamel may obscure the zone of decalcification
  - The presence of caries adjacent to restorations may be completely obscured by the restoration (see Fig. 17.12).

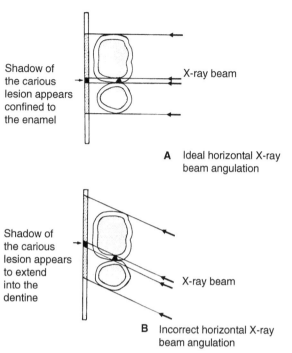

A Ideal horizontal X-ray beam angulation

B Incorrect horizontal X-ray beam angulation

Fig. 17.10 Diagrams showing how the appearance and extent of a caries lesion confined to enamel alter with different horizontal X-ray beam angulations.

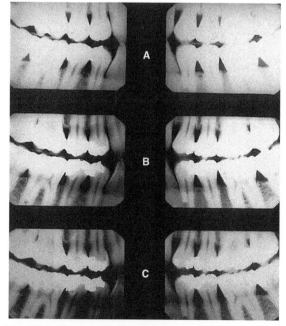

Fig. 17.11 Three pairs of bitewing radiographs taken on the same patient but with varying exposure factors. **A** Considerably reduced exposure. **B** Slightly reduced exposure. **C** Slightly increased exposure. Note the varying contrast between enamel, dentine and the pulp.

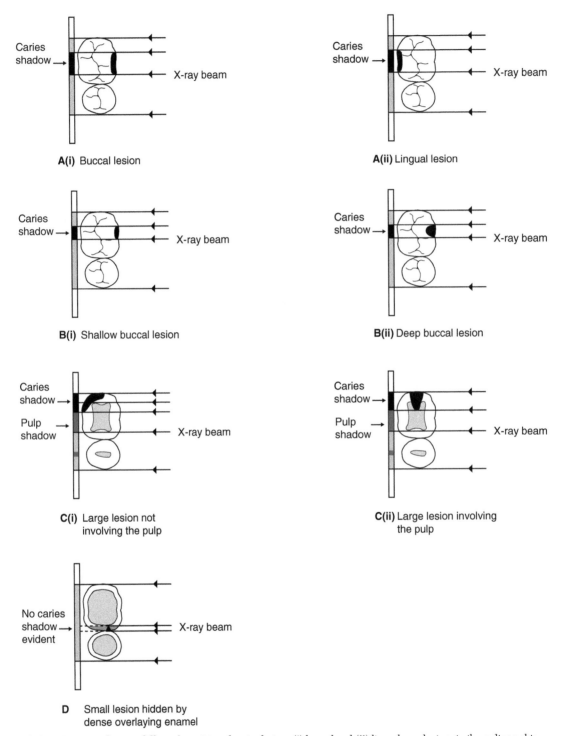

Fig. 17.12 A Diagrams showing differently positioned caries lesions (**i**) buccal and (**ii**) lingual, producing similar radiographic shadows. **B** Diagrams showing different sized buccal lesions (**i**) shallow and (**ii**) deep, producing similar radiographic shadows. **C** Diagrams showing (**i**) a large approximal lesion superimposed over, but not involving, the pulp and (**ii**) a large approximal lesion involving the pulp, both producing similar radiographic shadows. **D** Diagram showing how a small lesion may not be evident radiographically if dense radiopaque enamel shadows are superimposed.

Radiographic assessment of restorations

Critical assessment of the restoration

The important features to note include:

- The type and radiodensity of the restorative material, e.g.
  - amalgam
  - cast metal
  - tooth-coloured materials, such as composite or glass ionomer (see earlier and Fig. 17.5)
- Overcontouring
- Overhanging ledges
- Undercontouring
- Negative or reverse ledges
- Presence of contact points
- Adaptation of the restorative material to the base of the cavity

- Marginal fit of cast restorations
- Presence or absence of a lining material
- Radiodensity of the lining material.

Assessment of the underlying tooth

The important features to note include:

- Recurrent caries
- Residual caries (see earlier and Fig. 17.4)
- Radiopaque shadow of released tin and zinc ions (see earlier and Fig. 17.9)
- Size of the pulp chamber
- Internal resorption
- Presence of root-filling material in the pulp chamber
- Presence and position of pins or posts.

Examples showing several of these features are shown in Fig. 17.13.

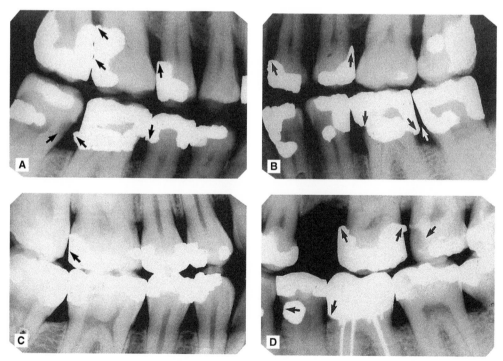

Fig. 17.13 Bitewing radiographs showing examples of heavily restored teeth. The major areas of concern – overhanging ledges, poor contour, defective contact points and recurrent caries – are arrowed.

Limitations of the radiographic image

Once again, the radiographic image provides only limited information when assessing restorations. The main problems include:

- Technique variations in X-ray tubehead position may cause recurrent caries lesions to be obscured (see Fig. 17.14)
- Cervical *burn-out* shadows tend to be more obvious when their upper borders are demarcated by dense white restorations because of the increased contrast differences (see Fig. 17.8)
- Superimposition and a two-dimensional image mean that:
  - Only part of a restoration can be assessed radiographically
  - A dense radiopaque restoration may totally obscure a caries lesion in another part of the tooth
  - Recurrent caries at the base of an interproximal box may not be detected (see Fig. 17.15).

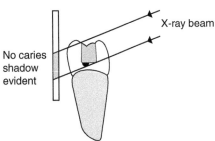

A Incorrect vertical X-ray beam angulation

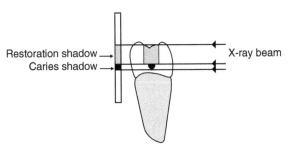

A (i) Lesion beneath the restoration

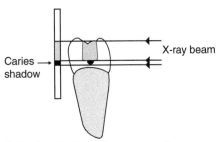

B Ideal vertical X-ray beam angulation

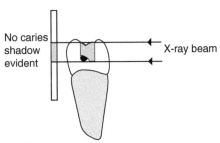

A (ii) Lesion hidden by the restoration

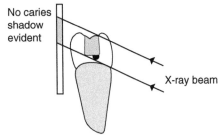

C Incorrect vertical X-ray beam angulation

Fig. 17.14 Diagrams illustrating the effect of incorrect vertical X-ray beam angulation in diagnosing recurrent lesions at the base of a restoration box.

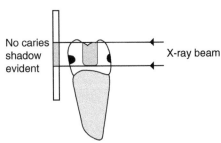

B Buccal and lingual lesions hidden by the restoration

Fig. 17.15 A Diagrams illustrating the difficulty of assessing caries beneath a restoration. **B** Diagram showing the difficulty of assessing buccal and lingual lesions in restored teeth.

Suggested guidelines for interpreting bitewing radiographs

Overall critical assessment

A typical series of questions that should be asked about the quality of a bitewing image based on the *ideal quality criteria* described in Chapter 8 include:

Technique (film OR digitally captured images)

- Are all the required teeth shown?
- Are the crowns of upper and lower teeth shown?
- Is the occlusal plane horizontal?
- Are the contact areas overlapped?
- Has there been any *coning off or cone cutting*?
- Are the buccal and lingual cusps overlapped?
- Is it geometrically comparable to previous films?

Exposure factors (film-captured images)

- Is the image too dark – and so possibly overexposed?
- Is the image too light – and so possibly underexposed?
- Is the exposure sufficient to allow the enamel–dentine junction to be seen?
- What effect do the exposure factors have on the structures shown?
- How noticeable is the cervical *burn-out*?

Processing (film-captured images)

- Is the radiograph correctly processed?
- Is it overdeveloped?
- Is it underdeveloped?
- Is it correctly fixed?
- Has it been adequately washed?

Image processing (digitally-captured images)

- Is the contrast optimal?
- Is the brightness optimal?
- Is image enhancement optimal?
- Is magnification optimal?

Systematic viewing

Suggested systematic approaches to viewing bitewing radiographs are shown in Figs 17.16 and 17.17.

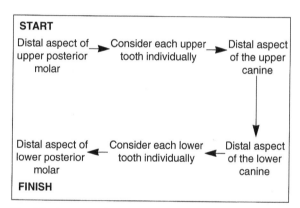

Fig. 17.16 Suggested sequence for examining a right bitewing radiograph.

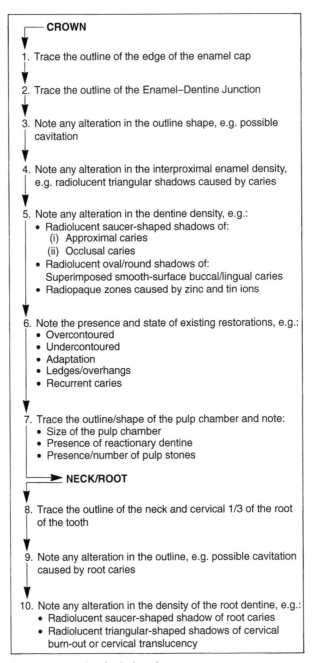

CROWN

1. Trace the outline of the edge of the enamel cap

2. Trace the outline of the Enamel–Dentine Junction

3. Note any alteration in the outline shape, e.g. possible cavitation

4. Note any alteration in the interproximal enamel density, e.g. radiolucent triangular shadows caused by caries

5. Note any alteration in the dentine density, e.g.:
   - Radiolucent saucer-shaped shadows of:
     (i) Approximal caries
     (ii) Occlusal caries
   - Radiolucent oval/round shadows of:
     Superimposed smooth-surface buccal/lingual caries
   - Radiopaque zones caused by zinc and tin ions

6. Note the presence and state of existing restorations, e.g.:
   - Overcontoured
   - Undercontoured
   - Adaptation
   - Ledges/overhangs
   - Recurrent caries

7. Trace the outline/shape of the pulp chamber and note:
   - Size of the pulp chamber
   - Presence of reactionary dentine
   - Presence/number of pulp stones

NECK/ROOT

8. Trace the outline of the neck and cervical 1/3 of the root of the tooth

9. Note any alteration in the outline, e.g. possible cavitation caused by root caries

10. Note any alteration in the density of the root dentine, e.g.:
   - Radiolucent saucer-shaped shadow of root caries
   - Radiolucent triangular-shaped shadows of cervical burn-out or cervical translucency

Fig. 17.17 Suggested sequence for examining each individual tooth.

To access the self assessment questions for this chapter please go to www.whaitesessentialsdentalradiography.com

18 The periapical tissues

Introduction

This chapter explains how to interpret the radiographic appearances of the periapical tissues by illustrating the various normal appearances, and describing in detail the typical changes associated with apical infection and inflammation following pulpal necrosis. To help explain the different radiographic appearances, they are correlated with the various underlying pathological processes. In addition, there is a summary of the other, sometimes sinister, lesions that can affect the periapical tissues and may simulate simple inflammatory changes.

Normal radiographic appearances

A reminder of the complex three-dimensional anatomy of the hard tissues surrounding the teeth in the maxilla and mandible, which contribute to the two-dimensional periapical radiographic image, is given in Fig. 18.1.

The appearances of normal, healthy, periapical tissues vary from one patient to another, from one area of the mouth to another and at different stages in the development of the dentition. These different normal appearances are described below.

The periapical tissues of permanent teeth
(Fig. 18.2)

The three most important features to observe are:

- The radiolucent line that represents the periodontal ligament space and forms a thin continuous black line around the root outline

- The radiopaque line that represents the lamina dura of the bony socket and forms a thin, continuous, white line adjacent to the black line
- The trabecular pattern and density of the surrounding bone:
  - In the mandible, the trabeculae tend to be relatively thick and close together, and are often aligned horizontally
  - In the maxilla, the trabeculae tend to be finer, and more widely spaced. There is no predominant alignment pattern.

These features hold the key to the interpretation of periapical radiographs, since changes in their thickness, continuity and radiodensity reflect the presence of any underlying disease, as described later.

Important points to note

- There is considerable variation in the definition and pattern of these features from one patient to another and from one area of the jaws to another, owing to variation in the density, shape and thickness of the surrounding bone.
- The limitations imposed by contrast, resolution and superimposition can make radiographic identification of these features particularly difficult, hence the need for ideal viewing conditions and digital image enhancement software.

The periapical tissues of deciduous teeth
(Fig. 18.3)

The important features of normality (thin lamina dura and periodontal ligament shadows) are the

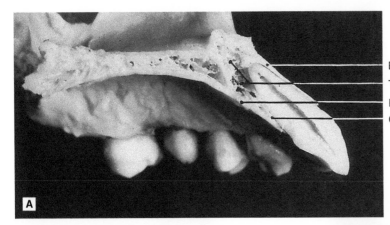

Buccal cortical plate of compact bone

Trabecular or cancellous bone

Palatal cortical plate of compact bone

Cortical bone of the socket

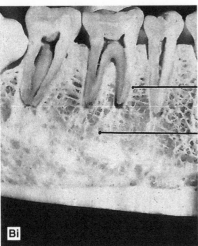

Cortical bone of the socket

Trabecular or cancellous bone

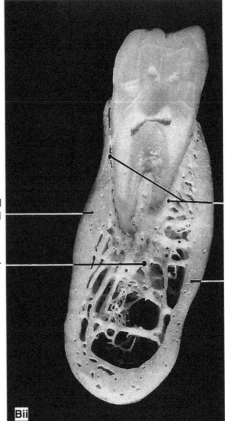

Lingual cortical plate

Trabecular or cancellous bone

Cortical bone of the socket

Buccal cortical plate

Fig. 18.1 A Sagittal section through the maxilla and central incisor showing the hard tissue anatomy. **B** (**i**) Sagittal and (**ii**) coronal sections through the mandible in the molar region showing the hard tissue anatomy.

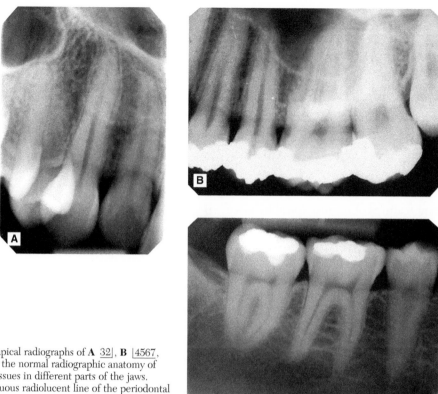

Fig. 18.2 Periapical radiographs of **A** 32|, **B** |4567, **C** 765| showing the normal radiographic anatomy of the periapical tissues in different parts of the jaws. Note the continuous radiolucent line of the periodontal ligament shadow and the radiopaque line of the lamina dura outlining the roots.

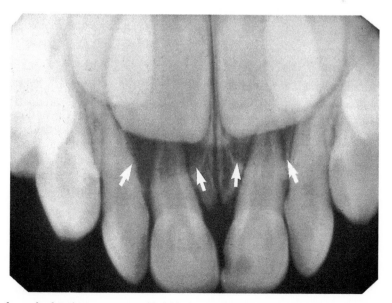

Fig. 18.3 Periapical radiograph of BA|AB in a 4-year-old child, showing normal periapical tissues. Note the confusing shadows created by the radiopaque crowns and radiolucent crypts (arrowed) of the developing permanent incisors.

same as for permanent teeth, but can be complicated by:

- The presence of an underlying permanent tooth and its crypt, the shadows of which may overlie the deciduous tooth apex
- Resorption of the deciduous tooth root during the normal exfoliation process.

The periapical tissues of developing teeth
(Fig. 18.4)

The important features of normal apical tissues where the root is partially formed and the radicular papilla still exists include:

- A circumscribed area of radiolucency at the apex
- The radiopaque line of the lamina dura is intact around the papilla
- The developing root is funnel-shaped

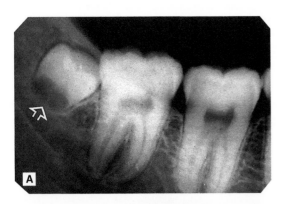

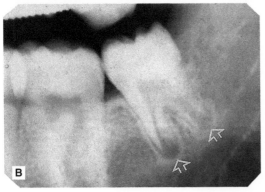

Fig. 18.4 Periapical radiographs showing the normal periapical tissues of developing teeth. **A** 8⌋, **B** ⌊7. Note the circumscribed areas of radiolucency of the radicular papillae (arrowed) and the funnel-shaped roots.

- Only after root development is complete does the thin continuous radiolucent line become evident.

The effects of normal superimposed shadows

Normal anatomical shadows superimposed on the apical tissues can be either *radiolucent* or *radiopaque*, depending on the structure involved.

Radiolucent shadows

Examples include:

- The maxillary antra
- The nasopalatine foramen
- The mental foramina.

Such cavities in the alveolar bone decrease the total amount of bone that would normally contribute to the final radiographic image, with the following effects:

- The radiolucent line of the periodontal ligament may appear MORE radiolucent or widened, but will still be continuous and well demarcated.
- The radiopaque line of the lamina dura may appear LESS obvious and may not be visible.
- There will be an area of radiolucency in the alveolar bone at the tooth apex (see Figs 18.5 and 18.6).

Important points to note

- The fact that the radiopaque lamina dura shadow may not be visible does not mean that the bony socket margin is not present clinically. It only means that there is now not enough total bone in the path of the X-ray beam to produce a visible opaque shadow. Since the bony socket is in fact intact, it still defines the periodontal ligament space. Thus, the radiolucent line representing this space still appears continuous and well demarcated.
- Although confusing, this effect of normal anatomical radiolucent shadows on the apical tissues is very important to appreciate, so as not to mistake a normal area of radiolucency at the apex for a pathological lesion.

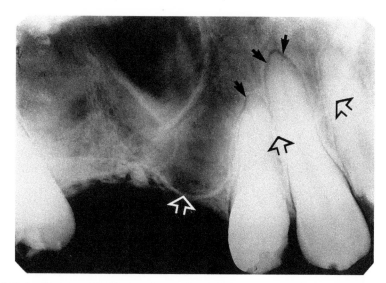

Fig. 18.5 Periapical of Q| showing normal healthy apical tissues but with the radiolucent shadow of the antrum superimposed (the antral floor is indicated by the open arrows). As a result the radiolucent line of the periodontal ligament appears widened and more obvious around the apices of the canine and premolar, but it is still well demarcated, while the radiopaque line of the lamina dura is almost invisible (solid arrows).

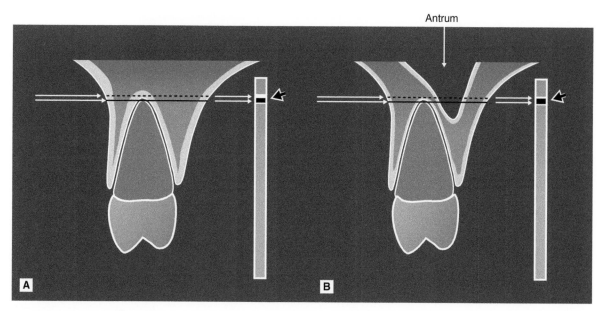

Fig. 18.6 Diagrams of 5| showing the anatomical tissues that the X-ray beam passes through to reach the image receptor. **A** Without a normal anatomical cavity superimposed. **B** With the antral cavity in the path of the X-ray beam. The different resultant radiopaque (white) and radiolucent (black) lines of the apical lamina dura and periodontal ligament are shown on the image receptor (arrowed).

Radiopaque shadows

Examples include:

- The mylohyoid ridge
- The body of the zygoma
- Areas of sclerotic bone (so-called *dense bone islands*).

Such radiopacities complicate periapical interpretation by obscuring or obliterating the detailed shadows of the apical tissues, as shown in Fig. 18.7.

Radiographic appearances of periapical inflammatory changes

Types of inflammatory changes

Following pulpal necrosis, either an acute or chronic inflammatory response is initiated in the apical tissues. The inflammatory response is identical to that set up elsewhere in the body from other toxic stimuli, and exhibits the same signs and symptoms.

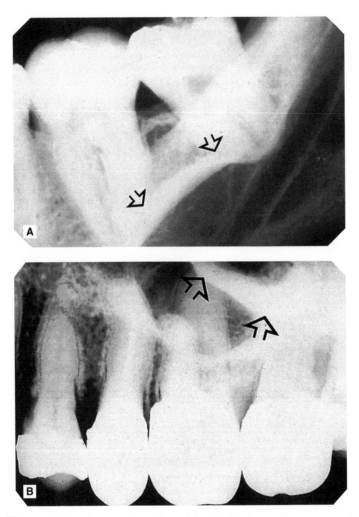

Fig. 18.7 A Periapical of ⌐78 showing the radiopaque line of the mylohyoid ridge (arrowed) superimposed over the apices.
B Periapical of ⌐4567 showing the radiopaque shadow of the zygomatic buttress (arrowed) overlying and obscuring the apical tissues of the molars.

Cardinal signs of acute inflammation

These include:

- Swelling – *tumor*
- Redness – *rubor*
- Heat – *calor*
- Pain – *dolor*
- Loss of function – *functio laesa*.

In the apical tissues, inflammatory exudate accumulates in the apical periodontal ligament space (*swelling*), setting up an **acute apical periodontitis**. The affected tooth becomes periostitic or tender to pressure (*pain*), and the patient avoids biting on the tooth (*loss of function*). *Heat* and *redness* are clinically undetectable. These signs are accompanied by destruction and resorption, often of the tooth root, and of the surrounding bone, as a **periapical abscess** develops, and radiographically a periapical radiolucent area becomes evident.

Hallmarks of chronic inflammation

These include the processes of *destruction* and *healing* which are going on simultaneously, as the body's defence systems respond to, and try to confine, the spread of the infection. In the apical tissues, a **periapical granuloma** forms at the apex and dense bone is laid down around the area of resorption. Radiographically, the apical radiolucent area becomes circumscribed and surrounded by dense sclerotic bone. Occasionally, under these conditions of chronic inflammation, the epithelial cell rests of Malassez are stimulated to proliferate and form an inflammatory **periapical radicular cyst** or there is an acute exacerbation producing another abscess (the so-called *phoenix abscess*).

The type and progress of the inflammatory response at the apex and the subsequent spread of apical infection is dependent on several factors relating to:

- The infecting organism including its virulence
- The body's defence systems.

The result is a wide spectrum of events ranging from a very rapidly spreading acute periapical abscess to a very slowly progressing chronic periapical granuloma or cyst. This variation in the underlying disease processes is mirrored radiographically, although it is often not possible to differentiate between an abscess, granuloma or cyst.

A summary of the different inflammatory effects and the resultant radiographic appearances is shown in Table 18.1. The effects are shown diagrammatically in Fig. 18.8. Various examples are shown in Figs 18.9–18.12.

Table 18.1 Summary of the effects of different inflammatory processes on the periapical tissues and the resultant radiographic appearances

State of inflammation	Underlying inflammatory changes	Radiographic appearances
Initial acute inflammation	Inflammatory exudate accumulates in the apical periodontal ligament space – *acute apical periodontitis*	Widening of the radiolucent line of the periodontal ligament space OR No apparent changes evident
Initial spread of inflammation	Resorption and destruction of the apical bony socket – *periapical abscess*	Loss of the radiopaque line of the lamina dura at the apex
Further spread of inflammation	Further resorption and destruction of the apical alveolar bone	Area of bone loss at the tooth apex
Initial low-grade chronic inflammation	Minimal destruction of the apical bone The body's defence systems lay down dense bone in the apical region	No apparent bone destruction but dense sclerotic bone evident around the tooth apex (*sclerosing osteitis*)
Latter stages of chronic inflammation	Apical bone is resorbed and destroyed and dense bone is laid down around the area of resorption – *periapical granuloma* or *radicular cyst*	Circumscribed, well-defined radiolucent area of bone loss at the apex, surrounded by dense sclerotic bone

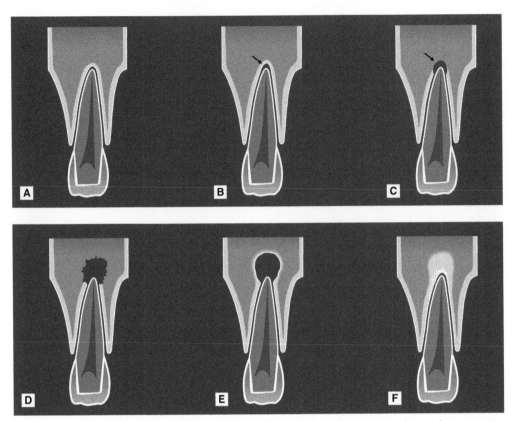

Fig. 18.8 Diagrams showing the various radiographic appearances of infection and inflammation in the apical tissues. **A** Normal. **B** Early apical change – widening of the radiolucent periodontal ligament space (*acute apical periodontitis*) (arrowed). **C** Early apical change – loss of the radiopaque lamina dura (*early periapical abscess*) (arrowed). **D** Extensive destructive acute inflammation – diffuse, ill-defined area of radiolucency at the apex (*periapical abscess*). **E** Longstanding chronic inflammation – well-defined area of radiolucency surrounded by dense sclerotic bone (*periapical granuloma or radicular cyst*). **F** Low-grade chronic inflammation – diffuse radiopaque area at the apex (*sclerosing osteitis*).

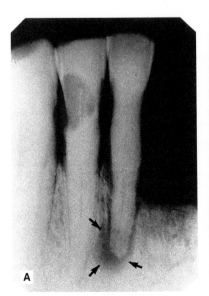

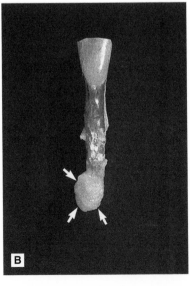

Fig. 18.9 A Periapical showing a well-defined area of radiolucency at the apex of $\overline{1|}$ (arrowed). The surrounding bone is relatively dense and opaque suggesting a chronic periapical granuloma or radicular cyst. **B** The extracted $\overline{1|}$, showing the granuloma attached to the root apex (arrowed).

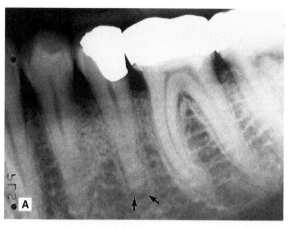
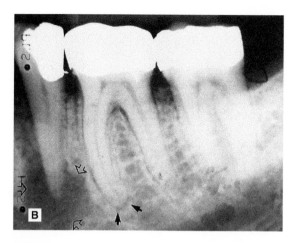

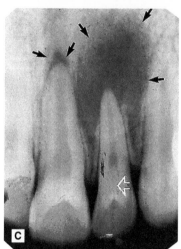
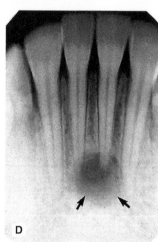

Fig. 18.10 Periapicals showing examples of inflammatory changes in the periapical tissues. **A** Early apical change on 5̅ showing widening of the periodontal ligament space and thinning of the lamina dura (*acute apical periodontitis*) (arrowed). **B** Same patient 6 months later – the area of bone destruction at the apex 5̅ has increased considerably (open arrows) and there is now early apical change associated with the mesial root 6̅ (solid arrows). **C** Large, diffuse area of bone destruction associated with |2 and a smaller area associated with |1 (black arrows) (*periapical abscess*). |2 shows evidence of a dens-in-dente (invaginated odontome) (open white arrow). **D** Reasonably well-defined area of bone destruction (arrowed) associated with 1̅ (*periapical abscess, granuloma or cyst*).

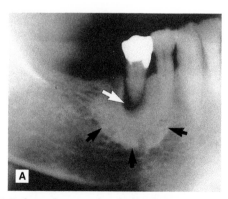
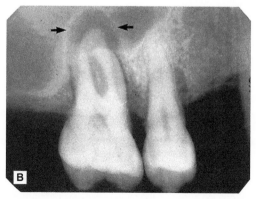

Fig. 18.11 Radiographic examples of other chronic inflammatory changes in the periapical tissues. **A** Long-standing low grade chronic infection associated with 5̅ resulting in a radiolucent periapical granuloma or radicular cyst (white arrow), surrounded by florid opaque sclerosing osteitis (black arrow). **B** Well-defined area of bone destruction associated with 1̲ which has resulted in remodelling of the antral floor, producing the so-called *antral halo* appearance (black arrow).

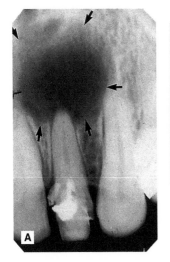

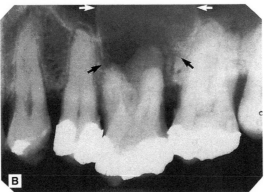

Fig. 18.12 Periapicals showing **A** inflammatory radicular cyst (arrowed) associated with 2| and **B** inflammatory radicular cyst (arrowed) associated with |6. The antrum has been displaced by the upper margin of the cyst, which is not evident on this radiograph.

Treatment and radiographic follow-up

Most inflammatory periapical lesions, and teeth damaged by minor trauma, are treated by conventional endondontic therapy. If endodontic treatment is clinically unsuccessful, subsequent treatment involves either:

- Repeat conventional endodontics
- Surgical exploration, curettage of the infected area and/or encleation of the cyst (if present), apicectomy and retrograde root filling
- Extrection of the tooth.

The main recommendations from the Faculty of General Dental Practice (UK)'s 2013 *Selection Criteria for Dental Radiography* booklet regarding imaging the periapical tissues in relation to endodontics are summarised in Table 18.2.

Table 18.2 Summary of the main recommendations for imaging the periapical tissues in relation to endodontics, based on the Faculty of General Dental Practice (UK)'s 2013 *Selection Criteria for Dental Radiography* (3rd Edn)

Recommendation	Evidence-based grading*
A good quality pre-operative paralleling technique periapical radiograph is essential for the diagnosis of endodontic problems	B
At least one good quality paralleling technique periapical radiograph is necessary to confirm working length(s)	B
If there are any doubts about the integrity of the apical constriction or resistance taper of the prepared root canal, a mid-fill periapical radiograph should be taken to confirm the position of the root filling before final compaction is carried out	C
At least one post-operative radiograph is necessary to assess the success of the obturation, and to act as a baseline for assessment of apical disease or healing	B
A further good quality follow-up paralleling technique periapical radiograph should be taken at one year after completion of treatment (see Fig. 18.13)	B
A good quality paralleling technique periapical baseline radiograph is essential in treatment planning in vital pulp procedures	C
A good quality paralleling technique periapical baseline radiograph is essential for the management of minor dental trauma	C
Post-trauma follow-up radiographs should be taken 6 months after treatment, and then annually until root formation is complete	C
While expert opinion supports the taking of review radiographs, there is no evidence to support any particular frequency or duration of review	C
CBCT is not indicated as a standard method for the demonstration of root canal anatomy but small volume, high resolution CBCT may be indicated in selected cases	C

*Evidence-based grading **B** = based on evidence from well conducted clinical studies but with no specific *in vitro* validation studies; **C** = based on evidence from expert committee reports or opinions and/or clinical experience of respected authorities and indicates an absence of directly applicable studies of good quality.

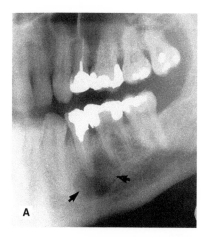
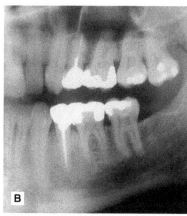

Fig. 18.13 A Part of a panoramic radiograph showing a round, well-defined area of radiolucency – a likely radicular cyst (arrowed), associated with the poorly root-filled ⌐5. **B** Same patient 6 months later following successful root filling at ⌐5. Note the bony fill-in in the apical area.

Other important causes of periapical radiolucency

Many of the conditions illustrated in Chapter 21 can present occasionally in the apical region of the alveolar bone. Some can simulate the simple inflammatory changes described above including:

- Benign and malignant bone tumours including secondary metastatic deposits (see Fig. 18.14)
- Lymphoreticular tumours of bone
- Langerhans cell disease
- Fibro-osseous lesions.

Although it is uncommon, dental care professionals should still be alert to the possibility that malignant lesions can present as apparently simple localized areas of infection. The signs of concern include:

- A vital tooth with minimal caries
- *Spiking* root resorption and an irregular radiolucent apical area with a ragged, poorly defined outline
- Tooth mobility in the absence of generalized periodontal disease
- Regional nerve anaesthesia
- Failure to respond to good endodontic therapy.

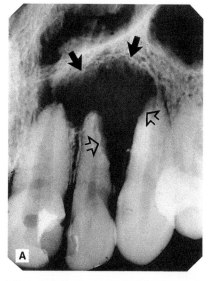
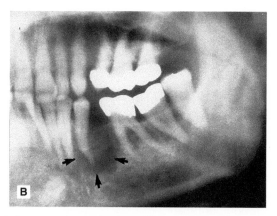

Fig. 18.14 A Periapical showing a poorly defined area of radiolucency in the apical region of ⌐123. Features of concern are the ragged bone margin (solid arrows) and the extensive resorption of ⌐2 and ⌐3 (open arrows). Initial treatment involved unsuccessful root treatment of ⌐1. Biopsy revealed an osteosarcoma. **B** Part of a dental panoramic tomograph showing a large poorly defined area of radiolucency in ⌐45 region (arrowed). Both premolars were caries-free and unrestored, but mobile. ⌐5 was extracted and histopathology revealed a secondary metastatic malignant tumour from a breast primary.

Suggested guidelines for interpreting periapical radiographs

Although somewhat repetitive, this methodical approach to radiographic interpretation is so important, and so often ignored, that it is described again.

Overall critical assessment

A typical series of questions that should be asked about the quality of a periapical radiographic image based on the *ideal quality criteria* described in Chapter 7 include:

Technique (film OR digitally captured images)

- Is the required tooth shown?
- Is the apical alveolar bone shown?
- Has the image been taken using the bisected angle or paralleling technique?
- How much distortion is present?
- Is the image foreshortened or elongated?
- Are the crowns overlapped?
- Has there been any *coning off or cone cutting*?

Exposure factors (film-captured images)

- Is the image too dark and so possibly overexposed?
- Is the image too light and so possibly underexposed?
- What effect do the exposure factors have on the appearance of the apical tissues?

Processing (film-captured images)

- Is the radiograph correctly processed?
- Is it overdeveloped?
- Is it underdeveloped?
- Is it correctly fixed?
- Has it been adequately washed?

Image processing (digitally captured images)

- Is the contrast optimal?
- Is the brightness optimal?
- Is image enhancement optimal?
- Is magnification optimal?

General overview of entire radiograph

1. Note the chronological and development age of the patient
2. Note the position, outline and density of all the normal superimposed anatomical shadows including any developing teeth

Examine each tooth on the radiograph and assess

3. **The crown**
   Note particularly:
   - The presence of caries
   - The state of existing restorations

4. **The root(s)**
   Note particularly:
   - The length of the root
   - The number(s)
   - The morphology
   - The size and shape of canals
   - The presence of:
     a. Pulp stones
     b. Root fillings
     c. Internal resorption
     d. External resorption
     e. Root fractures

5. **The apical tissues**
   Note particularly:
   - The integrity, continuity and thickness of:
     a. The radiolucent line of the periodontal ligament space
     b. The radiopaque line of the lamina dura
   - Any associated radiolucent areas
   - Any associated radiopaque areas
   - The pattern of the trabecular bone

6. **The periodontal tissues**
   Note particularly:
   - The width of the periodontal ligament
   - The level and quality of the crestal bone
   - Any vertical or horizontal bone loss
   - Any calculus deposits
   - Any furcation involvements

Fig. 18.15 A systematic sequence for viewing periapical radiographs.

Systematic viewing

A systematic approach to viewing periapical radiographs is shown in Fig. 18.15. This approach ensures that **all** areas of the image are observed and that the important features of the tooth apex are examined.

To access the self assessment questions for this chapter please go to www.whaitesessentialsdentalradiography.com

19 The periodontal tissues and periodontal disease

Introduction

An overall assessment of the periodontal tissues is based on both the clinical examination and radiographic findings – the two investigations complement one another. Unfortunately, like many other indicators of periodontal disease, radiographs only provide retrospective evidence of the disease process. However, they can be used to assess the morphology of the affected teeth and the pattern and degree of alveolar bone loss that has taken place. *Bone loss* can be defined as *the difference between the present septal bone height and the assumed normal bone height for any particular patient*, taking age into account. In fact radiographs actually show the amount of alveolar bone *remaining* in relation to the length of the root. But this information is still important in the overall assessment of the severity of the disease, the prognosis of the teeth and for treatment planning.

Radiographs are therefore used to:

- Assess the extent of bone loss and furcation involvement
- Determine the presence of any secondary local causative factors
- Assess root length and morphology
- Assist in treatment planning
- Evaluate treatment measures particularly following *guided tissue regeneration* (GTR).

Selection criteria

Several radiographic projections can be used to show the periodontal tissues. Those recommended by the Faculty of General Dental Practice (UK) in their 2013 booklet *Selection Criteria for Dental Radiography* (3rd Edn) are summarized in Table 19.1.

Table 19.1 Summary of the main recommendations for imaging the periodontal tissues based on the Faculty of General Dental Practice (UK)'s 2013 *Selection Criteria for Dental Radiography* (3rd Edn)

Recommendation	Evidence-based grading*
Horizontal bitewings if a patient has generalised pocketing <6 mm (BPE scores of Code 3) and little or no recession.	C
Vertical bitewings if a patient has pocketing 6 mm or more (BPE scores of Code 4), supplemented by paralleling technique periapicals at sites where the alveolar bone is not shown on the bitewings.	C
Bitewings (horizontal or vertical depending on pocket depth), supplemented by paralleling technique periapicals if necessary if a patient has localised pocketing	C
A paralleling technique periapical if a periodontal/endodontic lesion is suspected	C
CBCT is not indicated as a routine method of imaging periodontal bone support	C
Small volume, high resolution CBCT may be indicated in selected cases of infra-bony defects and furcation lesions, where clinical and conventional radiographic examination do not provide the information needed for patient management	C

* Evidence-based grading C = based on evidence from expert committee reports or opinions and/or clinical experience of respected authorities and indicates an absence of directly applicable studies of good quality.

In addition, digital radiography and image manipulation, including subtraction and densitometric image analysis (see Ch. 3), may assist in showing and measuring subtle changes in fine alveolar and crestal bone pattern. However, these techniques require the inclusion of a reference object of known density and a highly reproducible positioning technique to be helpful.

Important points to note

- In the interpretation of the periodontal tissues, images of excellent quality are essential – perhaps more so than in other dental specialties – because of the fine detail that is required.
- Exposure factors should be reduced when using film-based techniques to avoid *burn-out* of the interdental crestal bone

Radiographic features of healthy periodontium

A *healthy* periodontium can be regarded *as periodontal tissue exhibiting no evidence of disease.*

Unfortunately, *health* cannot be ascertained from radiographs alone, clinical information is also required.

However, to be able to interpret radiographs successfully observers need to know the usual radiographic features of healthy tissues where there has been no bone loss. The only reliable radiographic feature is the relationship between the crestal bone margin and the cemento-enamel junction (CEJ). If this distance is within normal limits (2–3 mm) and there are no clinical signs of loss of attachment, then it can be said that there has been no periodontitis.

The usual radiographic features of *healthy* alveolar bone are shown in Figs 19.1 and 19.2 and include:

- Thin, smooth, evenly corticated margins to the interdental crestal bone in the posterior regions.
- Thin, even, pointed margins to the interdental crestal bone in the anterior regions.

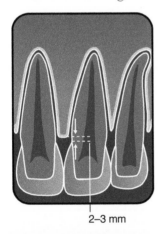

A   2–3 mm

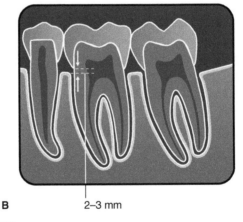

B   2–3 mm

Fig. 19.1 Diagrams illustrating the radiographic appearances of a healthy periodontium. **A** The upper incisor region. **B** The lower molar region. The normal distance of 2–3 mm from the crestal margin to the cemento-enamel junction is indicated.

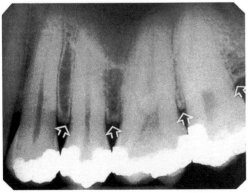

Fig. 19.2 Paralleling technique periapical radiograph of ⌊4567 (slightly reduced exposure) showing the radiographic features of a healthy periodontium (arrowed) before the onset of periodontitis.

- Cortication at the top of the crest is not always evident, owing mainly to the small amount of bone between the teeth anteriorly.
- The interdental crestal bone is continuous with the lamina dura of the adjacent teeth. The junction of the two forms a sharp angle.
- Thin even width to the mesial and distal periodontal ligament spaces.

Important points to note

- Although these are the usual features of a healthy periodontium, they are not always evident.
- Their absence from radiographs does not necessarily mean that periodontal disease is present.
- Failure to see these features may be due to:
  - Technique error
  - Overexposure

- Normal anatomical variation in alveolar bone shape and density.
- Following successful treatment, the periodontal tissues may appear healthy clinically, but radiographs may show evidence of earlier bone loss when the disease was active. Bone loss observed on radiographs is therefore not an indicator of the presence of inflammation.

Classification of periodontal disease

Various classifications of periodontal disease have been put forward over the years. The most comprehensive, although not universally agreed, was produced by the International Workshop of the American Academy of Periodontology and the European Federation of Periodontology in 1999. A simplified version is shown in Table 19.2.

Table 19.2 Simplified classification of periodontal diseases and conditions based broadly on that produced by the International Workshop of the American Academy of Periodontology and the European Federation of Periodontology

I	Gingival diseases	A. Plaque-induced gingival diseases
		  1. Gingivitis associated with dental plaque only
		    (a) Without local factors
		    (b) With local factors
		  2. Gingival diseases modified by systemic factors,
		    e.g. Smoking
		      Pregnancy
		      Uncontrolled diabetes
		  3. Gingival diseases modified by medications,
		    e.g. phenytoin, nifedipine
		  4. Gingival diseases modified by malnutrition,
		    e.g. Vitamin C deficiency
		B. Non-plaque-induced gingival lesions

II	Chronic periodontitis	A. Localized B. Generalized
III	Aggressive periodontitis	A. Localized B. Generalized

IV	Periodontitis as a manifestation of systemic disease	A. Associated with haematological disorders,
		  e.g. Leukaemia
		    Acquired neutropenia
		B. Associated with genetic disorders,
		  e.g. Down's syndrome
		    Papillon–Lefevre syndrome
		    Langerhans cell disease (histiocytosis X)
		C. Not otherwise specified, *e.g. HIV*

V	Necrotizing periodontal diseases	A. Necrotizing ulcerative gingivitis (NUG) B. Necrotizing ulcerative periodontitis (NUP)
VI	Abscesses of the periodontium	A. Gingival abscess B. Periodontal abscess C. Pericoronal abscess
VII	Periodontitis in association with endodontic lesions	
VIII	Developmental or acquired deformities and conditions	

Radiographic features of periodontal disease and the assessment of bone loss and furcation involvement

It is beyond the scope of this book to describe the features of all the periodontal diseases and conditions shown in the classification in Table 19.2. Discussion will be restricted to:

- Gingival diseases
- Periodontitis
  - Chronic
  - Aggressive
- Abscesses of the periodontium.

Gingival diseases

Radiographs provide no direct evidence of the soft tissue involvement in gingival diseases. However, in severe cases of necrotizing ulcerative gingivitis (NUG) or acute ulcerative gingivitis (AUG) where there has been extensive cratering of the interdental papilla, inflammatory destruction of the underlying crestal bone may be observed.

Periodontitis

Periodontitis is the name given to periodontal disease when *the superficial inflammation in the gingival tissues extends into the underlying alveolar bone and there has been loss of attachment*. The destruction of the bone can be either *localized*, affecting a few areas of the mouth, or *generalized*, affecting all areas. The rate of this progression and subsequent bone destruction is usually slow and continues intermittently over many years or it may be rapid. The radiographic features of the different forms of periodontitis are similar; it is the distribution and the rate of bone destruction that varies.

Terminology

The terms used to describe the various appearances of bone destruction include:

- Horizontal bone loss
- Vertical bone loss
- Furcation involvements.

The terms *horizontal* and *vertical* have been used traditionally to describe the direction or

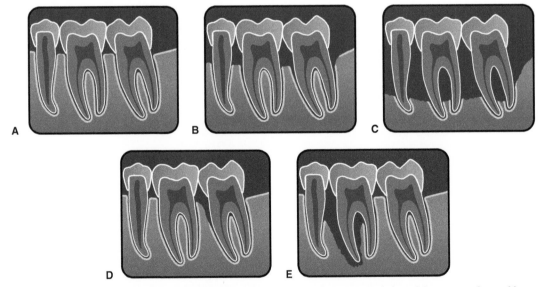

Fig. 19.3 Diagrams illustrating the various radiographic appearances *of periodontitis*. **A** Early loss of the corticated crestal bone, widening of the periodontal ligament and loss of the normally sharp angle between the crestal bone and the lamina dura. **B** Moderate horizontal bone loss. **C** Extensive generalized horizontal bone loss with furcation involvement. **D** Localized vertical bone loss affecting ⎡7. **E** Extensive localized bone loss involving the apex of ⎡6 – the so-called *perio-endo* lesion.

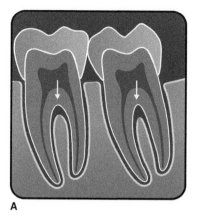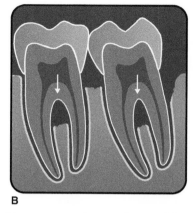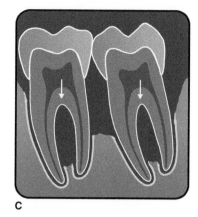

A B C

Fig. 19.4 Diagrams illustrating the radiographic appearances of varying degrees of furcation involvement in lower molars (arrowed). **A** Very early involvement showing widening of the furcation periodontal ligament shadow. **B** Moderate involvement. **C** Severe involvement.

pattern of bone loss using the line joining two adjacent teeth at their cemento-enamel junctions as a line of reference. The amount of bone loss is then assessed as mild, moderate or severe as shown diagrammatically in Fig. 19.3. Severe vertical bone loss, extending from the alveolar crest and involving the tooth apex, in which necrosis of pulp tissue is also believed to be a contributory factor, is described as *a perio-endo lesion* (see Figs 19.3E and 19.5).

The term *furcation involvement* describes the radiographic appearance of bone loss in the furcation area of the roots, which is evidence of advanced disease in this zone, as shown diagrammatically in Fig. 19.4. Although central furcation involvements are seen more readily in mandibular molars, they can also be seen in maxillary molars despite the superimposed shadow of the overlying palatal root. In addition, early maxillary molar furcation involvement between the mesiobuccal or distobuccal roots and the palatal root produces a characteristic triangular-shaped radiolucency at the edge of the tooth (see Figs 19.8C and 19.10A).

Chronic periodontitis (Figs 19.5–19.11)

This is the most common and important form of periodontal disease, affecting the majority of the dentate and partially dentate population. It is the main cause of loss of teeth in later adult life. The main pathological features of this disease are:

- Inflammation (usually a progression from chronic gingivitis)
- Destruction of periodontal ligament fibres
- Resorption of the alveolar bone
- Loss of epithelial attachment
- Formation of pockets around the teeth
- Gingival recession.

It is the resorption of the alveolar bone that provides the main radiographic features of chronic periodontitis. These include:

- Loss of the corticated interdental crestal margin – the bone edge becomes irregular or blunted
- Widening of the periodontal ligament space at the crestal margin
- Loss of the normally sharp angle between the crestal bone and the lamina dura – the bone angle becomes rounded and irregular
- Localized or generalized loss of the alveolar supporting bone
- Patterns of bone loss – *horizontal* and/or *vertical* – resulting in an even loss of bone or the formation of complex intrabony defects
- Loss of bone in the furcation areas of multirooted teeth – this can vary from widening of the furcation periodontal ligament to large zones of bone destruction
- Widening of the interdental periodontal ligament spaces
- Associated complicating *secondary local factors*.

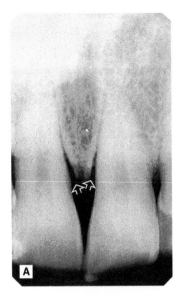 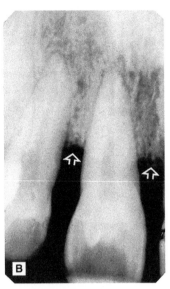

Fig. 19.5 Periapical radiographs showing the typical radiographic features of horizontal bone loss (arrowed) in periodontitis affecting maxillary incisors. **A** Moderate bone loss. **B** Severe bone loss.

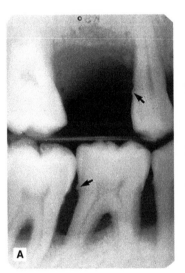 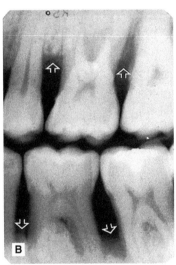

Fig. 19.6 A RIGHT and **B** LEFT vertical bitewings showing severe bone loss (open arrows) typical of chronic periodontitis. The black arrows indicate calculus deposits.

Secondary local factors

Although the primary cause of periodontal disease is bacterial plaque, many complicating secondary local factors may also be involved. Some of these factors can be detected on radiographs (see Fig. 19.11) and include:

- Calculus deposits
- Caries cavities
- Root resorption
- Overhanging filling ledges
- Poor restoration margins
- Lack of contact points
- Poor restoration contour
- Perforations by pins or posts
- Endodontic status in relation to perio-endo lesions
- Overerupted opposing teeth
- Tilted teeth
- Root approximation
- Gingivally fitting partial dentures
- Developmental grooves
- Dens-in-dente.

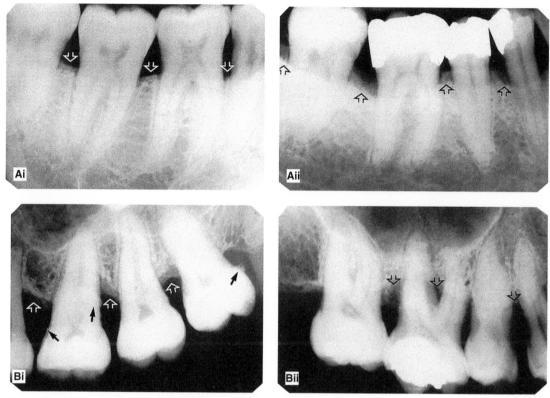

Fig. 19.7 Periapical radiographs showing the typical radiographic features of horizontal bone loss in chronic periodontitis affecting posterior teeth. **A** (**i**) Early or mild and (**ii**) moderate bone loss (arrowed) affecting mandibular molars. **B** (**i**) Moderate and (**ii**) severe bone loss (open arrows) affecting maxillary molars. The black arrows indicate calculus deposits.

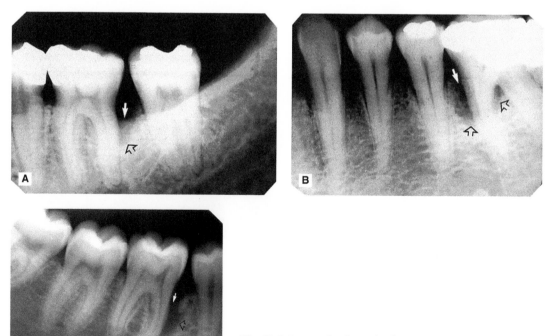

Fig. 19.8 Periapical radiographs showing examples of vertical bone loss in chronic periodontitis. **A** Mild/moderate. **B** Moderate. **C** Severe localized defect (arrowed).

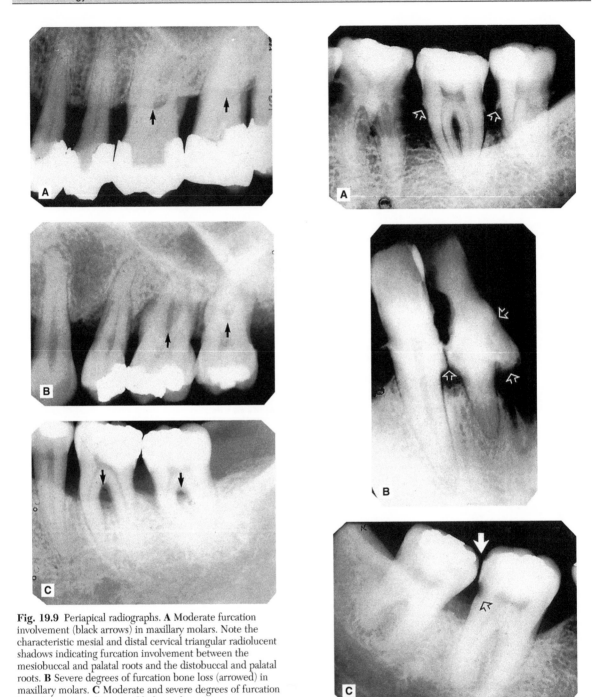

Fig. 19.9 Periapical radiographs. **A** Moderate furcation involvement (black arrows) in maxillary molars. Note the characteristic mesial and distal cervical triangular radiolucent shadows indicating furcation involvement between the mesiobuccal and palatal roots and the distobuccal and palatal roots. **B** Severe degrees of furcation bone loss (arrowed) in maxillary molars. **C** Moderate and severe degrees of furcation bone loss (arrowed) in mandibular molars.

Fig. 19.10 Radiographic examples of some secondary local causative factors (arrowed) associated with periodontal disease. **A** Small calculus deposits. **B** Gross calculus deposits. **C** Defective contact point and root caries.

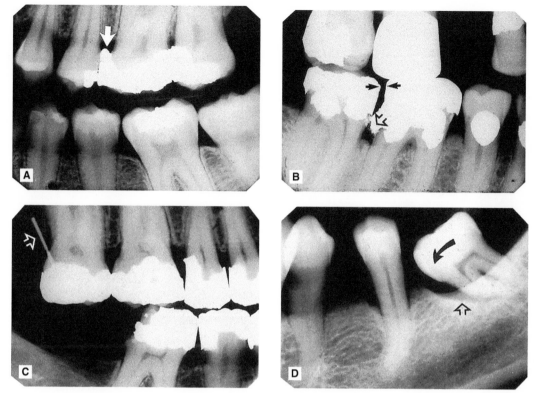

Fig. 19.11 Further radiographic examples of secondary local factors. **A** Overhanging filling ledge. **B** Defective contact point and overhanging filling ledge. **C** Pin perforated into the periodontal tissues. **D** Tilted tooth.

Aggressive periodontitis
(Figs 19.12 and 19.13)

As mentioned earlier, in aggressive periodontitis the progression of the disease and subsequent bone destruction is rapid and can be either generalized or localized. One example is *early onset periodontitis* which includes *localized juvenile periodontitis* and *prepubertal periodontitis*. Radiographic features include:

- Severe vertical bone defects affecting the first molars and/or incisors
- Arch- or saucer-shaped defects
- Sometimes the bone loss is more generalized
- Migration of the incisors with diastema formation
- Rapid rate of bone loss.

Abscesses of the periodontium

- Gingival abscess
- Periodontal abscess
  - Lateral periodontal abscess
  - Perio-endo lesion
- Pericoronal abscess.

Typically the patient presents with a localized acute exacerbation of underlying periodontal disease, usually originating in a deep soft tissue pocket which may have become occluded. The diagnosis of an abscess is made clinically where the signs of acute inflammation and infection are evident. Vitality testing helps to differentiate between the lateral periodontal abscess and the perio-endo lesion. The underlying radiographic bone changes may be indistinguishable from other forms of periodontal bone destruction, as shown in Fig. 19.14.

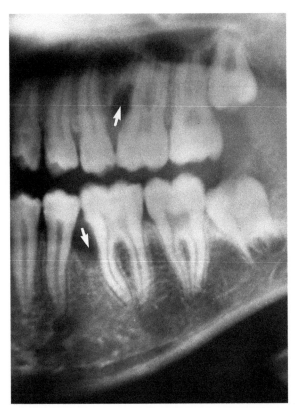

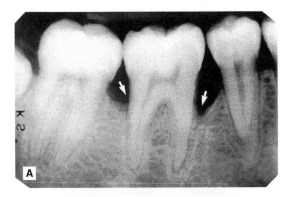

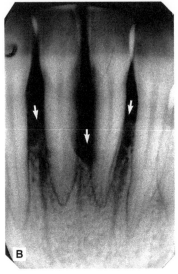

Fig. 19.12 Part of a panoramic radiograph showing the typical localized bone defects affecting the first molars (arrowed) of aggressive localized juvenile periodontitis.

Fig. 19.13 Periapicals showing the typical localized bone defects (arrowed) of aggressive localized juvenile periodontitis affecting **A** the mandibular molars and **B** the mandibular incisors in an 18-year-old.

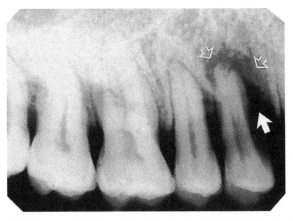

Fig. 19.14 Periapical radiograph showing an extensive area of bone loss (arrowed) associated with 4| – a so-called perio-endo lesion. The patient had presented clinically with a periodontal abscess.

Evaluation of treatment measures

Traditional treatment of periodontal disease involves improving oral hygiene, scaling, polishing and root planing of affected teeth surfaces and the removal of any other secondary local factors in an attempt to slow down or arrest the disease process. In recent years, there has been an attempt to achieve the ultimate treatment aim of regeneration of lost tissue by the development of the procedure called *guided tissue regeneration*. This favours regeneration of the attachment complex to denuded root surfaces by allowing selective regrowth of periodontal ligament cells while excluding the gingival tissues from reaching contact with the root during wound healing. This is achieved by surgically interposing a barrier membrane between the gingiva and the root surface.

The success or otherwise of these treatment measures can be assessed by a combination of clinical examination, including probing and attachment loss measurements, and periodic radiographic investigation, as shown in Figs 19.15 and 19.16.

Note: To provide useful information sequential radiographs ideally should be comparable in both technique and exposure factors.

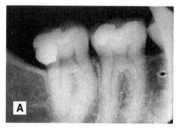 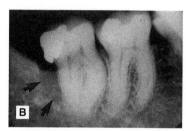 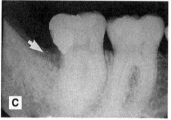

Fig. 19.15 Periapicals showing evaluation of treatment. **A** Initial film. **B** Nine years later showing overhanging filling margin and distal bony defect on 7| (arrowed). **C** Follow-up film 3 years later following guided tissue regeneration showing the reduced defect (arrowed) and the bone in-fill. (Kindly supplied by Dr A. Sidi.)

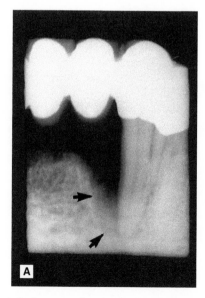 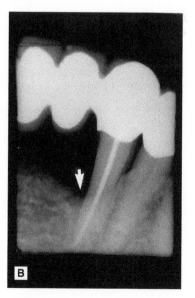

Fig. 19.16 Periapicals showing evaluation of treatment. **A** Preoperative film showing a perio-endo lesion affecting |3 with severe bony defect on the mesial aspect of the root (arrowed). **B** Follow-up film 2 years later following successful endodontic therapy and guided tissue regeneration. Note the reduced bony defect (arrowed). (Kindly supplied by Dr A. Sidi.)

Limitations of radiographic diagnosis

Radiographic evaluation of the periodontal tissues is somewhat limited. The main limitations include:

- Superimposition and a two-dimensional image bringing about the following problems:
  - It is difficult to differentiate between the buccal and lingual crestal bone levels.
  - Only part of a complex bony defect is shown.
  - One wall of a bone defect may obscure the rest of the defect.
  - Dense tooth or restoration shadows may obscure buccal or lingual bone defects, and buccal or lingual calculus deposits.
  - Bone resorption in the furcation area may be obscured by an overlying root or bone shadow.
- Information is provided only on the hard tissues of the periodontium, since the soft tissue gingival defects are not normally detectable.
- Bone loss is detectable only when sufficient calcified tissue has been resorbed to alter the attenuation of the X-ray beam. As a result, the histological front of the disease process cannot be determined by the radiographic appearance.
- Technique variations in image receptor and X-ray beam positions can considerably affect the appearance of the periodontal tissues; hence the need for accurate, reproducible techniques as described in Chapter 8.
- Exposure factors can have a marked effect on the apparent crestal bone height – overexposure causing *burn-out* when using film-based imaging.
- Complete reliance cannot be placed on the inherently inferior images of panoramic radiographs although they do provide a reasonable overview of the periodontal status (see Fig. 19.17 and Ch. 12).
- Some of the limitations of two-dimensional conventional radiography, in visualizing three-dimensional periodontal bone defects, can be overcome by high-resolution cone beam CT (see Ch. 13).

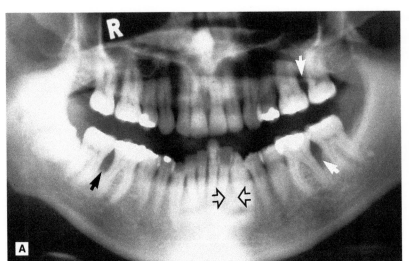
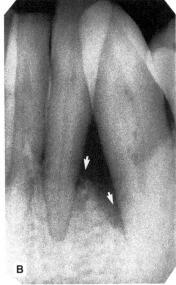

Fig. 19.17 A Panoramic radiograph showing bony defects in the molar regions (arrowed) but no evidence of a similar defect in the $\overline{23}$ region (open arrows) owing to superimposition of the radiopaque artefactual shadow of the cervical vertebrae. **B** Periapical of $\overline{23}$ region taken at the same time showing the severe bony defect (arrowed) that was actually present.

To access the self assessment questions for this chapter please go to www.whaitesessentialsdentalradiography.com

20 Implant assessment

Introduction

The restoration of edentulous and partially dentate jaws using a variety of implant-retained prostheses has become a relatively common clinical procedure in dental practice in recent years and therefore frequently encountered by dental care professionals. This chapter provides an introductory overview of implants and the role of radiography in implant assessment.

The implants are usually made of titanium and are described as either:

- Endosteal – placed **in** the bone. These are manufactured in a variety of shapes – screw, smooth-sided or plate-form, and essentially replace the roots of one or more teeth
- Subperiosteal – placed **on** the bone, under the periosteum and secured in place with screws.

This chapter concentrates on endosteal dental implants which are more commonly used, particularly since P. I. Brånemark's clinical research on the concept of *osseointegration* which he defined as *a direct connection between living bone and a load-carrying endosseous implant at the light microscopic level*. There are many different endosteal implant systems available, and it is beyond the scope of this book to discuss all the systems and their various advantages and disadvantages. The Brånemark system, described here, is probably the best known and has been researched over the longest period demonstrating acceptable 20-year success rates. However, whatever the system used, radiology plays an essential role in preoperative treatment planning, postoperative follow-up and success evaluation.

The Brånemark system

Treatment usually involves either a two-stage or a one-stage (non-submerged) surgical procedure followed by the restorative phase. Initially, in the two-stage technique the *fixture* is placed in vital bone ensuring a precision fit. The *cover screw* is screwed into the top of the *fixture* to prevent downgrowth of soft and hard tissue into the internal threaded area. The fixture is then left buried beneath the mucosa for 3–6 months. (It is important during this initial healing period to avoid loading the fixture although early loading protocols are being used in certain clinical circumstances.) The *fixture* is then surgically uncovered, the *cover screw* removed and the *abutment* (the transmucosal component) connected to *the fixture* by the *abutment screw*. An *hexagonal anti-rotation device* is incorporated into the top of the fixture. The *gold cylinder*, an integral part of the final restorative prosthesis, is finally connected to the abutment by the *gold screw*. A standard Brånemark implant is illustrated in Fig. 20.1.

Modifications to this basic design include slightly roughened implant surfaces to improve bone to implant contact and more stable, secure abutment/implant connection systems employing internal connections rather than the classic flattop hexagon described above. A variety of different abutments and connecting restorative elements are available for different clinical situations.

Main indications

Replacement of missing teeth in patients with:

- Healthy dentitions that have suffered tooth loss because of trauma

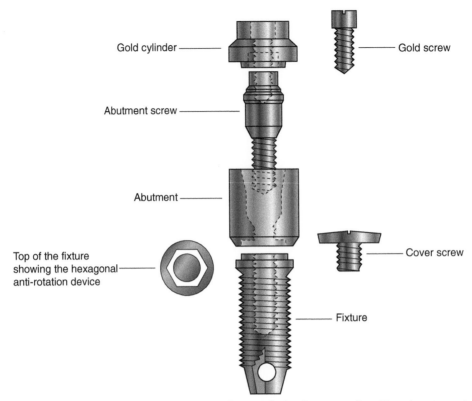

Gold cylinder

Gold screw

Abutment screw

Abutment

Top of the fixture showing the hexagonal anti-rotation device

Cover screw

Fixture

Fig. 20.1 Diagram showing the Brånemark system components for a standard endosseous implant. Note: there is a variety of different abutments and restorative elements available that attach to the hexagonal top of the standard fixture.

- Free-end saddles
- Developmentally missing teeth
- Remaining teeth not suitable as bridge abutments
- Severe ridge resorption making the wearing of dentures difficult
- Severe gag reflex
- Cleft palate and insufficient remaining teeth to support a denture/obturator
- Reconstruction following radical ablative jaw surgery
- A desire to avoid wearing a removable prosthesis.

Treatment planning considerations

Clinical examination

A thorough clinical examination using study casts, and overall evaluation of the patient are essential, as good case selection is imperative for the long-term success of implants. A multidisciplinary approach involving surgeons, prosthodontists and dental technicians is often adopted because of the many important factors that need to be taken into account, including:

- The patient's age, general health and motivation
- The condition and position of the remaining teeth (if present), including their occlusion
- The status of the periodontal tissues and the level of oral hygiene
- The condition – quality and quantity – of the edentulous mandibular or maxillary alveolar bone
- The condition of the oral soft tissues.

Radiographic examination

In recent years various guidelines have been published in both the USA and in Europe recommending the most appropriate radiographic examination(s) to use in preoperative treatment planning. However, the reliable evidence base on which to base recommendations is still limited. In addition, other variables contribute to disagreement on selection criteria in individual clinical situations. Examples of these include:

- The experience of the operator
- The thoroughness of the clinical examination including the use of ridge-mapping techniques
- The proposed anatomical site.

There are a range of investigations that are suitable in different clinical situations. Clinical choice may well depend on availability of facilities. Investigations include:

- Periapical radiography
- Panoramic radiography (see Fig. 20.2A)
- Lower 90° occlusal radiography (see Fig. 20.2B)

- Lateral cephalometric radiography (see Fig. 20.2C)
- Cross-sectional linear tomography programmes available with some modern panoramic machines
- Cone beam CT. This is ideal for implant assessment and is likely to become the imaging modality of choice when cross-sectional imaging is required (see Figs 20.3 and 20.4). Computer manipulation enables the production of panoramic and cross-sectional (transaxial) images. CBCT data can be imported into specially designed implant planning software programs, such as Simplant® or NobelGuide®, to create 3-D reconstructions of the jaws and to plan the placement of implants in three dimensions. The software can also be used to design a drill guide so that the implant

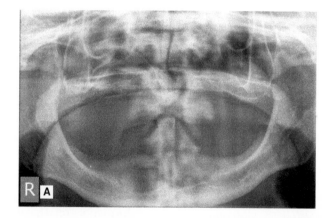

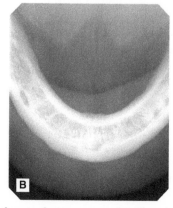
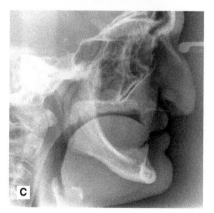

Fig. 20.2 Examples of pre-implant assessment plain films. **A** Panoramic radiograph. **B** Lower 90° occlusal radiograph. **C** Cephalometric radiograph (this view only supplies information on the morphology of the ridges in the anterior region).

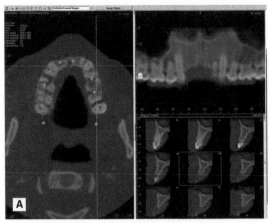 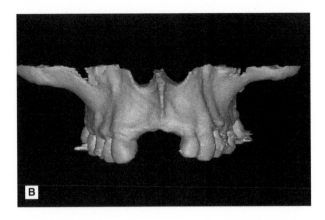

Fig. 20.3 Examples of pre-implant assessment CBCT images of the maxilla. **A** Axial, panoramic and a series of cross-sectional images (or transaxial) images. **B** 3-D surface-rendered reconstruction (© Materialise Dental NV-SimPlant®).

fixtures can be placed accurately at the proposed sites (see Fig. 20.4).

- Computed tomography (CT). Specific dental computer programs, designed for implant planning, have been written that are compatible with medical CT. This usually involves about 30 axial scans per jaw, each 1.5 mm thick. This information can then undergo computer manipulation to produce reformatted cross-sectional, panoramic and three-dimensional reconstructed images as shown in Fig. 20.5. The CT data can also be imported into implant planning software.
- Magnetic resonance (MR). This offers the advantages of not using ionizing radiation and producing sections in any desired plane without reformatting, as shown in Fig. 20.6.

These various radiographic investigations are used to show:

- The position and size of relevant normal anatomical structures, including the:
  - inferior dental canals
  - mental foramina
  - submandibular fossae
  - incisive or nasopalatine foramen and canal
  - nasal floor
- The shape and size of the antra, including the position of the antral floor and its relationship to adjacent teeth

- The presence of any underlying disease
- The presence of any retained roots or buried teeth
- The quantity of alveolar crest/basal bone, allowing direct measurements of the height, width and shape
- The quality (density) of the bone, noting:
  - the amount of cortical bone present
  - density of the cancellous bone
  - size of the trabecular spaces.

Important points to note

- Cross-sectional imaging is important to provide information on the width and quality of the alveolar bone and the location of anatomical structures. The choice of imaging modality will obviously depend on the availability of facilities. The more complex the clinical case, the more comprehensive the radiographic assessment needs to be.
- Plastic stents containing radio-opaque markers are often required for accurate localization of cross-sectional images. Gadolinium markers are used with MR (see Fig. 20.6).
- Radiation dose from medical CT imaging is typically higher than from cone beam CT.
- CT and cone beam CT data can be imported into specially designed implant planning software as described earlier.

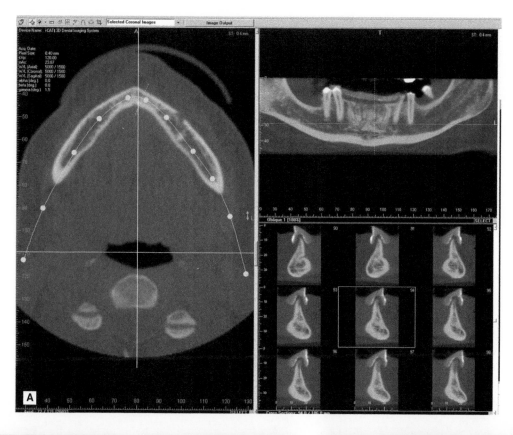

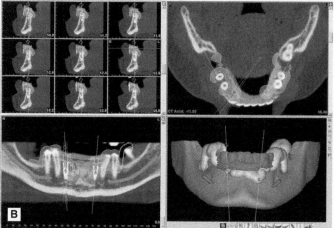

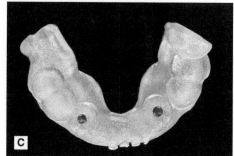

Fig. 20.4 Examples of pre-implant assessment CBCT images of the mandible. **A** Axial, panoramic and a series of cross-sectional images (or transaxial) images. **B** Example of an implant planning software program being used to plan the placement of implants in the lower right and left canine regions. Using the software the ideal position of the implants can be planned in three dimensions. The software is then used to design a drill guide, so the implant fixtures can be placed at the proposed sites (© Materialise Dental NV-SimPlant®). **C** The tooth-borne drill guide constructed to place implants in the lower canine regions. (Kindly provided by Dr Matthew Thomas.) (*See colour plates section*)

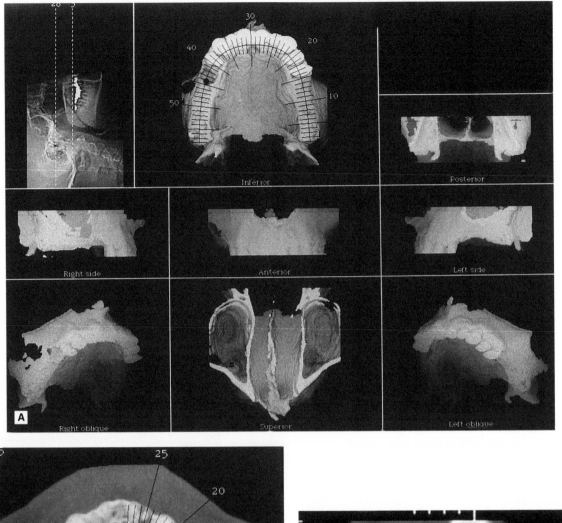

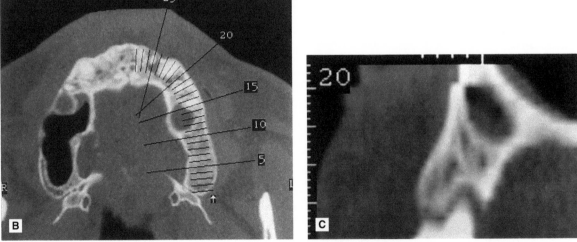

Fig. 20.5 Examples of CT images created by multiplanar reformatting used for pre-implant assessment in the maxilla. **A** Set of three-dimensional reconstructed images. **B** One axial slice showing the position of the various reconstructed cross-sectional images (kindly supplied by Dr A. Sidi). **C** One reconstructed cross-sectional slice – number 20 from the axial slice shown in **B.**

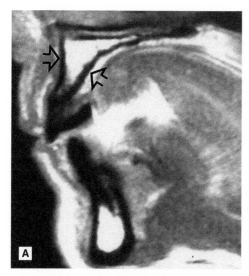
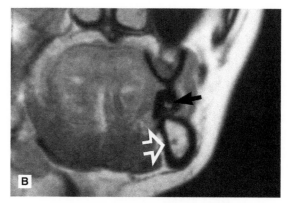

Fig. 20.6 A Sagittal section MRI scan showing the buccopalatal width and height of the edentulous anterior maxilla (arrowed).
B Cross-sectional MRI image showing an edentulous left mandible (open arrow) and the stent containing the gadolinium marker (black arrow). The inferior dental canal is clearly evident. (Images kindly supplied by Mr Crawford Gray.)

Postoperative evaluation and follow-up

Postoperative evaluation can be carried out immediately after surgery and usually after the initial 4–6 months healing period. Further clinical evaluation of the success or otherwise of the implant, including radiographic assessment, should be carried out on an annual basis for the first few years and then bi-annually. Geometrically accurate paralleling technique periapicals (either film-based or digital) are most commonly used.

Note: The accuracy can be checked by examining the geometric thread pattern of the fixture.

Criteria for success

Ideally, implants should be evaluated against standardized success criteria and not simply assessed for their survival. Several *criteria for success* have been put forward over the years for the different implant systems. Those favoured by the author, and cited frequently in the literature, are those proposed by Albrektsson in 1986. These include:

1. That an individual, unattached implant is immobile when tested clinically.

2. That a radiograph does not demonstrate any evidence of peri-implant radiolucency.
3. That vertical bone loss be less than 0.2 mm annually following the implant's first year of service.
4. That individual implant performance be characterized by an absence of signs and symptoms such as pain, infection, neuropathies, paraesthesia or violation of the inferior dental canal.
5. That, in the context of the above, a success rate of 85% at the end of a 10-year period be the minimum criterion for success.

Radiographic evaluation See (Figs 20.7 –20.9)

Radiographs allow evaluation of criteria 2 and 3, but also are used to assess:

- The position of the fixture in the bone and its relation to nearby anatomical structures
- Healing and integration of the fixture in the bone
- The peri-implant bone level and any subsequent vertical bone loss – threaded fixtures allow easy measurement if radiographs are geometrically accurate

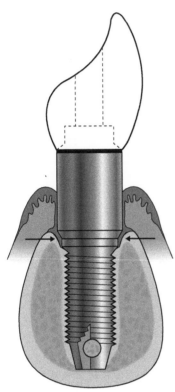

Fig. 20.7 Diagram showing (1) successful osseointegration – the bone/implant interface does not have fibrous tissue interposed, it is a direct contact and attachment between bone and the metallic implant surface, (2) minimal bone loss around the top of the implant, (3) no evidence of peri-implantitis and (4) a close fit of the abutment to the fixture (arrowed). These ideal features apply to the fixture and the surrounding tissues whatever type of abutment and restorative elements are chosen.

- Development of any associated disease, e.g. *perimplantitis*
- The fit of the abutment to the fixture
- The fit of the abutment to the crown/prosthesis
- Possible fracture of the implant/prosthesis.

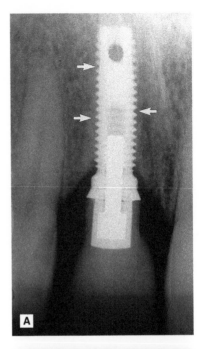

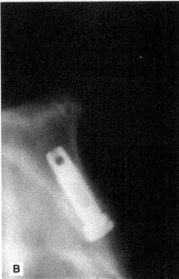

Fig. 20.8 A Periapical showing successful osseointegration, 2 years after implant placement. Note the bone/implant interface (arrowed), there is no radiolucency in between. (Kindly supplied by Mr L. Howe.) **B** Cross-sectional tomographic slice in the |1 region immediately after surgery showing the buccopalatal position and angulation of the implant.

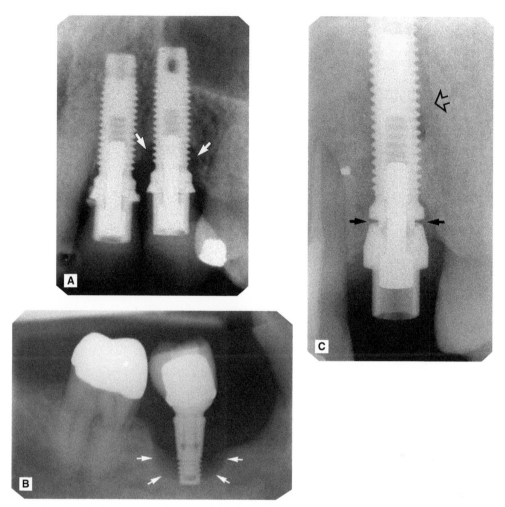

Fig. 20.9 A Periapical showing vertical bone loss (arrowed) around the thread of the implant replacing ⌊4 , but virtually no bone loss around the implant replacing ⌊3 . **B** Periapical showing unsuccessful osseointegration. Note the radiolucency surrounding the implant (arrowed). **C** Periapical showing incorrect seating of the abutment on the fixture (solid arrows) and residual radiolucency from previous periapical area (open arrow). (Examples kindly supplied by Professor R. Palmer, Mr W. McLaughlin and Mr L. Howe.)

Footnote

The limited nature of the information provided by conventional two-dimensional radiographs on the width or thickness of the alveolar bone cannot be overemphasized. Inadequate clinical and radiographic assessment by dentists of possible implant sites, before surgery, may lead to implant failure and, more seriously, to temporary or permanent nerve damage and possible litigation.

To access the self assessment questions for this chapter please go to www.whaitesessentialsdentalradiography.com

21 Atlas of diseases and abnormalities affecting the jaws

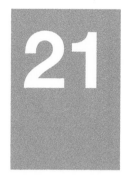

Dental care professionals should be aware of the more common diseases and important abnormalities that can affect the jaws. Detailed interpretative skills are not required, more the ability to recognize the abnormal. This chapter is therefore designed like an atlas to show examples of some of the conditions that have characteristic radiographic features. The lesions shown can be broadly grouped into:

- Developmental abnormalities
- Cysts
- Tumours – odontogenic and non-odontogenic
- Fibro-osseous lesions

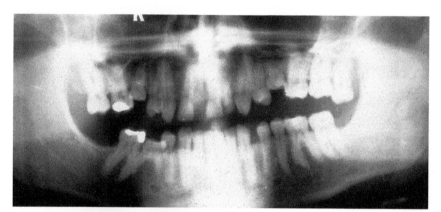

Fig. 21.1 Panoramic radiograph showing hypodontia

8	5	2	5		
8	7	5			8

are congenitally missing and |2 is rudimentary and peg-shaped.

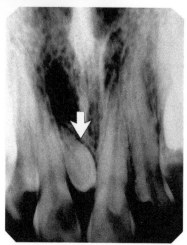

Fig. 21.2 Periapical showing a supernumerary or mesiodens (arrowed) between 1|1 .

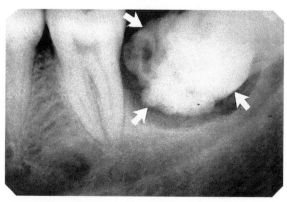

Fig. 21.3 Periapical showing a complex odontome, a disorganized mass of dental tissues in |7 region (arrowed).

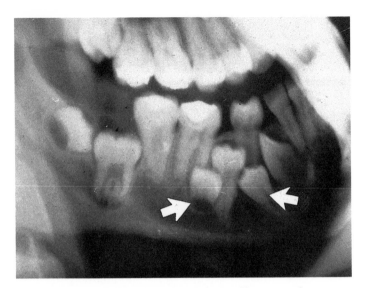

Fig. 21.4 Oblique lateral showing two supplemental lower premolars (arrowed) and a developing 9̅ .

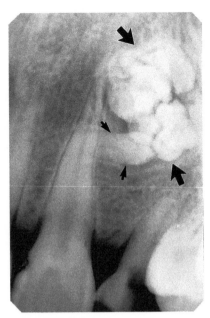

Fig. 21.5 Periapical showing a compound odontome in the anterior maxilla – several small discrete denticles are evident (arrowed) (right).

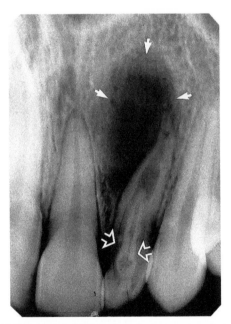

Fig. 21.6 Periapical showing a dens-in-dente or invaginated odontome involving ⌊2 . (open arrows). There is an associated periapical area of infection (solid arrows) – a common occurrence with dens-in-dente.

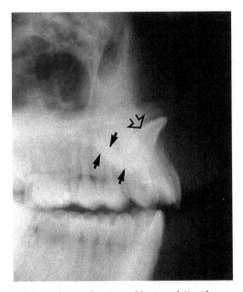

Fig. 21.7 Lateral view showing a dilacerated ⌊1 . The crown (open arrow) and the root (solid arrows) are in different planes as a result of the near right angle bend in the root.

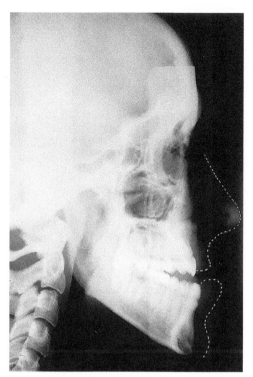

Fig. 21.8 True cephalometric lateral skull showing macrognathia (overgrowth of the mandible) in skeletal Class III. The soft tissue profile has been drawn in.

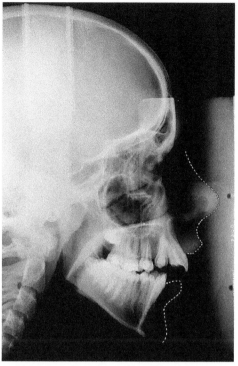

Fig. 21.9 True cephalometric lateral skull showing micrognathia (underdeveloped mandible) in skeletal Class II. The soft tissue profile has been drawn in.

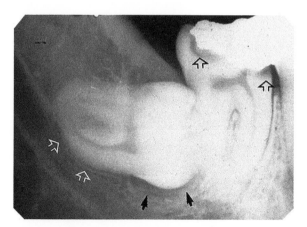

Fig. 21.10 Horizontally impacted 8⌋. Note the pincer-shaped roots and their indentation of the upper margin of the inferior dental canal (open white arrows) and radiolucency beneath the crown (solid black arrows) caused by the follicle. In addition, note the caries in 7⌋ (open black arrows).

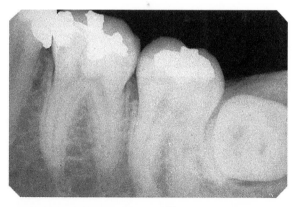

Fig. 21.11 Transversely positioned ⌈8. The crown is viewed end-on. Note that the bucco/lingual obliquity of the tooth cannot be determined from this radiograph.

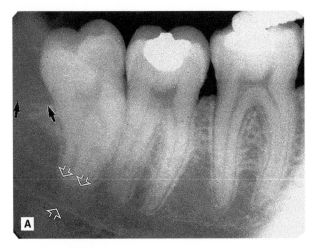
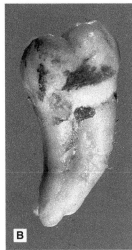
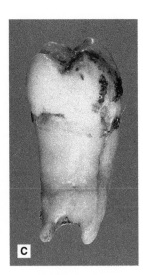

Fig. 21.12 A Slightly distoangularly impacted $\overline{8|}$. Note the extensive area of bone resorption distal to the crown (black arrows) caused by previous pericoronal infection. There is a radiolucent band across the tooth apex which is also hazy in outline (open white arrows) caused by the inferior dental canal, implying an intimate relationship. **B** The extracted $\overline{8|}$, viewed as in the radiograph from the buccal aspect. **C** The extracted tooth viewed from the distal aspect showing clearly the notching of the tooth apex by the inferior dental canal. This explains the radiolucent band across the apex – there is simply less tooth tissue in this zone, because of the position of the inferior dental canal. (Specimen and radiograph kindly supplied by Dr A. Sidi.)

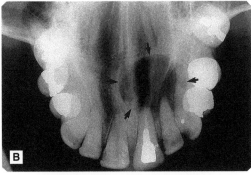
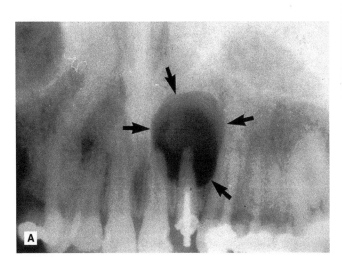
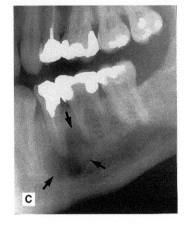

Fig. 21.13 A Static panoramic (Panoral) radiograph showing a typical radicular (dental) cyst (arrowed) associated with the non-vital $\underline{|2}$. **B** Upper standard occlusal showing a large radicular cyst associated with the root-filled $\underline{|1}$. **C** Part of a panoramic radiograph showing a typical monolocular radicular cyst associated with the non-vital $\overline{|5}$.

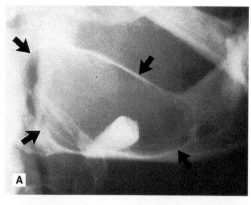

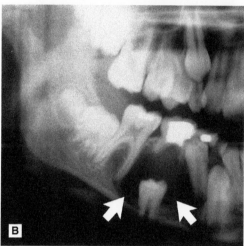

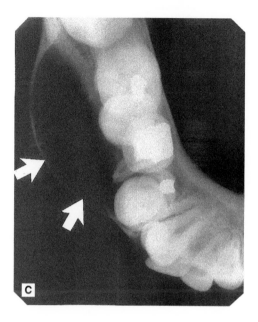

Fig. 21.14 **A** Oblique lateral of the right side of the mandible showing a typical circumferential dentigerous cyst (arrowed) associated with the unerupted and displaced $\overline{8|}$. **B** Part of a panoramic radiograph showing a unilocular central dentigerous cyst (arrowed) associated with the unerupted and inferiorly displaced $\overline{5|}$. **C** Right side of a lower 90° occlusal of the same patient showing the typical buccal expansion (arrowed).

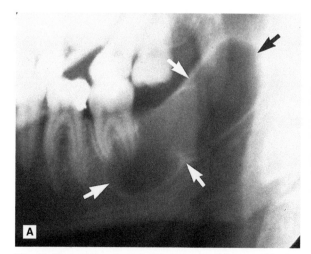

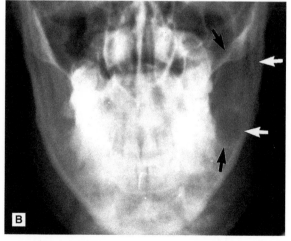

Fig. 21.15 **A** Oblique lateral of the left side of the mandible showing a typically extensive pseudolocular odontogenic keratocyst (arrowed) which has apparently developed instead of $\overline{|8}$. **B** PA jaws of the same patient showing that it has caused minimal mediolateral expansion (arrowed).

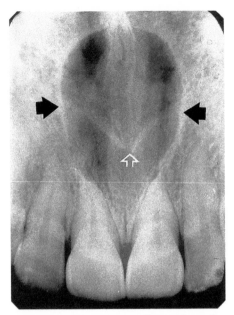

Fig. 21.16 Periapical showing a typical nasopalatine duct cyst (solid arrows) in the midline between the upper central incisors. Note the superimposed shadow of the anterior nasal spine (open white arrows) causing the cyst to appear heart-shaped.

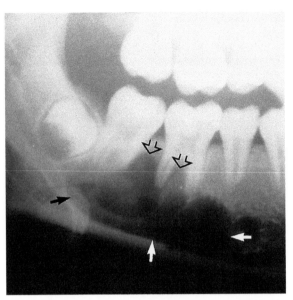

Fig. 21.17 Oblique lateral of the right side of the mandible of a teenager showing a typical solitary bone cyst (solid arrows) in the body of the mandible. Note the upper border arching up between the roots of the molar teeth (open arrows).

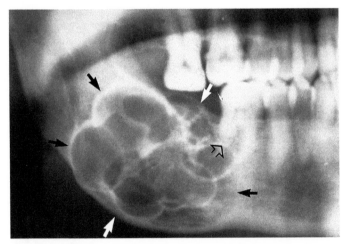

Fig. 21.18 Part of a panoramic radiograph showing the typical multilocular appearance of a large ameloblastoma at the angle of the mandible, with extensive expansion (solid arrows) and resorption of adjacent teeth (open arrow).

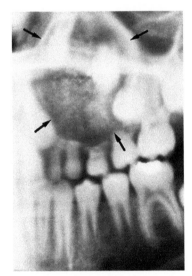

Fig. 21.19 Part of a panoramic radiograph showing a unilocular adenomatoid odontogenic tumour in the anterior maxilla (arrowed) surrounding the unerupted |3 . Internal calcification is evident.

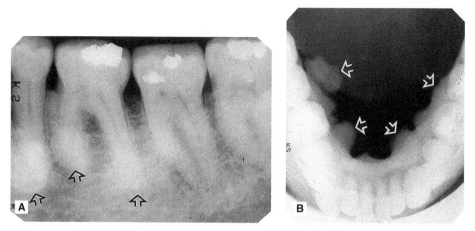

Fig. 21.20 A Periapical of $\overline{5678}$ showing ill-defined areas of radiopacity (arrowed) overlying the teeth. **B** Lower 90° occlusal of the same patient showing the large irregular exostoses (mandibular tori) on the lingual aspect of the mandible (arrowed).

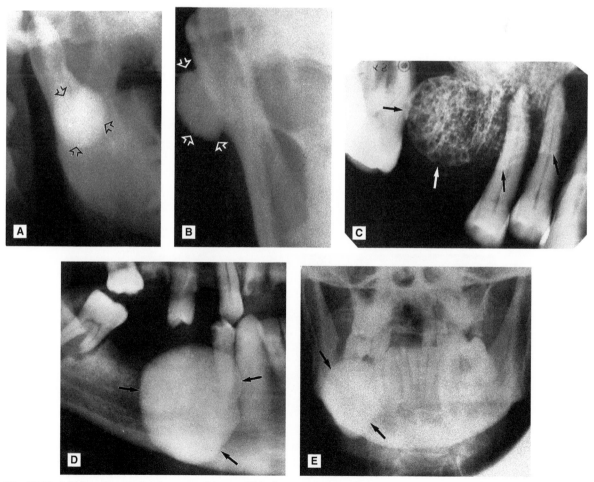

Fig. 21.21 A Oblique lateral of right ramus of the mandible showing a round radiopaque compact osteoma (arrowed). **B** Part of a PA jaws of the same patient showing the lesion (arrowed) arising from the lateral surface of the mandible confirming a periosteal osteoma. **C** Periapical showing a periosteal cancellous osteoma (arrowed). **D** Part of a panoramic radiograph and **E** PA jaws of the same patient showing a very large endosteal compact osteoma (arrowed) in the body of the mandible.

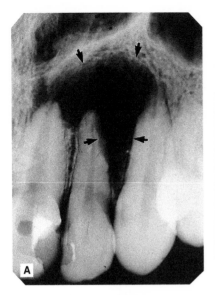

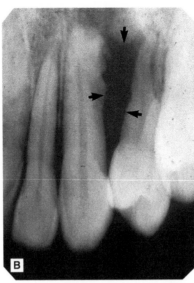

Fig. 21.22 A Periapical of |123 showing a poorly defined ragged area of radiolucency (arrowed) with resorption of the lateral aspect of |2 root. Biopsy revealed an osteolytic osteosarcoma. **B** Periapical showing a similar smaller poorly defined area of bone destruction between |34 (arrowed) which was again shown to be an osteosarcoma.

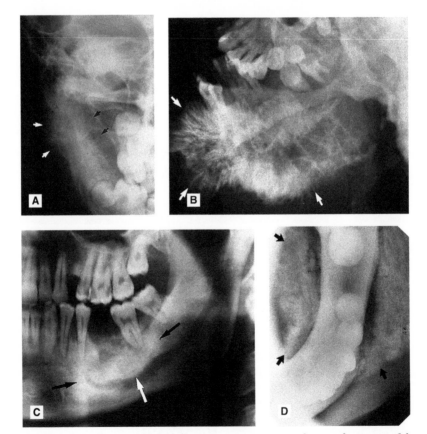

Fig. 21.23 A Right side of a PA jaws of a 7-year-old child showing an osteosarcoma in the ascending ramus of the mandible. The *sunray* or *sunburst* appearance is evident medially and laterally (arrowed). **B** Oblique lateral showing a very extensive osteogenic osteosarcoma of the mandible with obvious *sunray* or *sunburst* bone formation. **C** Left side of a panoramic radiograph showing an irregular, poorly defined area of radiopacity (arrowed) in the body of the mandible. **D** Lower 90° occlusal of the same patient showing extensive buccal and lingual abnormal bone formation (arrowed) of another osteogenic osteosarcoma.

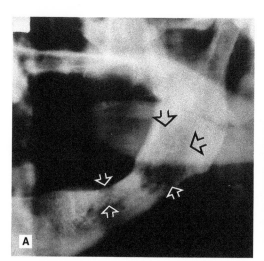

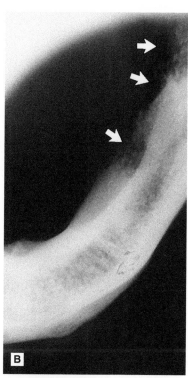

Fig. 21.24 A Part of a panoramic radiograph of a patient who presented with a large squamous cell carcinoma on the left ventral surface of his tongue and the floor of his mouth. The radiograph shows two areas of poorly defined radiolucency (arrowed) with a ragged or moth-eaten appearance. **B** Left side of a lower 90° occlusal of the same patient showing the bony destruction (arrowed) of the lingual surface of the mandible as the soft tissue tumour invades the bone.

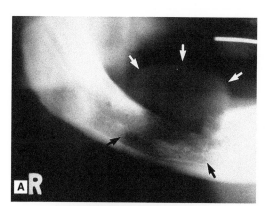

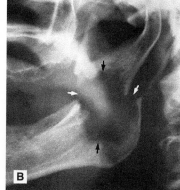

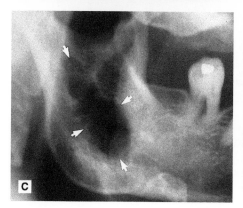

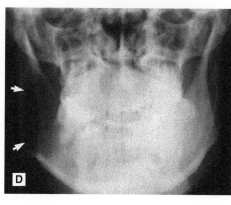

Fig. 21.25 A Right side of a panoramic radiograph showing the typical destructive, *moth-eaten* radiolucency of a malignant lesion (black arrows). Overlying soft tissue involvement is also evident (white arrows). Subsequent investigation showed this to be a secondary metastatic tumour from the breast. **B** Left side of a panoramic radiograph showing a large irregular destructive secondary metastatic tumour in the ascending ramus (black arrows). There is an associated pathological fracture (white arrows). **C** Right side of a panoramic radiograph and **D** PA jaws of the same patient showing a poorly defined radiolucent secondary metastatic deposit, from the lung, presenting centrally in the ramus (arrowed).

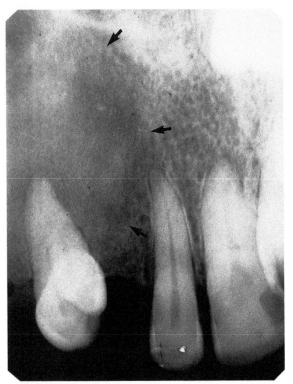

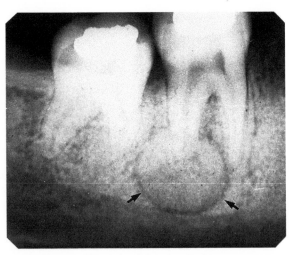

Fig. 21.27 Periapical showing the typical radio-opaque mass at the apex of the 6̄| of a benign cementoblastoma, the so-called *golf ball* appearance. The mass is attached to the root and has a thin radiolucent line around it (arrowed).

Fig. 21.26 Periapical of the upper right maxilla showing the generalized radiolucency with the fine internal trabeculation of monostotic fibrous dysplasia, giving a *ground glass* appearance. The almost imperceptible junction between abnormal and normal bone is arrowed.

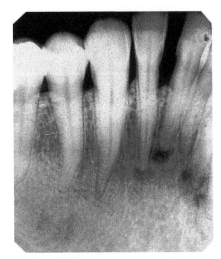

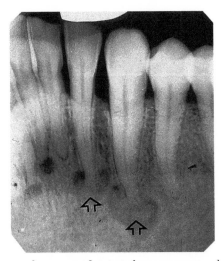

Fig. 21.28 Periapicals of the lower incisors showing the early and intermediate stages of periapical cemento-osseous dysplasia. Several, small, discrete radiolucencies are evident at the apices. The more mature lesions at the apices |23 show evidence of internal calcification (open arrows).

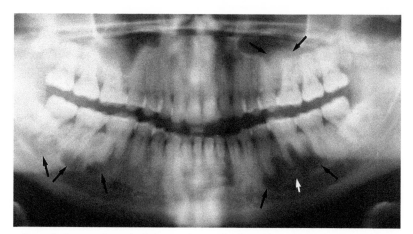

Fig. 21.29 Panoramic radiograph showing the multiple lesions (arrowed) of variable radiodensity of florid cemento-osseous dysplasia.

To access the self assessment questions for this chapter please go to www.whaitesessentialsdentalradiography.com

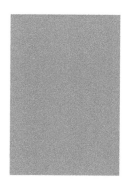

Bibliography and suggested reading

Part 1

Introduction (Ch. 1)

Coren S, Porac C, Ward LM 1979 Sensation and perception. Academic Press, New York

Cornsweet TN 1970 Visual perception. Academic Press, New York

Lindsay PH, Norman DA 1977 Human information and processing. 2nd edn. Academic Press, New York

Part 2

Radiation physics, equipment and radiation protection (Chs 2–7)

Allisy-Roberts P, Williams J 2008 Farr's physics for medical imaging. 2nd ed. Saunders Elsevier, Edinburgh

Berkhout WE, Beuger DA, Sanderink GC, van der Stelt PF 2004 The dynamic range of digital radiographic systems: dose reduction or risk of overexposure? Dentomaxillofacial Radiology 33:1–5

Bury B, Hufton A, Adams J 1995 Radiation and women of childbearing potential. British Medical Journal 310:1022–1023

Dendy PP, Heaton B 1999 Physics of diagnostic radiology. 2nd edn. Taylor and Francis, New York

EC 2004 European guidelines on radiation protection in dental radiology – the safe use of radiographs in dental practice. European Commission, Radiation Protection No. 136

Farman AG, Farman TT 2005. A comparison of 18 different X-ray detectors currently in use in dentistry. Oral Surgery, Oral Medicine, Oral Pathology, Oral Radiology and Endodontics 99:485-489

FGDP (UK) 2013 Selection criteria for dental radiography. 3rd edn. Faculty of General Dental Practice (UK) of the Royal College of Surgeons of England

Frederiksen NL, Benson BW, Sokolowski TW 1994 Effective dose and risk assessment from film tomography used for dental implant diagnostics. Dentomaxillofacial Radiology 23:123–127

Goulson AD, Knapp TA, Ramsden PG 2007 Doses to patients arising from dental X-ray examinations in the UK 2002–2004. A review of Dental X-ray Protection Service data. HPA-RPD-022. Health Protection Agency, Chilton

Graham D, Cloke P, Vosper MP 2007 Principles of radiological physics. 5th edn. Churchill Livingstone Elsevier, Edinburgh

Hart D, Wall BF, Miller MC, Shrimpton PC 2008 Frequency and collective dose for medical and dental X-ray examinations in the UK, HPA-CRCE-12. Health Protection Agency, Chilton

Hart D, Hillier MC, Shrimpton PC 2012 Doses to patients from Radiographic and Fluoroscopic X-ray Imaging procedures in the UK – 2010 review. HPA-CRCE-034. Health Protection Agency, Chilton

Health and Safety at Work, etc. Act 1974. HMSO, London

Horner K, Drage N, Brettle D 2007 21st century imaging. Quintessence, London

HSE 1992 Fitness of equipment used for medical exposure to ionising radiation. Health and Safety Guidance Note PM77. Health & Safety Executive, London

ICRP 1982 Protection of the patient in diagnostic radiology. ICRP publication 34. Pergamon, Oxford

ICRP 1990 Recommendations of the International Commission on Radiological Protection. ICRP publication 60. Annals ICPR 21(Nos 1–3)

ICP 2007 Recommendations of the International Commission on Radiological Protection. ICRP publication 103 Annals ICRP 37:1-332

Ionising Radiation (Medical Exposure) (Amendment) Regulations 2006. SI 2006 No. 2523. HMSO, London

Ionising Radiation (Medical Exposure) (Amendment) Regulations 2011. SI 2011 No. 1567. HMSO, London

Ionising Radiation (Medical Exposure) Regulations 2000. SI 2000 No. 1059. HMSO, London

Ionising Radiations Regulations 1999. SI 1999 No. 3232. HMSO, London

IPEM 2004 Guidance on the establishment and use of diagnostic reference levels for medical X-ray examinations. IPEM Report No. 88. Institute of Physics and Engineering in Medicine, York

IPEM 2005 Recommended standards for the routine performance testing of diagnostic X-ray imaging systems. IPEM Report No. 91. Institute of Physics and Engineering in Medicine, York

Lecomber AR, Downes SL, Mokhtari M, Faulkner K 2000 Optimisation of patient doses in programmable dental panoramic radiography. Dentomaxillofacial Radiology 29:107–112

Ludlow JB, Davies-Ludlow LE, White SC 2008 Patient risk related to common dental radiographic examinations: the impact of 2007 International Commission on Radiological Protection recommendations regarding dose calculation. Journal of American Dental Association 139:1237-1243

Mason RA, Bourne S 1998 A guide to dental radiography. 4th edn. Oxford University Press, Oxford

Mobbs SF, Muirhead CR, Harrison JD 2010 Risks from ionizing radiation, HPA-RPD-066. Health Protection Agency, Chilton

Napier ID. 1999 Reference doses for dental radiography. British Dental Journal 186(8):392–396

NCRP 2003 Radiation protection in dentistry. National Council on Radiation Protection and Measurements, Report No. 145

NCRP 2009 Ionizing radiation exposure of the population of the United States. National Council on Radiation Protection and Measurements, Report No. 160

NRPB 1994 Guidelines on radiology standards in primary dental care. National Radiological Protection Board, Vol. 5, No. 3

NRPB 1999 Guidelines on patient dose to promote the optimisation of protection for diagnostic medical exposures. National Radiological Protection Board, Vol. 10, No. 1

NRPB/DH 2001 Guidance notes for dental practitioners on the safe use of X-ray equipment. National Radiological Protection Board/Department of Health, London

Pittayapat P, Oliveira-Santos C, Thevissen P et al. 2010 Image quality assessment and medical physics evaluation of different portable dental X-ray units. Forensic Science International 201:112-117

SEDENTEX CT Guidelines – EC 2012 Guidelines on Cone Beam CT for Dental and Maxillofacial Radiology. European Commission, Radiation Protection 172. Available from http://ec.europa.eu/energy/nuclear/radiation_protection/doc/publication/172.pdf

Sherer MAS, Visconti PJ, Ritenour ER 2002 Radiation protection in medical radiography. 4th edn. Mosby, London

Smith NJD 1989 Dental radiography. 2nd edn. Blackwell Scientific, Oxford

Wall BF, Meara JR, Muirhead CR et al. 2009 Protection of pregnant patients during diagnostic medical exposures to ionizing radiation RCE 9. Advice from the Health Protection Agency, The Royal College of Radiologists and the College of Radiographers. Chilton, Health Protection Agency

Watson SJ, Jones AL, Oatway WB, Hughes JS 2005 Ionising radiation exposure of the UK population. 2005 Review. HPA-RPD-001. Health Protection Agency, Chilton

White SC 1992 Assessment of radiation risk from dental radiography. Dentomaxillofacial Radiology 21:118–126

Part 3
Radiography (Chs 8–16)

Armstrong P, Wastie ML, Rockall AG 2009 Diagnostic imaging. 6th edn. Wiley–Blackwell, Chichester

British Orthodontic Society 2008 Guidelines for the use of radiographs in clinical orthodontics. 3rd edn. London

BSI 1983 The British Standards glossary of dental terms BS 4492. British Standards Institute, London

Cobourne MT, DiBiase AT 2010 A handbook of orthodontics. Mosby Elsevier, Edinburgh

Core curriculum in cone beam computed tomography (CBCT) for dentists and dental care professionals 2009. Available from the British Society of Dental and Maxillofacial Radiology website from www.bsdmfr.org.uk/

Farman AG 2010 Panoramic radiology: seminars on maxillofacial imaging and interpretation. Springer-Verlag, Berlin

Horner K 1992 Quality assurance: 1 Reject analysis, operator technique and the X-ray set. Dental Update 19:75–80

Horner K 1992 Quality assurance: 2. The image receptor, the darkroom and processing. Dental Update 19:120–122

Horner K, Islam M, Flygare L, Tsiklakis K, Whaites E 2009 Basic principles for the use of cone beam computed tomography: consensus guidelines of the European Academy of Dental and Maxillofacial Radiology. Dentomaxillofacial Radiology 38:187-195

HPA 2010 Guidance notes for dental practitioners on the safe use of dental cone beam computed tomography (CBCT) equipment 2010 HPA-CRCE-010. Health Protection Agency, Chilton

Iannucci, Howerton LJ 2012 Dental radiography: principles and techniques. 4th edn. Saunders Elsevier, St Louis

IPEM 2005 Recommended stardards for the routine performance testing of diagnostic X-ray imaging systems. IPEM Report No 91. Institute of Physics and Engineering in Medicine, York

Jacobson A, Jacobson RL 2006 Radiographic cephalometry from basics to 3-D imaging. 2nd edn. Quintessence, Chicago

Jones ML, Oliver RG 1994 Walther and Houston's orthodontic notes. 5th edn. Butterworth–Heinemann, Oxford

Kidd EAM 2005 Essentials of dental caries. 3rd edn. Oxford University Press, Oxford

Langland OE, Langlais RP, McDavid WD, Delbalso AM 1989 Panoramic radiology. Lea and Febiger, Philadelphia

Langland OE, Langlais RP, Preece J 2002 Principles of dental imaging. 2nd edn. Lippincott Williams and Wilkins, Baltimore

Ludlow JB, Davies-Ludlow LE, Brooks SL 2003 Dosimetry of two extra-oral direct digital imaging devices: NewTom cone beam CT and Orthophos Plus DS panoramic unit. Dentomaxillofacial Radiology 32:229–234

Mason RA, Bourne S 1998 A guide to dental radiography. 4th edn. Oxford University Press, Oxford

McDonald F, Ireland AJ 1998 Diagnosis of the orthodontic patient. Oxford University Press, Oxford

NRPB/DH 2001 Guidance notes for dental practitioners on the safe use of X-ray equipment. National Radiological Protection Board/Department of Health, London

Scarfe WC, Farman AG 2008 What is cone beam CT and how does it work? Dental Clinics of North America 52:707-730

SEDENTEX CT Guidelines – EC 2012 Guidelines on Cone Beam CT for Dental and Maxillofacial Radiology. European Commission, Radiation Protection 172. Available from

http://ec.europa.eu/energy/nuclear/radiation_protection/doc/
publication/172.pdf

Smith NJD 1989 Dental radiography. 2nd edn. Blackwell
Scientific, Oxford

White SC, Pharoah MJ 2009 Oral radiology principles and
interpretation. 6th edn. Mosby Elsevier, St Louis

World Health Organization 1982 Quality assurance in
diagnostic radiology. WHO, Geneva

Part 4
Radiology (Chs 17–22)

Albrektson T, Zarb GA 1989 The Branemark osseointegrated
implant. Quintessence, Chicago

Brocklebank L 1996 Dental radiology (understanding the
X-ray image). Oxford University Press, Oxford

Browne RM, Edmondson HD, Rout PGJ 1995 Atlas of dental
and maxillofacial radiology. Mosby–Wolfe, London

Cawson RA, Odell EW 2008 Cawson's essentials of oral
pathology and oral medicine. 8th edn. Churchill Livingstone
Elsevier, Edinburgh

FGDP (UK) 2013 Selection criteria for dental radiography.
3rd edn. Faculty of General Dental Practice (UK) of the
Royal College of Surgeons of England

Horner K, Rout J, Rushton V 2002 Interpreting dental
radiographs. Quintessence, London

Hutchinson IL, Hopper C, Conar HS 1990 Neoplasia
masquerading as periapical infection. British Dental Journal
168:228–294

Kidd EAM 2005 Essentials of dental caries. 3rd edn. Oxford
University Press, Oxford

Logan BM, Reynolds PA, Hutchings RT 2010 McMinn's
colour atlas of head and neck anatomy. 4th edn.
Mosby Elsevier, Philadelphia

Macdonald D 2011 Oral and maxillofacial radiology: a
diagnostic approach. Wiley–Blackwell, Chichester

Palmer RM 2000 A clinical guide to implants in dentistry.
British Dental Association, London

Rout PGJ, Browne RM 1997 Self-assessment picture tests.
Oral radiology. Mosby–Wolfe, London

Rudolphy MP, van Amerongen JP, ten Cate JM 1994
Radiopacities in dentine under amalgam restorations.
Caries research 28:240–245

Tyndall AA, Brooks SL 2000 Selection criteria for dental
implant site imaging: a position of the American Academy
of Oral and Maxillofacial Radiology. Oral Surgery Oral
Medicine Oral Pathology Oral Radiology Endodontics
89(5):630–637

White SC, Pharaoh MJ 2009 Oral radiology – principles and
interpretation. 6th edn. Mosby Elsevier, St Louis

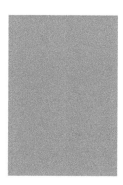

Index

Page numbers in **BOLD** indicate illustrations/images.